Pulmonary Hypertension

Editors

AARON B. WAXMAN
INDERJIT SINGH

CLINICS IN
CHEST MEDICINE

www.chestmed.theclinics.com

March 2021 • Volume 42 • Number 1

ELSEVIER

1600 John F. Kennedy Boulevard • Suite 1800 • Philadelphia, Pennsylvania, 19103-2899

http://www.theclinics.com

CLINICS IN CHEST MEDICINE Volume 42, Number 1
March 2021 ISSN 0272-5231, ISBN-13: 978-0-323-73401-1

Editor: Joanna Collett
Developmental Editor: Karen Justine Solomon

Clinics in Chest Medicine (ISSN 0272-5231) is published quarterly by Elsevier Inc., 360 Park Avenue South, New York, NY 10010-1710. Months of issue are March, June, September, and December. Periodicals postage paid at New York, NY and additional mailing offices. Subscription prices are $396.00 per year (domestic individuals), $1009.00 per year (domestic institutions), $100.00 per year (domestic students/residents), $423.00 per year (Canadian individuals), $1075.00 per year (Canadian institutions), $484.00 per year (international individuals), $1075.00 per year (international institutions), $100.00 per year (Canadian Students), and $230.00 per year (International Students). International air speed delivery is included in all Clinics subscription prices. All prices are subject to change without notice. **POSTMASTER:** Send address changes to Clinics in Chest Medicine, Elsevier Health Sciences Division, Subscription Customer Service, 3251 Riverport Lane, Maryland Heights, MO 63043. **Customer Service: Telephone: 1-800-654-2452** (U.S. and Canada); **1-314-447-8871** (outside U.S. and Canada). **Fax: 1-314-447-8029. E-mail: journalscustomerservice-usa@elsevier.com (for print support); journalsonlinesupport-usa@elsevier.com (for online support).**

Reprints. For copies of 100 or more of articles in this publication, please contact the Commercial Reprints Department, Elsevier Inc., 360 Park Avenue South, New York, NY 10010-1710. Tel.: 212-633-3874; Fax: 212-633-3820; E-mail: reprints@elsevier.com.

Clinics in Chest Medicine is covered in *MEDLINE/PubMed (Index Medicus)*, *Current Contents/Clinical Medicine*, *EMBASE/ Excerpta Medica*, *Science Citation Index*, and *ISI/BIOMED*.

Printed in the United States of America.

Contributors

EDITORS

AARON B. WAXMAN, MD, PhD, FACP, FCCP
Pulmonary and Critical Care Medicine, Director, Pulmonary Vascular Disease Program, Executive Director, Center for Pulmonary-Heart Diseases, Brigham and Women's Hospital, Associate Professor of Medicine, Harvard Medical School, Boston, Massachusetts, USA

INDERJIT SINGH, MD, FRCP
Pulmonary Critical Care and Sleep Medicine Program, Director of Pulmonary Vascular Disease Program, Yale New Haven Hospital, Yale New Haven Health, Assistant Professor of Medicine, Yale School of Medicine, New Haven, Connecticut, USA

AUTHORS

JALIL AHARI, MD
Associate Professor of Medicine, George Washington University School of Medicine, Washington, DC, USA

ROZA BADR-ESLAM, MD
Department of Internal Medicine II, Division of Cardiology, Medical University of Vienna, Vienna, Austria

AKSHAY BHATNAGAR, MD
George Washington University School of Medicine, Washington, DC, USA

HARM J. BOGAARD, MD, PhD
Full Professor, Department of Pulmonary Medicine, Amsterdam UMC (Location VUMC), Amsterdam, the Netherlands

BARRY A. BORLAUG, MD
Department of Cardiovascular Medicine, Mayo Clinic, Rochester, Minnesota, USA

GHAZWAN BUTROUS, MB, ChB, PhD
Professor of Cardiopulmonary Sciences, Medway School of Pharmacy, The Universities of Greenwich and Kent at Medway, Chatham Maritime, Kent, United Kingdom

IOANA A. CAMPEAN, MD
Department of Internal Medicine II, Division of Cardiology, Medical University of Vienna, Vienna, Austria

VINICIO DE JESUS PEREZ, MD
Associate Professor, Division of Pulmonary, Allergy and Critical Care, Stanford University School of Medicine, Vera Moulton Wall Center for Pulmonary Vascular Disease, Stanford, California, USA

FRANCES S. DE MAN, PhD
Associate Professor, Department of Pulmonary Medicine, Amsterdam UMC (Location VUMC), Amsterdam, the Netherlands

NINA DENVER, PhD
Strathclyde Institute of Pharmacy and Biomedical Sciences, University of Strathclyde, Glasgow, Scotland

JAN FOUAD, MD
Fellow, Pulmonary, Critical Care, and Sleep Medicine, Yale New Haven Hospital/Yale School of Medicine, New Haven, Connecticut, USA

ROSEMARY GAW, MSc
Strathclyde Institute of Pharmacy and
Biomedical Sciences, University of
Strathclyde, Glasgow, Scotland

CHRISTIAN GERGES, MD, PhD
Department of Internal Medicine II, Division of
Cardiology, Medical University of Vienna,
Vienna, Austria

MARDI GOMBERG-MAITLAND, MD, MSc
George Washington University School of
Medicine, Professor of Medicine, Director of
the GW Pulmonary Hypertension Program,
George Washington University School of
Medicine and Health Sciences, Washington,
DC, USA

EILEEN M. HARDER, MD
Division of Pulmonary and Critical Care
Medicine, Department of Medicine, Brigham
and Women's Hospital, Boston,
Massachusetts, USA

JENNIFER HAYTHE, MD
Associate Professor of Medicine, Columbia
University Vagelos College of Physicians and
Surgeons, Director of Cardio-obstetrics and
Co-Director of the Women's Center for
Cardiovascular Health, NewYork-Presbyterian
– Columbia University Hospital, CUMC/Vivian
& Seymour Milstein Family, New York, New
York, USA

PAUL M. HEERDT, MD, PhD, FCCP
Department of Anesthesiology, Yale School of
Medicine, New Haven, Connecticut, USA

ANNA R. HEMNES, MD
Associate Professor, Department of Medicine,
Division of Allergy, Pulmonary and Critical Care
Medicine, Vanderbilt University Medical
Center, Nashville, Tennessee, USA

EVELYN HORN, MD
Professor of Medicine, Weill Cornell Medical
College, Director of Heart Failure, Pulmonary
Hypertension, and Mechanical Circulatory
Support Programs, NewYork-Presbyterian –
Weill Cornell Medical Center, New York, New
York, USA

ANNA JOHNSON, BS
George Washington Medical Faculty
Associates, Washington, DC, USA

PHILLIP JOSEPH, MD
Assistant Professor of Medicine, Pulmonary,
Critical Care, and Sleep Medicine, Yale New
Haven Hospital/Yale School of Medicine, New
Haven, Connecticut, USA

**KATHERINE KEARNEY, MBBS, MMed,
FRACP**
Cardiology Department, St Vincent's Hospital,
Darlinghurst, New South Wales, Australia; St
Vincent's Clinical School, University of New
South Wales, Sydney, Australia

EUGENE KOTLYAR, MBBS, MD, FRACP
St Vincent's Clinical School, University of New
South Wales, Sydney, Australia; Heart
Transplant Unit, St Vincent's Hospital,
Darlinghurst, New South Wales, Australia

USHA KRISHNAN, MD
Associate Director, Pediatric Pulmonary
Hypertension Center, Division of Pediatric
Cardiology, Professor of Pediatrics, Columbia
University Irving Medical Center – NewYork-
Presbyterian, New York, New York, USA

HICHAM LABAZI, PhD
Strathclyde Institute of Pharmacy and
Biomedical Sciences, University of
Strathclyde, Glasgow, Scotland

IRENE M LANG, MD
Professor of Vascular Biology, Department of
Internal Medicine II, Division of Cardiology,
Medical University of Vienna, Vienna, Austria

**EDMUND M.T. LAU, BSc, MBBS, PhD,
FRACP**
Department of Respiratory Medicine, Royal
Prince Alfred Hospital, Sydney Medical School,
University of Sydney, Camperdown, Australia

JANE A. LEOPOLD, MD
Associate Professor of Medicine, Division of
Cardiovascular Medicine, Brigham and
Women's Hospital, Harvard Medical School,
Boston, Massachusetts, USA

AIDA LLUCIÀ-VALLDEPERAS, PhD
Postdoctoral Researcher, Department of
Pulmonary Medicine, Amsterdam UMC
(Location VUMC), Amsterdam, the Netherlands

KIRSTY MAIR, PhD
Strathclyde Institute of Pharmacy and
Biomedical Sciences, University of
Strathclyde, Glasgow, Scotland

HARI R. MALLIDI, MD
Divisions of Cardiac Surgery and Thoracic
Surgery, Brigham and Women's Hospital,
Boston, Massachusetts, USA

MARGARET R. MacLEAN, PhD
Strathclyde Institute of Pharmacy and
Biomedical Sciences, University of
Strathclyde, Glasgow, Scotland

HANNAH MORRIS, MSc
Strathclyde Institute of Pharmacy and
Biomedical Sciences, University of
Strathclyde, Institute of Cardiovascular and
Medical Sciences, College of Medical
Veterinary and Life Sciences, University of
Glasgow, Glasgow, Scotland

CHRISTOPHER J. MULLIN, MD, MHS
Assistant Professor, Department of Medicine,
Brown University, Providence, Rhode Island,
USA

ROBERT NAEIJE, MD, PhD
Faculty of Medicine, Free University of
Brussels, Brussels, Belgium

LAURA M. PIECHURA, MD
Divisions of Cardiac Surgery and Thoracic
Surgery, Brigham and Women's Hospital,
Boston, Massachusetts, USA

SHAUN M. PIENKOS, MD
Department of Medicine, Stanford University
School of Medicine, Stanford, California, USA

FARBOD N. RAHAGHI, MD, PhD
Division of Pulmonary and Critical Care
Medicine, Department of Medicine, Brigham
and Women's Hospital, Boston,
Massachusetts, USA

RAMON L. RAMIREZ III, MD
Division of Pulmonary, Allergy and Critical
Care, Stanford University School of Medicine,
Stanford, California, USA

YOGESH N.V. REDDY, MBBS, MSc
Department of Cardiovascular Medicine, Mayo
Clinic, Rochester, Minnesota, USA

DANIEL E. RINEWALT, MD
Division of Cardiac Surgery, Brigham and
Women's Hospital, Boston, Massachusetts,
USA

ERIKA B. ROSENZWEIG, MD
Director, Adult and Pediatric Pulmonary
Hypertension Comprehensive Care Center,
Director, CTEPH Program, Vice Chair for
Clinical Research, Department of
Pediatrics, Division of Pediatric Cardiology,
Professor of Pediatrics (in Medicine),
Columbia University Irving Medical Center –
NewYork-Presbyterian, New York, New York,
USA

NICOLE F. RUOPP, MD
Assistant Professor of Medicine, Division of
Pulmonary, Critical Care, and Sleep Medicine,
Tufts Medical Center, Boston, Massachusetts,
USA

ROELA SADUSHI-KOLICI, MD
Department of Internal Medicine II, Division of
Cardiology, Medical University of Vienna,
Vienna, Austria

ANDREA M. SHIOLENO, MD
Assistant Professor of Medicine, Division of
Pulmonary and Critical Care Medicine,
University of Miami, Miami, Florida, USA

INDERJIT SINGH, MD, FRCP
Pulmonary Critical Care and Sleep Medicine
Program, Director of Pulmonary Vascular
Disease Program, Yale New Haven Hospital,
Yale New Haven Health, Assistant Professor of
Medicine, Yale School of Medicine, New
Haven, Connecticut, USA

NIKA SKORO-SAJER, MD
Department of Internal Medicine II, Division of
Cardiology, Medical University of Vienna,
Vienna, Austria

JOCHEN STEPPAN, MD, DESA, FAHA
Associate Professor, Director of Perioperative
Medicine, High Risk Cardiovascular Disease,
Department of Anesthesiology and Critical
Care Medicine, Divisions of Cardiac
Anesthesia and Pediatric Anesthesia, Johns

Hopkins University, School of Medicine, Baltimore, Maryland, USA

DAVID SYSTROM, MD
Brigham and Women's Hospital, Harvard Medical School, Boston, Massachusetts, USA

REBECCA VANDERPOOL, PhD
Division of Translational and Regenerative Medicine, Department of Medicine, University of Arizona, Tucson, Arizona, USA

COREY E. VENTETUOLO, MD, MS
Associate Professor, Departments of Medicine, and Health Services, Policy, and Practice, Brown University, Providence, Rhode Island, USA

ARABELLA WARREN
Brigham and Women's Hospital, Harvard Medical School, Boston, Massachusetts, USA

MARTIN R. WILKINS, MD, FMedSci
Professor, National Heart and Lung Institute, Imperial College London, Hammersmith Hospital, London, United Kingdom

ROHAM T. ZAMANIAN, MD
Associate Professor, Division of Pulmonary, Allergy and Critical Care, Stanford University School of Medicine, Vera Moulton Wall Center for Pulmonary Vascular Disease, Stanford, California, USA

Contents

Section 1: Introduction

The current description of pulmonary hypertension is a testament to the physicians and scientists who dedicated their lives to furthering understanding of the pulmonary circulation. This has spanned a millennium, from ancient Egyptian descriptions of human anatomy to the current molecular and hemodynamic phenotyping of pulmonary hypertension. The recent Sixth World Symposium on Pulmonary Hypertension is a direct result of these discoveries and reflects an evolution in a classification scheme that has spanned half a century. This provides a framework for future directions related to therapeutics and mechanisms of disease.

Section II: Different Pulmonary Hypertension Subtypes

Presently, with increasing survival of patients with congenital heart disease (CHD), pulmonary arterial hypertension (PAH) associated with CHD is commonly encountered in children and adults. This increased prevalence is seen despite significant advances in early diagnosis and surgical correction of patients with structural CHD. PAH is the cause of significant morbidity and mortality in these patients and comes in many forms. With the increased availability of targeted therapies for PAH, there is hope for improved hemodynamics, exercise capacity, quality of life, and possibly survival for these patients. There may also be opportunities for combined medical and interventional/surgical approaches for some.

Pulmonary arterial hypertension secondary to drugs and toxins is an important subgroup of group 1 pulmonary hypertension associated with significant morbidity and mortality. Many drugs and toxins have emerged as risk factors for pulmonary arterial hypertension, which include anorexigens, illicit agents, and several US Food and Drug Administration–approved therapeutic medications. Drugs and toxins are classified as possible or definite risk factors for pulmonary arterial hypertension. This article reviews agents that have been implicated in the development of pulmonary arterial hypertension, their pathologic mechanisms, and methods to prevent the next deadly outbreak of drug- and toxin-induced pulmonary arterial hypertension.

Pulmonary hypertension is common in left heart disease and is related most commonly to passive back transmission of elevated left atrial pressures. Some patients, however, may develop pulmonary vascular remodeling superimposed on their left-sided heart disease. This review provides a contemporary appraisal of existing criteria to diagnose a precapillary component to pulmonary hypertension in left heart disease as well as discusses etiologies, management issues, and future directions.

Group 3 pulmonary hypertension (PH) is a known sequelae of chronic lung disease. Diagnosis and classification can be challenging in the background of chronic lung disease and often requires expert interpretation of numerous diagnostic studies to ascertain the true nature of the PH. Stabilization of the underlying lung disease and adjunctive therapies such as oxygen remain the mainstays of therapy, as there are no Food and Drug Administration–approved therapies for group 3 PH. Referral to PH centers for individualized management and clinical trial enrollment is paramount.

A wide variety of infectious diseases are major contributors to the causation of pulmonary vascular disease and, consequently, pulmonary hypertension, especially in the developing world. Schistosomiasis and human immunodeficiency virus are the most common infections that are known to contribute to pulmonary hypertension worldwide. The resultant inflammation and immunologic milieu caused by infection are the main pathologic processes affecting the pulmonary vasculature.

Chronic thromboembolic pulmonary hypertension (CTEPH) and chronic thromboembolic pulmonary vascular disease (CTED) are rare manifestations of venous thromboembolism. Presumably, CTEPH and CTED are variants of the same pathophysiological mechanism. CTEPH and CTED can be near-cured by pulmonary endarterectomy, balloon pulmonary angioplasty, and medical treatment with Riociguat or subcutaneous treprostinil, which are the approved drugs.

Pregnancy in pulmonary hypertension (PH) is associated with a high maternal morbidity and mortality. The normal physiologic pulmonary and systemic hemodynamic alterations that occur during pregnancy are poorly tolerated during pregnancy, birth, and the immediate postpartum period. This article (a) highlights the normal anatomic and physiologic changes that accompany pregnancy and the potential deleterious consequences on the cardiopulmonary circulation in pregnant PH patients and (b) provides an in-depth approach in the management of the pregnant PH patient.

Section III: Advanced Diagnostics

Although the diagnosis of pulmonary hypertension requires invasive testing, imaging serves an important role in the screening, classification, and monitoring of patients with pulmonary vascular disease (PVD). The development of advanced imaging techniques has led to improvements in the understanding of disease pathophysiology, noninvasive assessment of hemodynamics, and stratification of patient risk. This article discusses the current role of advanced imaging and the emerging novel techniques for visualizing the lung parenchyma, mediastinum, and heart in PVD.

Exercise intolerance is the dominant symptom of pulmonary hypertension (PH). The gold standard for the estimation of exercise capacity is a cycle ergometer incremental cardiopulmonary exercise test (CPET). The main clinical variables generated by a CPET are peak oxygen uptake (Vo2peak), ventilatory equivalents for carbon dioxide (VE/Vco2), systolic blood pressure, oxygen (O2) pulse, and chronotropic responses. PH is associated with hyperventilation at rest and at exercise, and an increase in physiologic dead space. Maximal cardiac output depends on right ventricular function and critically determines a PH patient's exercise capacity. Dynamic arterial O2 desaturation can also depress the Vo2peak.

Section IV: Management of the Pulmonary Hypertension Patient

Since the 1973 World Symposium on Pulmonary Hypertension, advancements in the understanding of pathophysiology and pathobiology have led to a myriad of pharmacotherapies for the disease. This article journeys through the development of therapeutic approaches for pulmonary arterial hypertension.

The incidence of pulmonary hypertension (PH) in patients undergoing noncardiac surgery has increased steadily over the past decade. Patients with known PH have significantly higher perioperative morbidity and mortality than those without PH. Moreover, a substantial number of patients may have occult disease. It, therefore, is of paramount importance for perioperative providers to recognize high-risk patients and treat them appropriately. This review first provides an overview of PH pathophysiology, then estimates the perioperative incidence of PH and its impact on surgical outcomes, and finally outlines a perioperative management strategy.

ventriculoarterial coupling. RV hypertrophy is the first adaptation to diminish RV wall tension, increase contractility, and protect cardiac output. Unfortunately, RV hypertrophy cannot be sustained and progresses toward a maladaptive phenotype, characterized by dilation and ventriculoarterial uncoupling. The mechanisms behind the transition from RV adaptation to RV maladaptation and right heart failure are unraveled. Therefore, in this article, we explain the main traits of each phenotype, and how some early beneficial adaptations become prejudicial in the long-term.

Advances in high-throughput biotechnologies have facilitated omics profiling, a key component of precision phenotyping, in patients with pulmonary vascular disease. Omics provides comprehensive information pertaining to genes, transcripts, proteins, and metabolites. The resulting omics big datasets may be integrated for more robust results and are amenable to analysis using machine learning or newer analytical methodologies, such as network analysis. Results from fully integrated multi-omics datasets combined with clinical data are poised to provide novel insight into pulmonary vascular disease as well as diagnose the presence of disease and prognosticate outcomes.

Pulmonary hypertension is a convergent phenotype that presents late in the natural history of the condition. The current clinical classification of patients lacks granularity, and this impacts on the development and deployment of treatment. Deep molecular phenotyping using platform 'omic' technologies is beginning to reveal the genetic and molecular architecture that underlies the phenotype, promising better targeting of patients with new treatments. The future treatment of pulmonary hypertension depends on the integration of clinical and molecular information to create a new taxonomy that defines patient groups coupled to druggable targets.

Pulmonary arterial hypertension (PAH) occurs in women more than men whereas survival in men is worse than in women. In recent years, much research has been carried out to understand these sex differences in PAH. This article discusses clinical and preclinical studies that have investigated the influences of sex, serotonin, obesity, estrogen, estrogen synthesis, and estrogen metabolism on bone morphogenetic protein receptor type II signaling, the pulmonary circulation and right ventricle in both heritable and idiopathic pulmonary hypertension.

CLINICS IN CHEST MEDICINE

SERIES OF RELATED INTEREST

Cardiology Clinics

THE CLINICS ARE AVAILABLE ONLINE!
Access your subscription at:
www.theclinics.com

Preface
Pulmonary Hypertension: An Integrative Approach to Assessment and Management

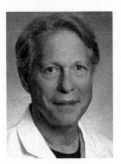

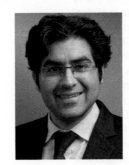

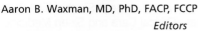

Aaron B. Waxman, MD, PhD, FACP, FCCP   Inderjit Singh, MD, FRCP
Editors

Pulmonary vascular disease (PVD), including precapillary and postcapillary pulmonary hypertension, is a spectrum of progressive, symptomatic, and ultimately fatal disorders for which substantial advances in treatment have been made. Despite advances in the management of PVD, the mortality remains excessive. All too often, evaluation and treatment are often delayed until serious complications develop. Effective management requires timely recognition, accurate diagnosis, and appropriate selection of the various therapeutic options. Almost all diseases that culminate in pulmonary hypertension can cause right heart failure. Right ventricular failure can either occur as an acute event in scenarios where the pulmonary hypertension develops acutely as with sepsis/acute lung injury, pulmonary embolism, cardiac surgery, and cardiopulmonary bypass, or as a chronic condition. Chronic pulmonary hypertension is manifested as pulmonary arterial hypertension (PAH), chronic thromboembolic pulmonary hypertension, chronic obstructive pulmonary disease, interstitial lung disease, and sleep disorder breathing.

Early detection and appropriate management can improve quality of life and may improve survival. The window of opportunity to potentially reverse or alter the course of pulmonary hypertension is thought to be early in the disease before irreversible vascular remodeling is advanced and right heart failure is established. The initial stages of disease are often clinically silent without symptoms; therefore, patients at risk should be screened at

regular intervals. Guidelines-mandated noninvasive tests are often underperformed. Medical therapy has come a long way toward decreasing symptoms, enhancing performance, and improving prognosis, but there is still a long way to go, especially for diagnoses other than PAH.

The response of the right ventricle to increased afterload produced by pulmonary vascular remodeling is a key factor in the development of symptoms and in determining survival. Given the central role that right ventricular failure plays in PVD and the fact that right ventricular failure remains the most common cause of death in patients with PVD, further understanding of both the assessment and the management of right ventricular failure is imperative.

Although a variety of treatments for pulmonary hypertension are available, most agents target a limited number of existing disease and pharmacologic categories. Newer therapeutic avenues are being investigated and contemplated. This expanding armamentarium of therapies has added to the complexity of therapeutic decision making. Recent guidelines may help but provide no specific recommendations on approved agents. Currently, there is no convincing evidence to support treating World Health Organization (WHO) functional class I patients. Most clinicians use an oral therapy to initiate therapy for WHO class II or III patients, but decision making behind which treatment should be initiated, and what combinations to use is currently a matter of debate. Many questions remain unanswered,

Clin Chest Med 42 (2021) xiii–xiv
https://doi.org/10.1016/j.ccm.2020.11.011
0272-5231/21/© 2020 Published by Elsevier Inc.

chestmed.theclinics.com

such as whether all patients should be initiated on combination therapy, what to do when patients fail to respond adequately to initial therapy, and when to use inhaled or parenteral therapies. New delivery systems are also expanding the options for treatment. Because of the complexity of managing PAH patients, referral to centers specializing in pulmonary hypertension is recommended, partly to give them the opportunity to participate in clinical trials. Importantly, there are no approved therapies for the vast majority of patients with PVD, although a number of new clinical trials are ongoing.

Evidence demonstrates that patients at a relatively early stage of PAH are subject to hemodynamic and clinical deterioration over a relatively short timeframe. These findings provide important insight into the disease progression in PAH, confirming the suspicions of many clinicians experienced at treating PAH, that once diagnosed, PAH should be aggressively treated because relative preservation of functional capacity can provide false reassurance.

For clinicians, these complex scenarios present challenges to understanding existing and new treatments, identifying appropriate patients for the various treatments, and understanding the potential role for new combination therapies. While there are published evidence-based guidelines for the management of PAH, practicing physicians appreciate reinforcement of these guidelines and updates on the approaches to treatment. Despite

the fact that in recent years, earlier disease recognition and new treatment modalities have improved, the outlook for patients with PAH remains poor. PAH and pulmonary hypertension remain deadly diseases with an unacceptably high mortality.

Aaron B. Waxman, MD, PhD, FACP, FCCP
Pulmonary and Critical Care Medicine
Pulmonary Vascular Disease Program
Center for Pulmonary-Heart Diseases
Brigham and Women's Hospital Heart
and Vascular Center
Harvard Medical School
Brigham and Women's Hospital
75 Francis Street
PBB Clinics-3
Boston, MA 02115, USA

Inderjit Singh, MD, FRCP
Pulmonary Critical Care and Sleep Medicine
Program
Pulmonary Vascular Disease Program
Yale New Haven Hospital
Yale School of Medicine
333 Cedar Street
New Haven, CT 06510, USA

E-mail addresses:
abwaxman@bwh.harvard.edu (A.B. Waxman)
Inderjit.Singh@Yale.edu (I. Singh)

Section I: Introduction

The Evolution in Nomenclature, Diagnosis, and Classification of Pulmonary Hypertension

Jan Fouad, MD[a], Phillip Joseph, MD[b,*]

KEYWORDS

• Nomenclature • Classification • Diagnosis • Pulmonary hypertension

KEY POINTS

• Outline the history of key discoveries related to the pulmonary circulation.
• Describe the evolution of the current classification scheme for pulmonary hypertension.
• Introduce future directions related to the diagnosis and classification of pulmonary hypertension.

INTRODUCTION

The current description and understanding of pulmonary hypertension reflect research that has spanned many centuries. Scientists' characterization of cardiopulmonary pathophysiology has morphed wildly over millennia; what initially was described is seemingly a small iota of what has come to be known today. Each fundamental discovery, however small or deranged relative to current understanding, has played a pivotal role in the construct of current practices. The authors hope to describe some of the many champions of the principles that have helped create the modern concept of pulmonary vascular disease.

CARDIOPULMONARY CIRCULATION—AN EVOLUTION OF PERSPECTIVE

The concept of circulatory anatomy has roots that far predate current standards of modern medicine and seems now as many parts spiritual as it does scientific. Although ancient Egyptians considered the heart to play a paramount role in human anatomy and spirituality, it was not until Praxagoras of Cos (340 BC) that medicine began to expand understanding to include anatomic differences between arteries and veins.[1] While adopting the 4 humors of medicine previously outlined by Hippocrates (460 BC–377 BC), that is, the balance of blood, black bile, yellow bile, and phlegm, he moved the needle forward in hypothesizing that pneuma (Greek for breath or soul) was taken by arteries from the heart and carried forward, whereas veins originated in the liver.

Although others, such as Herophilus and Erasistratus, followed him with postulates of cardiovascular models, Claudius Galenus (Galen) (129 AD) has been credited by many as the largest contributor to understanding during that era. A Greek philosopher and physician, he eventually was appointed as surgeon to Roman gladiators and ultimately physician to the emperor. Between his animal models and field experience with his patients, he formulated an array of observations, describing an open-ended system, with independent networks of arteries and veins.[2] In his design, food in the gut underwent concoction and eventually found its way to the liver, where blood was formed and served as the antecedent of all veins. This blood then would travel to the right ventricle (RV), where a small fraction supplied the lungs via the

a Pulmonary, Critical Care, and Sleep Medicine, Yale New Haven Hospital/Yale School of Medicine, 300 Cedar Street, New Haven, CT 06520, USA; b Pulmonary, Critical Care, and Sleep Medicine, Yale New Haven Hospital/Yale School of Medicine, 20 York Street, New Haven, CT 06519, USA
* Corresponding author.
E-mail address: phillip.joseph@yale.edu

0272-5231/21/© 2020 Elsevier Inc. All rights reserved.

chestmed.theclinics.com

pulmonary artery, and the rest would transit to the left ventricle (LV) via invisible pores in the interventricular septum.[3] This blood then was mixed with pneuma from inhaled air and appropriated to the body via arteries based on the demand of various tissues. This general concept of an open-ended vascular system (**Fig. 1**) persisted for hundreds of years, seemingly unchallenged until the era of Arab scholars in the thirteenth century and, even then, left in flux until the Renaissance, when there became a growing acknowledgment of pulmonary

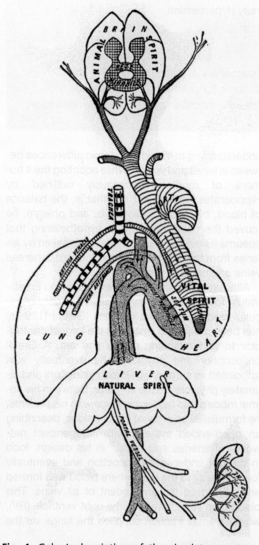

Fig. 1. Galen's description of the circulatory system. (*Reprinted from* Welcome Library, London. (Oct 22, 2014). Diagram illustrating Singer's 1925 interpretation of Galen's view of the human "Physiological system". Wikimedia Commons. https://commons.wikimedia.org/wiki/File:Galen%27s_%22Physiological_system%22_Wellcome_M0000376.jpg. License: https://creative commons.org/licenses/by/4.0/deed.en.)

circulation serving as an interventricular transit rather than as an isolated destination.

Until the work of Ibn al-Nafis (1213–1288), it was not conceptualized that blood from the lung returned to the heart. This Damascene physician was the first who posited that blood traveled through the pulmonary artery, mixed with air, and then returned to the heart via the pulmonary veins. Sadly, his work on cardiopulmonary circulation was lost to the Western world until the early twentieth century, and thus independent works of later scientists, such as Michael Servetus (1511–1553) in *Christianismi Restitutio* and Realdus Columbus (1516–1559) in *De Humani Corporis Fabrica*, were thought to be the first descriptions of the pulmonary circulation. The next sequential leap in logic came via William Harvey (1578–1657) who, in his publication, *Exercitatio Anatomica de Motu Cordis et Sanguinis in Animalibus*, was the first to illustrate a theory on a truly closed circulatory system. Blood flowed seamlessly from the heart to peripheral tissues via an arterial system and returned via a venous one, including passage through the lungs via pores, later described by his contemporaries to be vascular capillaries. He further theorized on the differing functions of the RV and LV. Given its drastic transformation from existing dogma, his theory was met with a large sum of doubt.[1]

A TRUE MEASURE OF PRESSURE

Although the scientific community was slowly but surely gaining momentum in conceptualizing cardiopulmonary circulation, there became an impetus to more objectively quantify what previously had been only qualified. One of the first to do so by means of measuring blood pressure was Stephen Hales (1677–1761), initially by way of placing a tube into a horse's femoral artery and noting the rise in elevation of blood up the tube.[3] In his book, *Haemastaticks*, he described this experience: "I caused a mare to be tied down alive on her back-…having laid open the left crural artery about 3 inches from her belly, I inserted into it a brass pipe whose bore was 1/6 of an inch in diameter; and to that, by means of another brass pipe which was fitly adapted to it, I fixed a glass tube, of nearly the same diameter, which was 9 feet in length; then untying the ligature on the artery, the blood rose in the tube 8 feet 3 inches perpendicular above the level of the left ventricle of the heart…when it was at its full height, it would rise and fall at and after each pulse 2, 3, or 4 inches…" This minister-turned-scientist also developed the U-tube manometer, the basis of which was utilized by Jean Poiseuille (1799–1869) to accurately measure blood pressure by a mercury-based device of the same premise. Perhaps his most famous contribution is the law by his own name, which describes the velocity of flow of a fluid as it relates to the radius, pressure differential, and length of the system by which it is contained. The correlate to this is the ability to measure pulmonary pressures, a unique task given the lack of direct access to this part of the circulation.

Fortunately, this is exactly what was done in the laboratory of German scientist Carl Ludwig (1816–1895). By directly opening the chest and cannulating the pulmonary arteries of various animals, he was able to describe the first pulmonary artery pressures and observed that pulmonary pressures were less than systemic pressures. Following in his footsteps were Jean-Baptiste Chauveau (1827–1917) and Etienne Marey (1830 –1904), who, by advancing catheters into the jugular vein and carotid artery, could effectively transduce and compare pressures between the RV and LV. These applications would have been meaningless if not for the standardization of pressure measurements, which in large part can be attributed to Otto Frank (1865–1944). His work in circulatory physiology, as well as that of Ernest Starling (1866–1927), who helped define the regulation of the pulmonary circulation, helped establish the Frank-Starling law of the heart.[4] This law describes the relationship between cardiac output, myocyte stretch, and ventricular filling pressure.

THE RIGHT HEART CATHETERIZATION

These advances were historic in their era but limited when translating these seemingly primitive procedures to humans. As with many moments of major medical advancement, the innovation of cardiac catheterization took the bold efforts of an individual willing to put his own well-being and reputation on the line. In this case, it was German physician Werner Forssmann (1904–1979). As a 25-year-old surgical trainee in 1929, Dr Forssmann took interest in the potential of directly accessing the cardiac chambers but was forced into self-experimentation given the profession's innate fear of such a concept. After trialing similar interventions on a cadaver, he was able to convince a colleague to first puncture his antecubital vein with a needle, and thereafter, pass an oiled ureteral catheter into it. After advancing it 35 cm, however, his colleague feared that further advancement would be too dangerous, so the procedure was terminated. One week later, he was forced to pursue this experiment in solitude. As Dr Forssmann put it, "I used a local anesthetic, and since it proved too difficult to do a venipuncture upon myself with a large needle, I did a venesection at my left elbow and passed the catheter without any resistance to its full length, 65 cm. This distance appeared to me, after having measured on the body surface, to correspond to the distance from the left elbow to the heart." He was able to prove this after obtaining a chest radiograph with the catheter still hanging from his extremity. Despite his ability to demonstrate the safety of his intervention by walking around his own institution with the catheter in place, he was subject to much contempt and mockery.[5]

For years, he received no recognition for his work and was quite surprised to be a recipient for the Nobel Prize in Physiology or Medicine in 1956.[6] Despite this, he laid the groundwork for invasive hemodynamic monitoring. In the early 1940s at Bellevue Hospital in New York City, André Cournand and Dickinson Richards made major strides in hemodynamic evaluation by using modified techniques of Forssmann's approach to introduce a catheter into a peripheral vein and sequentially measuring pressures in the right atrium, RV, and pulmonary artery. For this, they were able to join Forssmann as recipients of the 1956 Nobel Prize. This was followed by the work of Lewis Dexter, who was able to describe in detail the final step in modern catheterization in the article, "Pulmonary Capillary Pressure in Man."[7] From Forssmann's archaic methodology grew many stepwise technologic iterations in developing flow-directed catheters with an inflatable balloon. This culminated in 1970, when William Ganz and Harold Swan were able to introduce a multilumen balloon-tipped catheter amenable to bedside or fluoroscopic introduction.[8]

A DISEASE WITH A NAME

Prior to the hemodynamic research of the aforementioned scientists and physicians, pulmonary hypertension was being recognized based on a clinical syndrome rather than a set of invasive pressure parameters. This manifested as a cyanotic individual with or without RV hypertrophy, in conjunction with LV disease, congenital heart disease, chronic pulmonary disorders, or diffuse thromboembolic phenomena.[9] It soon became recognized, however, that such an entity of cyanosis and RV remodeling could exist without the concomitant diseases described. This was reported by German physician Ernst von Romberg, in 1891, when he noted post mortem pulmonary vascular pathologic changes without a clear etiology. He effectively coined this, *pulmonary vascular sclerosis*.

In 1901, this syndrome was defined further by Argentinean physician Abel Ayerza, who specified *cardíaco negro* (black heart) to indicate a sum of signs and symptoms including cough, dyspnea, cyanosis, polycythemia, and atypical pulmonary vascular histopathology. He also suggested that pulmonary artery sclerosis could be an isolated primary process or secondary to another chronic pulmonary process. There were multiple efforts at to determine the etiology of this novel disease process. Ayerza theorized that this was due to pulmonary endarteritis from syphilis, with the disease called Ayerza disease. Decades later, British physician Oscar Brenner concluded that this syndrome was in fact a disease of heart failure secondary to pulmonary disease, with morphologic and pathologic findings of pulmonary atherosclerosis and RV hypertrophy, although the correlation between these 2 was not yet recognized. His apt description of what he saw to be more muscular arteries and arterioles in diseased vessels, however, lay the groundwork for years to come.[10]

By the middle of the twentieth century, the advent of invasive pulmonary pressure monitoring, combined with histopathologic data, led to an explosion of progress in the field. In 1951, David Dresdale broadened the understanding of this disease to its dynamic physiologic underpinnings. He first illustrated a hemodynamic profile of pulmonary hypertension without an obvious secondary cause and termed this, *primary pulmonary hypertension*. His second contribution was by way of appreciating the role of vasoconstriction in disease state and progression and the corollary that pulmonary vasodilators may play a beneficial role in treatment. In Dresdale and colleagues publication in the *American Journal of Medicine*,[11] he described multiple cases, and included electrocardiogram findings suggestive of RV hypertrophy, radiography with prominent pulmonary arteries and enlarged hilar vascular shadows, autopsies showing markedly dilated right atria and ventricles, RV hypertrophy, and intimal sclerosis of intrapulmonary artery histology. He noted that in the hemodynamic studies of the patients he presented, "All had greatly elevated pulmonary artery pressures, elevated RV end diastolic pressure, diminished cardiac outputs... [and] a seven-to nine-fold increase in pulmonary resistance." He was able to perform dynamic studies on animal models, wherein he elicited acute pulmonary vasoconstriction via hypoxemia and mitigated these effects with the pulmonary vasodilator tolazoline.[11]

PULMONARY HYPERTENSION SYMPOSIUMS

Despite the progressive steps taken toward insight into this new disease, it took a crisis to raise the urgency of the medical community to come together and quickly advance its understanding and approach to pulmonary hypertension. This came by way of aminorex (2-amino-5-phenyl-2-oxazoline), an appetite suppressant, which was introduced in Switzerland and sold in Europe from November 1965 to October 1968. By the late part of this interval, it was observed that there was a 20-fold increase in the incidence of primary pulmonary hypertension in a Swiss medical clinic, with comparable findings in Austria and Germany. The unifying underpinning was that many of the patients identified had taken this drug to lose weight.[12] Post mortem studies in those who died from aminorex-associated pulmonary hypertension showed similar plexiform vascular lesions as those previously described in primary pulmonary hypertension. This led to questions about the possibility of a genetic predisposition, because not everyone who took aminorex developed the disease, as well as questions related to the pathophysiology of pulmonary hypertension.

Ultimately, this actuated the First Pulmonary Hypertension Symposium in 1973 in Geneva, Switzerland. This was the first attempt at uniformly qualifying the current state of knowledge on the subject matter and systematizing the nomenclature used. The primary outcome was in hemodynamically defining primary pulmonary hypertension by an elevated pulmonary arterial pressure (mean pressure not normally exceeding 15 mm Hg at rest while lying down; hypertension definitely present when exceeding 25 mm Hg) with a normal pulmonary capillary wedge pressure (PCWP) (at that time described to be 6–9 mm Hg and up to 12 mm Hg), while representing a disease of unknown cause. Another outcome was in delineating 2 known histopathologic patterns associated with the disease: plexogenic pulmonary arteriopathy, pulmonary venoocclusive disease, and chronic thromboembolic disease.[13] Although this meeting also called for an international registry of primary pulmonary hypertension patients, this only came to fruition in a parallel national registry formulated in 1981 by the National Heart, Lung, and Blood Institute.

Similar to aminorex, fenfluramine/phentermine became the next source of further advancement in the field. Despite some staunch opposition to its release due to links with primary pulmonary hypertension in animal models and epidemiologic studies, the US Food and Drug Administration approved fenfluramine and dexfenfluramine as appetite suppressants in April 1996. Soon thereafter, there was a reported 23-fold increase in pulmonary hypertension in those using 1 of these agents for more than 3 months. These drugs were removed from market within 18 months of release. In 1998, the Second Pulmonary Hypertension Symposium was held in Evian, France. There were many targeted goals of this meeting, including a review of pathologic endothelial dysfunction of the pulmonary vasculature, known or hypothetical risk factors related to development of the disease, the genetic relationship of pulmonary hypertension in described familial disorders, and possible novel therapeutics. Perhaps most enduring was the derivation of a clinical classification system known as the Evian classification. Previously, a pathologic classification was used but was impractical to consistently utilize in a diagnostic algorithm. This new 5-tier classification system was derived for a standardized approach. The term, *secondary pulmonary hypertension*, was abandoned due to its nondescript inclusion of intrinsic vascular lesions that may have been associated with infections, toxins, left-sided heart failure, respiratory failure, or thromboembolic phenomena.

Group 1 encompassed *pulmonary arterial hypertension (PAH)*, whose criteria included a resting mean pulmonary artery pressure (mPAP) greater than or equal to 25 mm Hg, PCWP less than or equal to 15 mm Hg, and a pulmonary vascular resistance (PVR) greater than or equal to 3 Wood units. This entity was characterized by small pulmonary arterial and arteriolar constrictive (concentric laminar intimal proliferation) and complex (plexiform lesions, dilation, and arteritis) lesions. In addition to the utility of calcium channel blockers in vasoreactive patients, epoprostenol became the first known targeted therapy with survival benefit for PAH. Group 2 was named *pulmonary venous hypertension*, defined by its passive transmission of elevated left-sided pressure due to LV or valvular disease. Because no gross gradient exists between mPAP and pulmonary wedge pressure, treatment was aimed at improving LV performance or correcting valvular abnormalities. Group 3 was termed, *pulmonary hypertension associated with disorders of the respiratory system or hypoxemia*, whose categories of disease caused vasoconstriction of the small pulmonary arteries and whose survival was most predicated on improved oxygenation. Group 4 was defined by recurrent embolic or in situ thrombosis of pulmonary arteries, with pathologic findings including intravascular fibrous septa or eccentric intimal fibrosis. This group was dubbed *pulmonary hypertension from chronic thrombotic or embolic disease*. Finally, group 5 basketed a compilation of diseases otherwise thought to injure and/or remodel the pulmonary vasculature

---

Box 1
Updated clinical classification of pulmonary hypertension from the Sixth World Symposium on Pulmonary Hypertension

1. PAH

   Idiopathic PAH

   Heritable PAH

   Drug-induced and toxin-induced PAH

   PAH associated with

      Connective tissue disease

      HIV infection

      Portal hypertension

      Congenital heart disease

      Schistosomiasis

   PAH long-term responders to calcium channel blockers

   PAH with overt features of venous/capillaries (PVOD/PCH) involvement

   Persistent PH of the newborn syndrome

2. PH due to left heart disease

   PH due to heart failure with preserved LVEF

   PH due to heart failure with reduced LVEF

   Valvular heart disease

   Congenital/acquired cardiovascular conditions leading to postcapillary PH

3. PH due to lung diseases and/or hypoxia

   Obstructive lung disease

   Restrictive lung disease

   Other lung disease with mixed restrictive/obstructive pattern

   Hypoxia without lung disease

   Developmental lung disorders

4. PH due to pulmonary artery obstructions

   Chronic thromboembolic PH

   Other pulmonary artery obstructions

5. PH with unclear and/or multifactorial mechanisms

   Hematologic disorders

   Systemic and metabolic disorders

   Others

   Complex congenital heart disease

Abbreviations: LVEF, LV ejection fraction; PCH, pulmonary capillary hemangiomatosis; PH, pulmonary hypertension; PVOD, pulmonary venoocclusive disease. *Adapted from* Galie N, et al. An overview of the 6th World Symposium on Pulmonary Hypertension. *Eur Respir J.* 2019;53(1).

and was termed, *pulmonary hypertension from disorders affecting the pulmonary vasculature.*

The Third Pulmonary Hypertension Symposium took place in Venice, Italy, in 2003, and was used predominantly to evaluate and modify the Evian classification system. Given overwhelmingly positive feedback, the task force opted to preserve the classification's structure, albeit with some important changes. The first was the withdrawal of the term, primary pulmonary hypertension, one that existed in medical nomenclature for half a century, namely because it was becoming more obvious that the clinical and histopathologic findings under its definition actually were inclusive of an aggregate of different processes, such as human immunodeficiency infection, connective tissue disease, or specific drugs. In its place was a separately defined *idiopathic PAH.* Other changes included reclassifying pulmonary venoocclusive disease and pulmonary capillary hemangiomatosis into group 1, and adding a miscellaneous category to group 5, which included sarcoidosis and lymphangiomatosis.[14]

The major point of intersection between the Third and Fourth World Symposia on Pulmonary Hypertension in Dana Point, California, in 2008, was in the identification and discussion of the BMPR2 gene, whose loss-of-function mutation promoted cell proliferation and suppressed apoptosis. It was described in 4 out of 5 familial cases and as many as 3 out of 10 sporadic cases. Specifically, in the fourth symposium, the term, *familial PAH,* was replaced with *heritable*

PAH, because the mutation to this gene was thought to involve as many as 40% of idiopathic PAH cases without known familial involvement.[15] Other genes, including those of the ALK-1 and EGN proteins, also were deemed to be deserving of attention in hereditary cases. Other notable movements in the classification system included schistosomiasis to group 1, given similar histologic lesions, and a newly defined subcategory of hemolytic anemias, previously defined under "other." New drugs were identified under PAH risk factors, including St. John's wort, phenylpropanolamine, and selective serotonin reuptake inhibitors. Group 2 was subdivided further into systolic dysfunction, diastolic dysfunction, and valvular disease. Group 3 now included a new mixed obstructive-restrictive subcategory, whereas group 4 eliminated the delineation between proximal and distal thrombotic disease. Group 5, given its multifactorial nature, also was redivided into 4 new umbrella categories.[16]

The foreground of the Fifth Pulmonary Hypertension Symposium in Nice, France, in 2013, was further insight into the molecular genetics of heritable PAH. Aside from those previously described, other mutations that were thought to account for a minority of this disease were included, such as SMAD9, CAV1, KCNK3, and EIF2AK4, the details of which are beyond the scope of this article. Another important focus was that of the transforming growth factor β pathway, involved in cell proliferation, differentiation, and apoptosis. Because many of these mutations are not closely related,

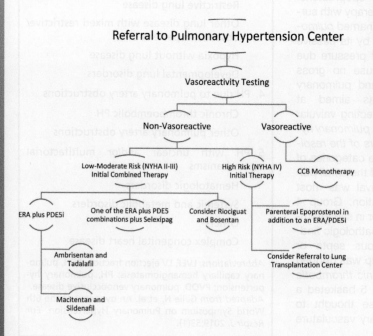

Fig. 2. Proposed algorithm for PAH management based on the 6th World Symposium on Pulmonary Hypertension. (*Adapted from* Condon, D. F., et al. (2019). "The 6th World Symposium on Pulmonary Hypertension: what's old is new." F1000Res. 2019;8.

Already underway is the planning for the Seventh Pulmonary Hypertension Symposium, tentatively scheduled for early 2023 in Orlando, Florida).

it provided new insight into mechanisms of pathogenesis not understood previously. In addition, several other drugs were added to the definitely, likely, and possible associations of PH lists, including benfluorex, dasatinib, and interferon alpha, respectively. Updates in congenital heart disease also were used to better categorize this diverse phenotype, and a better understanding of hemodynamic and autopsy-based profiles moved sickle cell disease from group 1 to group 5.

The Sixth World Symposium on Pulmonary Hypertension in 2018 (again in Nice, France) featured what may only be described as a small revolution of diagnostic and therapeutic formulae.[17] Aside from an updated schema (**Box 1**), in defining pulmonary hypertension, the suggestion was to change the mPAP criteria from 25 mm Hg to 20 mm Hg, because the former number did not represent the upper limit of normal in the general population, with a healthy individual mPAP approximately 14 mm Hg ± 3.3 mm Hg across available studies.[18] Furthermore, published data were suggestive that those in the mPAP category of 21 mm Hg to 24 mm Hg were at increased risk of poor outcomes and often progressed to "overt pulmonary hypertension."[19] A more universal role was given in the inclusion of PVR as a diagnostic factor (previously considered most important only in PAH). In those with an elevated PCWP, a PVR less than or greater than 3 Wood units delineated between combined precapillary and postcapillary pulmonary hypertension and isolated postcapillary pulmonary hypertension. These categories were in addition to isolated precapillary pulmonary hypertension (mPAP >20 mm Hg; PCWP ≤15 mm Hg; and PVR ≥3 WU).

The other major outcome was a revised treatment algorithm in PAH, which now takes into account functional classes as well as a recognition of upfront initiation of dual-combination therapy (**Fig. 2**).[20]

A REVOLUTION TO COME

The field of pulmonary hypertension is one of constant progression and transformation. As knowledge of molecular science and genetics has grown at an unprecedented rate, it comes with the ability to characterize known diseases into previously unfamiliar constructs. Described in this text are decades of effort at explaining pulmonary vascular disease with regard to specific etiologies. There now is an emerging field of pulmonary vascular disease phenomics (PVDOMICS), however, that is working to reclassify this disease based on molecular or cellular pathobiology.[21] If effective, there may be an opportunity to create a new classification scheme altogether. With this move toward genotype-phenotype characterizations, it may be possible to identify previously unappreciated relationships between molecular profiles and clinical manifestations, potentially leading to new therapeutics. Ultimately, it is hypothesized that the initial identification of disease to active management could be completely reformed (**Box 2**).

As of the time of publication in October 2017, the National Institutes of Health/National Heart, Lung and Blood institute declared its efforts at directing a multicenter, multidisciplinary collaboration. The specified goal was to establish 1500 participants with pulmonary hypertension as well as healthy comparators. After undergoing

---

Box 2
Specific hypotheses as addressed by the pulmonary vascular disease phenomic study protocol

- The molecular basis of pulmonary vascular disease of all etiologies will be discovered by integration of biological markers, with careful phenotyping of all patients with PH and comparing these data with healthy subjects and with non-PH patients as diseased comparators, such as emphysema and interstitial lung disease.

- Racial and gender-related (or ancestry) genetic variations in phenotype, natural history, and responses to therapy will be discovered and lead to more precise diagnostic and therapeutic approaches.

- The response, adaptation, and dysfunction of the RV will be elucidated by careful phenotyping, including specialized imaging and –omic correlations.

- Exercise pathophysiology will lead to improved early diagnosis of PVD, elucidation of RV–pulmonary vascular interactions, RV functional reserve, failure, and response to therapies.

- The biological and genetic features of patients with combined pulmonary venous hypertension and PAH will lead to better differentiation of these 2 etiologies of PH and of shared biological mechanisms.

- Epigenetic and RNA variants will influence the development, severity, and type of PVD and reveal therapeutic responses and form a basis for new therapies.

Adapted from Hemnes, A. R., et al. (2017). "PVDOMICS: A Multi-Center Study to Improve Understanding of Pulmonary Vascular Disease Through Phenomics." Circ Res 121(10): 1136-1139.

intensive phenotypic classification, high-dimensional model-based clustering methods will be utilized to derive molecular-based subtypes of pulmonary vascular disease, which would result in the formulation of new classification based on endophenotypes.[21]

SUMMARY

The field of pulmonary hypertension has been defined by its exponential growth. On the shoulders of inquisitive philosophers and scientists who dared to hypothesize, experiment, and ultimately redefine understanding of anatomy, physiology, and histopathology, patients with complex and heterogeneous disease have been able to be more readily identified and cared for. Although many questions have been answered, a whole host of questions has appeared. Understanding the historical basis of pulmonary hypertension helps define a road map for the future. The authors hope that this introductory piece is instructional as a foundation for what lies ahead.

CLINICS CARE POINTS

- The current understanding of pulmonary hypertension is a result of research that has spanned centuries.
- Future research using omics is underway, with the goal of refining the classification of pulmonary hypertension.

DISCLOSURE

The authors have nothing to disclose.

REFERENCES

1. ElMaghawry M, Zanatta A, Zampieri F. The discovery of pulmonary circulation: from Imhotep to William Harvey. Glob Cardiol Sci Pract 2014;2014(2): 103–16.
2. Maron BA, Zamanian RT, Waxman AB. Pulmonary hypertension: basic science to clinical medicine. 2016.
3. Yuan JXJ. Textbook of pulmonary vascular disease. New York (NY): Springer; 2011.
4. Hill NS, Farber HW. Pulmonary hypertension. Totowa (N.J.): Humana Press; 2008.
5. Meyer JA. Werner Forssmann and catheterization of the heart, 1929. Ann Thorac Surg 1990;49(3):497–9.
6. Nicholls M. Werner Forssmann nobel prize for physiology or medicine 1956. Eur Heart J 2020;41(9): 980–2.
7. Hellems HK, Haynes FW, Dexter L. Pulmonary capillary pressure in man. J Appl Physiol 1949;2(1):24–9.
8. Swan HJ, Ganz W, Forrester J, et al. Catheterization of the heart in man with use of a flow-directed balloon-tipped catheter. N Engl J Med 1970; 283(9):447–51.
9. Foshat M, Boroumand N. The evolving classification of pulmonary hypertension. Arch Pathol Lab Med 2017;141(5):696–703.
10. Brenner O. Pathology of the vessels of the pulmonary circulation: Part I. Arch Intern Med 1935; 56(2):211–37.
11. Dresdale DT, Schultz M, Michtom RJ. Primary pulmonary hypertension. I. Clinical and hemodynamic study. Am J Med 1951;11(6):686–705.
12. Kay JM, Smith P, Heath D. Aminorex and the pulmonary circulation. Thorax 1971;26(3):262–70.
13. Hatano S, Strasser T, Organization WH. Primary pulmonary hypertension: report on a WHO meeting. Geneva (Switzerland): World Health Organization; 1975. p. 15–7.
14. Proceedings of the 3rd world symposium on pulmonary arterial hypertension. Venice, Italy, June 23-25, 2003. J Am Coll Cardiol 2004;43(12 Suppl S): 1S–90S.
15. International PPHC, Lane KB, Machado RD, et al. Heterozygous germline mutations in BMPR2, encoding a TGF-beta receptor, cause familial primary pulmonary hypertension. Nat Genet 2000;26(1):81–4.
16. Proceedings of the 4th world symposium on pulmonary hypertension, February 2008, Dana Point, California, USA. J Am Coll Cardiol 2009;54(1 Suppl): S1–117.
17. Galie N, McLaughlin VV, Rubin LJ, et al. An overview of the 6th world symposium on pulmonary hypertension. Eur Respir J 2019;53(1).
18. Kovacs G, Berghold A, Scheidl S, et al. Pulmonary arterial pressure during rest and exercise in healthy subjects: a systematic review. Eur Respir J 2009; 34(4):888–94.
19. Valerio CJ, Schreiber BE, Handler CE, et al. Borderline mean pulmonary artery pressure in patients with systemic sclerosis: transpulmonary gradient predicts risk of developing pulmonary hypertension. Arthritis Rheum 2013;65(4):1074–84.
20. Condon DF, Nickel NP, Anderson R, et al. The 6th world symposium on pulmonary hypertension: what's old is new. F1000Res 2019;8. F1000 Faculty Rev-888.
21. Hemnes AR, Beck GJ, Newman JH, et al. PVDOMICS: a multi-center study to improve understanding of pulmonary vascular disease through phenomics. Circ Res 2017;121(10):1136–9.

Section II: Different Pulmonary Hypertension Subtypes

Congenital Heart Disease-Associated Pulmonary Hypertension

Erika B. Rosenzweig, MD*, Usha Krishnan, MD

KEYWORDS

- Pulmonary arterial hypertension • Congenital heart disease • Eisenmenger syndrome
- Pulmonary vascular disease

KEY POINTS

- Pulmonary arterial hypertension (PAH) is a frequent complication of congenital heart disease (CHD), most commonly occurring with moderate to large unrepaired systemic-to-pulmonary shunt lesions.
- Given similar histopathologic changes, clinical presentation, and response to targeted therapy, PAH associated with CHD is classified with other forms of World Symposium on Pulmonary Hypertension group 1 PAH.
- Prognosis varies depending on the type and size of the congenital heart defect, the timing of the development of PAH, and the response to treatment.
- Pulmonary vascular disease associated with univentricular heart (both before and after total cavopulmonary connection) forms a unique and challenging subgroup of APAH-CHD, with different diagnostic and prognostic criteria and therapeutic indications.

EPIDEMIOLOGY AND PATHOPHYSIOLOGY OF PULMONARY ARTERIAL HYPERTENSION ASSOCIATED WITH CONGENITAL HEART DISEASE

Data from the Registry to Evaluate Early and Long-Term Pulmonary Arterial Hypertension Disease Management (REVEAL) and the French registry estimate the prevalence of pulmonary arterial hypertension associated with congenital heart disease (APAH-CHD) to be between 10% and 11% of all patients with pulmonary hypertension.[1–6] This number is likely to continue to grow as the number of patients with congenital heart disease (CHD) surviving to adulthood increases. In the pediatric age group, CHD forms a much larger proportion of patients with PAH.[7] PAH is hemodynamically characterized by mean pulmonary artery pressure (PAPm) $\geq$25 mm Hg (and more recently PAPm >20 mm Hg)[8] with a mean pulmonary arterial wedge pressure (PAWP) of 15 mm Hg or less and pulmonary vascular resistance (PVR) $\geq$3 Woods units (WU). This proposed incorporation of PVR into the recent hemodynamic definition is a further reminder of how important PVR is for the hemodynamic assessment of the APAH-CHD patient. In patients with CHD, it is essential to distinguish between PAH with low PVR versus high PVR, which is typically associated with vasoconstriction and changes at the pulmonary arteriolar level. For example, patients with large posttricuspid shunts can have elevated pulmonary arterial pressures (PAPs) without elevation of PVR, because of increased pulmonary blood flow (PBF) from large systemic-to-pulmonary shunts typically with a Qp:Qs >1.5:1. However, with prolonged exposure of the pulmonary circulation to increased flow, vasoconstriction, intimal proliferation, and in situ thrombosis, impaired apoptosis, vascular remodeling, and inflammation ensue, all of which contribute to increasing PVR and irreversible vascular disease.[9]

Division of Pediatric Cardiology, Columbia University Irving Medical Center – New York Presbyterian Hospital, 3959 Broadway–CH-2N, New York, NY 10032, USA
* Corresponding author.
E-mail address: esb14@cumc.columbia.edu

Clin Chest Med 42 (2021) 9–18
https://doi.org/10.1016/j.ccm.2020.11.005

These histopathologic changes are very similar to those seen in the lungs of patients with idiopathic pulmonary arterial hypertension (IPAH). However, there are important differences in the natural history, clinical presentation, physiology, and outcome of the 2 conditions.[10] Despite similar changes at the level of the lung microvasculature and the endothelium, the effect of these changes on the right ventricle (RV) are different in APAH-CHD versus other forms of World Symposium on Pulmonary Hypertension (WSPH) group 1 PAH. Despite hypertrophy and dilatation, the RV systolic function can remain normal for decades in the patient with classic Eisenmenger syndrome (ES) phenotype is due to the ability of the RV to unload itself with a right-to-left shunt, reducing the pressure overload on the RV at the expense of cyanosis. Another hypothesis proposed in these patients to account for the relatively preserved RV function is that these RVs are subjected to systemic pressures from fetal life and have never undergone the postnatal regression that normally occurs in other forms of PAH. This RV phenotype may be better able to work against higher PVR for a longer time. Whether there are other molecular adaptations that help to preserve RV function in the Eisenmenger patient remain to be seen.

Manes and colleagues[11] analyzed data from 192 patients with APAH-CHD collected over 13 years and compared the outcomes of different subtypes of APAH-CHD with patients with IPAH. The investigators demonstrated that patients with ES had the highest baseline PVR and lowest exercise capacity. They also found a 20-year Kaplan-Meier survival estimate of 87% for ES compared with 36% in postoperative APAH-CHD. Other studies have also shown a favorable prognosis for patients with APAH-CHD. Evaluation to determine operability is critical before repair in patients with APAH-CHD (**Table 1**).[10,12–14] However, in 2010 the REVEAL study analyzed long-term outcomes specifically with APAH-CHD and found that the survival in patients with APAH-CHD was not significantly different than those with IPAH. Unfortunately, these patients included all types of APAH-CHD and were not likely representative of the pure Eisenmenger patient phenotype; patients with classic type 1 Eisenmenger syndrome appear to have a survival advantage over IPAH and postoperative APAH-CHD.[15] Management of patients with the first 2 categories, those with ES and those with PAH in the setting of unrepaired moderate to large defects, pose added challenges and is the focus of the remainder of this article. Management of groups 3 and 4 is similar to the management of other forms of WSPH group 1 PAH.

Table 1
Guidance for assessing operability in pulmonary arterial hypertension associated with congenital heart disease

PVR Index (WUm^2)	PVR (WU)	Correctability/ Favorable Long-Term Outcome
<4	<2.3	Yes
4–8	2.3–4.6	Individual patient evaluation in tertiary centers
>8	>4.6	No

Special considerations include age of patient, type of defect, comorbidities, resting or exercise-induced desaturation and PAH therapy (treat with intent-to-repair approach has not been proven).

Adapted from Rosenzweig EB, Abman SH, Adatia I, Beghetti M, Bonnet D, Haworth S, Ivy DD, Berger RMF. Paediatric pulmonary arterial hypertension: updates on definition, classification, diagnostics and management. European Respiratory Journal, 2019.

A more recent study was the first to extensively investigate the prognostic value of serial changes in standard clinical parameters in PAH-CHD showing that serial changes in World Health Organization Functional Class (WHO-FC), peak systemic arterial oxygen saturation (Sao_2), 6-minute walk distance (MWD), NTproBNP, and tricuspid annular plane systolic excursion (TAPSE) predict mortality and were more potent compared with baseline parameters. Moreover, serial changes in these parameters each have a specific impact on the length of survival. Mortality is highest in patients who deteriorate to WHO-FC IV, followed by those with NTproBNP increase of +1000 ng/L and a TAPSE decrease of −0.5 cm. Mortality is lowest in patients with a −50-m change in 6-MWD and −5% change in peak Sao_2. In addition, *multivariate analysis* showed that serial changes in peak Sao_2, NTproBNP, and TAPSE independently predict mortality.[16]

ANATOMIC AND CLINICAL CLASSIFICATION

Even among patients with APAH-CHD, there are several clinical phenotypes with important differences in clinical manifestations and outcomes leading to further subclassification of patients with APAH-CHD at the WSPH in 2013[17] (**Box 1**). There are 4 important broad classifications, including (1) classic ES, (2) left-to-right shunts ("correctable" and "noncorrectable"), (3) PAH with coincidental CHD (ie, small defects), and (4) CHD is repaired but PAH either persists immediately after surgery or recurs/develops months or years after surgery in the absence of significant postoperative hemodynamic lesions. These subtypes may also have very varied natural history. For example, patients with large unrestrictive posttricuspid shunts, such as a ventricular septal defect (VSD) or an aortopulmonary shunt, begin developing pulmonary vascular disease in early childhood as compared with pretricuspid defects, such as atrial septal defects (ASD), which can exist for decades without the development of pulmonary vascular disease.

Before considering closure of a defect with borderline pulmonary hypertension in the second group, one can easily test the directionality of shunting at rest and with exertion by using pulse oximetry and/or echocardiographic imaging. One should also perform full hemodynamics if correctability is in question and can follow guidance outlined from the WSPH 2018 meetings[8] (see **Table 1**). The repair status of the defect is also important, as patients with severe residual PAH after closure of shunts may have more rapid progression of disease and worse outcome, similar to IPAH, versus those with unrepaired shunts and ES physiology who have the ability to unload the RV.

PULMONARY ARTERIAL HYPERTENSION ASSOCIATED WITH UNRESTRICTED SHUNTS

The clinical presentation of APAH-CHD depends on the status of pulmonary vascular disease at the time of evaluation. In patients with large shunts and normal PVR, such as the infant with a large, nonrestrictive VSD, increased PBF, and congestive heart failure, the presentation is usually of failure to thrive, feeding intolerance, resting tachypnea, and recurrent respiratory infections. In these patients, surgical therapy after medical stabilization is the treatment of choice. Even within this group, in about 2% of children with large systemic-to-pulmonary shunts present, postoperative PAH occurs.[18] Children at increased risk for postoperative PAH crises are those with Down syndrome, with complex CHD (atrioventricular canal defects, aortopulmonary window, transposition of the great arteries, and truncus arteriosus), and with very reactive PAH in the preoperative period.[19]

In older patients (beyond infancy), careful evaluation to determine operability is critical before repair. Patients with APAH-CHD with modestly elevated PVR and moderate systemic-to-pulmonary shunts (type 2) are also quite challenging to manage.[20] Despite the lack of evidence-based guidelines, an assessment for operability should include a discussion about pretreatment with targeted PAH therapies and fenestrated closure of a defect to leave a "pop-off" should the patient have postoperative residual PAH. Closing a defect should not be performed just because it can be, but rather only when the PAH is likely to improve after surgical intervention. This point is important, particularly now that data have shown that patients with postoperative APAH-CHD fare worse than other forms of APAH-CHD. Cardiac catheterization and acute vasodilator testing (AVT) remain important tools to help determine safe operability in these patients. Although no validated criteria exist for predicting long-term postsurgical morbidity and mortality, a complete set of hemodynamics should be obtained; vasodilator testing and temporary balloon occlusion of the defect may also be helpful. Obtaining resting room air oxygen saturations and then oxygen saturation following exertion can be helpful in the assessment of operability. For a patient with resting cyanosis or even cyanosis with exertion, closing the defect can lead to worsening right heart failure by removing the pressure/volume "pop-off" that the defect affords the RV. Other important elements of the history include age at diagnosis, current age, and type and size of CHD. The importance of the type of CHD has been previously discussed, and, in general, the earlier a shunt lesion is diagnosed, the more likely the patient is operable. A history suggestive of initial congestive heart failure, including recurrent respiratory infection and effort intolerance, which improves over time to a "honeymoon period" of symptomatic relief, is suspicious of the development of irreversible pulmonary vascular disease with less net left-to-right shunting. In this situation, exercise testing may reveal latent cyanosis. Elevated hemoglobin in an iron-replete patient, suggesting erythrocytosis in response to hypoxia, may also indicate intermittent right-to-left shunting through the course of the day.

INTERPRETATION OF HEMODYNAMIC DATA

Indices of right heart function, including right atrial pressure and cardiac index, are important determinants of prognosis in IPAH.[21] In patients with APAH-CHD, PVR also becomes an important assessment of the PAH patient. It is essential to understand that PAH in patients with large systemic-to-pulmonary shunts can be due to an increase in PBF or to an increase in the PVR. In patients with large unrestrictive VSD or patent ductus arteriosus, PAP will be at systemic levels regardless of the PVR because of the increase in PBF (PBF [Qp]: systemic blood flow [Qs]). In contrast, elevation in the PVR is determined by the extent of the pulmonary vascular obstructive disease. Therefore, in patients with APAH-CHD, calculation of the PVR is critical as well. In a patient with a large shunt and normal PVR index (PVRi) less than 3 WUm^2, complete repair of the defect is usually not associated with residual PAH. However, when there is elevation of PVR > 6 WUm^2, completely repairing the defect can be dangerous and associated with residual PAH and postoperative PH crises and RV strain. During the hemodynamic evaluation of a systemic-to-pulmonary shunt, baseline room air hemodynamics should include 3 complete oxygen saturation runs and pressure measurements in the superior vena cava, right atrium (RA), RV, pulmonary artery, and pulmonary capillary wedge pressures. Once baseline data are collected, if there is no significant elevation of PAWP and PVRi is greater than 3 WUm^2, AVT preferably with inhaled nitric oxide (iNO) should be performed and another full assessment should be performed. Data should be obtained in the absence of respiratory or metabolic acidosis, hypoxia, anemia, or agitation. Nevertheless, the issue of determining operability is not straightforward and has been highlighted in several recent articles.[14,22–24] Lopes and O'Leary[25] proposed the following hemodynamic criteria for operability based on existing literature and surveying centers of excellence with experience in the treatment of pulmonary hypertensive patients: baseline PVRi less than 6 WUm^2 and PVR:SVR ratio less than 0.3. AVT was suggested if PVR at baseline was 6 to 9 WUm^2 with a PVR:SVR ratio of 0.3 to 0.5. In these patients, a favorable outcome is considered likely if with AVT, the following criteria are met: (1) a decrease of PVRi by greater than 20%, (2) a decrease in PVR:SVR ratio by 20%, (3) a final PVR less than 6 WUm^2, and (4) a final PVR:SVR ratio less than 0.3. Other centers have reported higher baseline PVRi values for operability PVRi less than or equal to 7 to 8 WUm^2 and PVR:SVR ratios of less than or equal to 0.4.[26,27] None of these studies report long-term outcomes following closure of the defects, and the question of the benefits of pretreating with targeted PAH therapies before surgical repair remains unanswered.

Cardiac catheterization alone, however, is usually not sufficient to determine operability. The hemodynamic findings taken at rest must be taken in the context of the medical history, physical examination, and results of all invasive and noninvasive testing. For example, in a case of borderline PVR at rest in the catheterization laboratory, but with significant exertional cyanosis, shunt repair may be more harmful than beneficial.

In patients with "borderline" hemodynamics (eg, PVRi 3–6 WUm^2), there may be an evolving role for a combined medical-surgical approach. Although this has not been proven to provide long-term benefit, there have been anecdotal cases, including at the authors' own institution, of being able to partially repair after using targeted PAH therapy in borderline cases. It may be reasonable to treat with targeted PAH therapies for a period of months and serially reevaluate by catheterization to determine operability or partial operability with intentional creation of a small residual defect as a "pop-off."[24] In rare borderline patients, medical therapy may drop the PVR enough to increase the left-to-right shunt to such an extent that there is significantly elevated PBF and the patient develops signs and symptoms of high-output failure.[22] As a result, surgical shunt closure should be expeditiously performed to protect the pulmonary vasculature from high-flow shear stress–related damage.

Surgery on a patient with borderline PAH should be undertaken after careful consideration of all these factors, and there should be a multidisciplinary team approach involving the pulmonary hypertension specialist, cardiologist, surgeon, intensivists, anesthesiologists, and the postoperative intensive care unit team. Care should be taken to anticipate and avoid PAP swings during induction of anesthesia and during recovery. Circulating vasoactive factors from blood products, particularly from platelets, are known to precipitate PAH crises and should be avoided if possible. In the postoperative period, use of pulmonary vasodilators, including iNO and adequate oxygenation, as well as avoidance of respiratory acidosis, is essential. Some patients may require sedation (and/or paralysis) and mechanical ventilation for several days if they have labile PH in the postoperative period. The use of sildenafil while weaning iNO has been found to be effective in preventing rebound PH in some cases.[28]

EISENMENGER SYNDROME

The term "Eisenmenger syndrome" (ES) was coined by Paul Hamilton Wood in 1958 to define the condition of increased PAP and PVR in relation to a VSD with resultant shunt reversal and cyanosis. Currently, the term Eisenmenger physiology has been expanded to include any reversed shunt secondary to elevated PVR, including shunts associated with complex CHD.[29] With timely CHD diagnosis and cardiac surgery, especially during infancy, survival of patients into adulthood is commonplace, and the worldwide incidence of ES has declined by 50%.[30,31] However, ES still remains a significant problem in the developing world, where patients with large shunts are unable to undergo repair before the development of pulmonary vascular disease. The worldwide prevalence of PAH in adults with CHD has recently been estimated at between 1.6 and 12.5 million, with 25% to 50% presenting with ES.[32]

Although life expectancy is reduced in ES, it is significantly better than IPAH, with many patients with ES surviving into their third and fourth decades, and even some surviving into their seventh decade.[30,31] More than 40% of subjects are expected to be alive 25 years after diagnosis.

Patients with complex lesions have a much worse prognosis than those with simple shunts. However, with advances in targeted therapies, the outlook for patients with ES may improve, as a recent study predicted Kaplan-Meier survival estimate at 20 years of 87% in patients with ES.[11] The presentation and clinical course of ES are a result of chronic hypoxia and are different from those of IPAH. Patients with ES often have objective evidence of significant effort intolerance, but may not perceive their limitation because of the chronicity of their disease. Their symptoms and complications are secondary to the cyanosis, erythrocytosis, and end-organ damage. On physical examination, central cyanosis with clubbing may be present; RV heave and a prominent second heart sound are often present, and hepatomegaly and peripheral edema may be appreciated in more advanced cases. Patients may also present with serious complications, such as cerebral abscess or stroke, pulmonary arterial thrombosis, massive hemoptysis, owing to rupture of thin-walled pulmonary vessels, bacterial endocarditis, or severe myocardial dysfunction with low-cardiac output.

MANAGEMENT STRATEGIES FOR EISENMENGER SYNDROME

In the past, treatment options for patients with ES had been limited to palliative therapies and heart-lung transplantation or lung transplantation with repair of the CHD. However, over the past decade, there has been growing experience using both conventional and targeted PAH therapies in patients with ES. Commonly used conventional therapies include digoxin, diuretics, and antiarrhythmics, although none of these have been shown to improve survival in ES. Anticoagulation in patients with ES remains controversial because of increased risks of pulmonary artery thrombosis, as well as hemoptysis, stroke, and hemorrhage. Given the potential complications, the decision to anticoagulate should be made carefully on an individual case-by-case basis. In general, oral anticoagulation is recommended for ES patients with intrapulmonary thrombi, confirmed paradoxic embolism, in the presence of atrial flutter or fibrillation, and for patients requiring indwelling lines for medication administration or intracardiac pacing leads.[33] Oxygen is often used long term in patients with ES, and although it may be associated with improvement in subjective status, no survival benefit has been seen. Although secondary erythrocytosis is commonly seen, current practice has moved away from phlebotomy, which should only be used for patients with signs of severe hyperviscosity symptoms.[34] Maternal mortality in patients with ES is reported at approximately 50%, with death usually occurring during delivery or the first postpartum week because of hypervolemia, thromboembolism, or preeclampsia. In addition, spontaneous abortion rates are quite high, and for infants carried to term, there are high rates of infant mortality. As a result, pregnancy is contraindicated in ES.[34–36]

Targeted Therapies for Eisenmenger Syndrome

There are 3 main classes of targeted PAH therapies initially used in patients with group 1 PAH, and currently, all have been used in the treatment of patients with ES. These therapies include prostanoids, endothelin receptor antagonists (ERAs), and phosphodiesterase-5 (PDE5) inhibitors. The aim of targeted therapies in patients with ES is to improve exercise tolerance by improving pulmonary blood flow, hypoxemia, physical capacity, and, ultimately, survival.

Prostanoids

The use of intravenous epoprostenol in ES was first described by Rosenzweig and colleagues[37] in 1999, with subjects showing improvements in functional capacity, hemodynamics, and survival. Because intravenous epoprostenol is chemically unstable at neutral pH/room temperature and has a short half-life (1–2 minutes), a continuous intravenous delivery system is needed to maintain stability. An indwelling central venous line is necessary, with associated potential complications, including thrombosis/emboli and line occlusion, local and systemic infection, and catheter breakage. The risk of thromboembolism is of particular concern in patients with ES with right-to-left shunts, and the use of a subcutaneous prostanoid analogue is preferred if there is a concern for potential central venous catheter complications. In addition, pump malfunction may rarely lead to administration of a sudden bolus of epoprostenol (leading to systemic hypotension) or interruption of the medication, which can cause severe rebound PAH. Therefore, a search for alternate routes of drug delivery has led to the approval of inhaled (iloprost, treprostinil), subcutaneous (treprostinil), and more stable and longer-acting intravenous prostacyclin analogues (veletri, treprostinil). Treprostinil sodium is a prostacyclin analogue with a neutral pH, longer half-life, which is stable at room temperature, and shares the same pharmacologic actions as epoprostenol with potential advantages by

being able to deliver the agent via inhalation or subcutaneous infusion, thus eliminating the risk of thromboembolic events in patients with ES.[38] The use of oral prostanoids has not been well studied for ES. In 1 case report, it was successfully initiated, but follow-up data were not available.[39] However, in concept, the use of an oral route for a prostanoid may be preferred if it is demonstrated to be effective.

Endothelin receptor antagonists

Endothelin (ET)-1 is one of the most potent vasoconstrictors implicated in the pathobiology of PAH, and plasma ET-1 levels are increased in patients with IPAH (and other forms of PAH) and correlate inversely with prognosis. The first randomized, double-blinded, placebo-controlled study in patients with ES was the BREATHE-5 (Bosentan Randomized Trial of Endothelin Antagonist Therapy-5) trial investigating the efficacy and safety of the dual ERA bosentan in patients with ES.[40,41] During the 16-week study, bosentan significantly reduced PVR and improved PAP and exercise capacity compared with placebo without worsening oxygenation, and longer-term data from the follow-up portion of the study demonstrated continued improvements in the exercise capacity over an additional 24 weeks.[41] The study also demonstrated a worsening of PVR in the placebo group, which underscores the progressive nature of untreated ES. Risks associated with ERAs include acute hepatotoxicity (bosentan), teratogenicity, and possibly male infertility. The selective ERA ambrisentan may offer potential advantages over bosentan, given its selectivity for the ET-A receptor, which demonstrates vasoconstrictor effects, although this remains controversial. Ambrisentan, which can be administered once a day, was also found to be efficacious in a series of patients with ES with an acceptable safety profile.[42] Macitentan did not show superiority over placebo on the primary end point of change from baseline to week 16 in exercise capacity in patients with ES.[43] Given the current experience with ERAs for ES, their role alone and in combination with other targeted PAH therapies seems to warrant further study.[44]

Phosphodiesterase-5 inhibitors PDE5 inhibitors prevent the inactivation of cyclic guanosine monophosphate (GMP), thereby raising cyclic GMP levels. Oral sildenafil is the most widely used of the PDE5 inhibitors in the treatment of PAH and has been used in children with APAH-CHD, with benefits on exercise capacity and hemodynamics.[45,46] In a recent prospective open-label, multicenter study, using sildenafil, patients with

ES demonstrated an acceptable safety profile and improved exercise capacity, oxygen saturation, and hemodynamics after 12 months of therapy.[47] A recent randomized, placebo-controlled, double-blinded crossover study using tadalafil in patients with ES also demonstrated safety and short-term improvements in exercise capacity, functional class, oxygen saturation, and hemodynamics after 6 weeks of therapy.[48]

Lung and heart lung transplantation Currently, the overall 1-, 5-, and 10-year survival for lung transplantation for patients with PAH is 64%, 44%, and 20%, respectively.[48–51] For patients with untreated ES, the 5- and 25-year survival is greater than 80% and 40%, respectively, as opposed to following lung transplantation (52% and 39%).[48–51] Thus, lung transplantation should be reserved for patients with WHO-FC IV symptoms with an estimated likelihood of survival of less than 50% at 5 years. Although lung and heart/lung transplantation are imperfect therapies for PAH, when offered to an appropriately selected population, transplantation may improve survival with an improved quality of life. The use of extracorporeal membrane oxygenation as a bridge to recovery (in acutely decompensated patients), as well as a bridge to transplantation, may also be a viable option in selected patients.[50]

PULMONARY HYPERTENSION IN THE UNIVENTRICULAR HEART: THE FAILING FONTAN

The Fontan (total cavopulmonary connection) circulation, which is surgically created for hypoplastic left heart syndrome, lacks a pumping subpulmonary ventricle and is dependent on the central venous pressure to perfuse the pulmonary circulation. Thus, changes in the PVR can have a tremendous impact on forward flow in this circulation. For patients with a single ventricle, the usual hemodynamic criteria used for shunt closure do not apply for predicting operability. Pre-Fontan PVRi should be normal in these patients, to sustain the cavopulmonary circulation (ie, <3 WUm^2). In these patients, a preoperative mean PAP of only 15 to 18 mm Hg is a risk factor for poor outcome after Fontan repair.[21,22] Postoperatively, even small increases in PAP can lead to low-cardiac output syndrome, even in the setting of a technically successful operation. Current medical management of Fontan failure aims mostly at treating manifestations, such as ventricular dysfunction and protein-losing enteropathy (PLE).

Most of the complications of failing Fontan circulation are attributed to structural changes (stenosis) in the pulmonary vascular tree or to pulmonary vascular disease. Late complications include ventricular dysfunction and low-cardiac output syndrome, PLE, hypoxemia, and decreased exercise intolerance, and all these are ultimately related to elevated PVR.[52,53] There are small case series reporting benefit of therapies, such as subcutaneous heparin, oral budesonide, spironolactone, bosentan, and sildenafil, in the treatment of PLE.[54] Because elevated PVR is implicated in failure of the Fontan circulation, targeted PAH therapies, including iNO, are sometimes used. In the immediate postoperative period, iNO in combination with milrinone has been found to be beneficial in improving hemodynamics.[54] Although prostacyclins are rarely used in the perioperative period, epoprostenol has been shown to prevent the rebound effects of NO cessation.[55] There is scant literature on the effects of targeted PAH therapies in patients with failing Fontan; however, sildenafil and bosentan have been used in the treatment of PLE and plastic bronchitis, and to improve hemodynamic response to exercise.[56–61] Because of the liver toxicity associated with nonselective ERAs and the potential for liver complications in patients with Fontan failure, there may be some hesitation to use bosentan in these patients. Postmarketing surveillance of bosentan found transaminase elevation to be less of a problem in patients with APAH-CHD than other types of PAH; however, these studies do not specifically discuss the Fontan subgroups. Currently, there are several ongoing clinical trials investigating the role of targeted therapies in patients with univentricular circulation.[61–65]

SUMMARY

Although PAH associated with CHD has common histopathologic and pathobiologic findings as other disorders clustered together under WHO group 1 pulmonary hypertension, this group is very heterogeneous in terms of anatomic, physiologic, and clinical features, as well as outcomes. With improved survival of patients with CHD, the number of patients with CHD and PAH seen in adult CHD clinics is increasing. This subgroup of patients has unique clinical features and potential complications compared with patients with other forms of WHO group 1 PAH. Targeted PAH therapies have clear short-term benefits in these patients, and their use in patients with borderline hemodynamics may pave the way for a combined medical-surgical approach to management in borderline cases in the future. However, further large studies are required to evaluate the long-term outcome using these strategies. A subpopulation of APAH-CHD that is growing rapidly includes those patients with complex single-ventricle anatomy, and large multicenter studies are required to better understand the Fontan physiology and evaluate potential benefits of targeted PAH therapies in these patients.

CLINICS CARE POINTS

- Understanding that not all APAH-CHD is physiologically the same is key to understanding how to best manage.
- Despite worse hemodynamics, the 20-yr survival for Eisenmenger patients is better than for those with postoperative APAH-CHD.
- Repair of a CHD in a patient with elevated PVR should be carefully assessed by a specialized team prior to closure even when PVR is only borderline elevated.(eg, > 2.3 WU).

REFERENCES

1. Rose ML, Strange G, King I, et al. Congenital heart disease-associated pulmonary arterial hypertension: preliminary results from a novel registry. Intern Med J 2012;42:874–9.
2. Gatzoulis MA, Alonso-Gonzalez R, Beghetti M. Pulmonary arterial hypertension in paediatric and adult patients with congenital heart disease. Eur Respir Rev 2009;18:154–61.
3. Fratz S, Geiger R, Kresse H, et al. Pulmonary blood pressure, not flow, is associated with net endothelin-1 production in the lungs of patients with congenital heart disease and normal pulmonary vascular resistance. J Thorac Cardiovasc Surg 2003;126:1724–9.
4. Arvind B, Relan J, Kothari SS. "Treat and repair" strategy for shunt lesions: a critical review. Pulm Circ 2020;10(2). 2045894020917885.
5. Humbert M, Sitbon O, Chaouat A, et al. Pulmonary arterial hypertension in France: results from a national registry. Am J Respir Crit Care Med 2006; 173:1023–30.
6. Badesch DB, Raskob GE, Elliott CG, et al. Pulmonary arterial hypertension: baseline characteristics from the REVEAL registry. Chest 2009;137:376–87.
7. Haworth SG, Hislop AA. Treatment and survival in children with pulmonary arterial hypertension: the UK pulmonary hypertension service for children 2001-2006. Heart 2009;95:312–7.
8. Simonneau G, Montani D, Celermajer DS, et al. Haemodynamic definitions and updated clinical classification of pulmonary hypertension. Eur Respir J 2019;53(1):1801913.
9. Durmowicz AG, Stenmark KR. Mechanisms of structural remodeling in chronic pulmonary hypertension. Pediatr Rev 1999;20:e91–102.
10. Hopkins WE, Ochoa LL, Richardson GW, et al. Comparison of the hemodynamics and survival of adults with severe primary pulmonary hypertension or Eisenmenger syndrome. J Heart Lung Transplant 1996;15:100–5.
11. Manes A, Palazzini M, Leci E, et al. Current era survival of patients with pulmonary arterial hypertension associated with congenital heart disease: a comparison between clinical subgroups. Eur Heart J 2014; 35(11):716–24.
12. Engelfriet PM, Duffels MG, Moller T, et al. Pulmonary arterial hypertension in adults born with a heart septal defect: the Euro Heart Survey on adult congenital heart disease. Heart 2007;93:682–7.
13. McLaughlin VV, Archer SL, Badesch DB, et al. ACCF/AHA 2009 expert consensus document on pulmonary hypertension. A report of the American College of Cardiology Foundation Task Force on Expert Consensus Documents and the American Heart Association developed in collaboration with the American College of Chest Physicians; American Thoracic Society, Inc.; and the Pulmonary Hypertension Association. J Am Coll Cardiol 2009;53: 1573–619.
14. Rosenzweig EB, Abman SH, Adatia I, et al. Paediatric pulmonary arterial hypertension: updates on definition, classification, diagnostics and management. Eur Respir J 2019;53(1):1801916.
15. Benza RL, Miller DP, Gomberg-Maitland M, et al. Predicting survival in pulmonary arterial hypertension: insights from the registry to evaluate early and long-term pulmonary arterial hypertension disease management (REVEAL). Circulation 2010; 122:164–72.
16. Schuijt MTU, Blok IM, Zwinderman AH, et al. Mortality in pulmonary arterial hypertension due to congenital heart disease: serial changes improve prognostication. Int J Cardiol 2017;243:449–53.
17. Simonneau G, Robbins IM, Beghetti M, et al. Updated clinical classification of pulmonary hypertension. J Am Coll Cardiol 2009;54(Suppl 1): S43–54.
18. Lindberg L, Olsson AK, Jogi P, et al. How common is severe pulmonary hypertension after pediatric cardiac surgery? J Thorac Cardiovasc Surg 2002;123: 1155–63.
19. Bando K, Turrentine MW, Sharp TG, et al. Pulmonary hypertension after operations for congenital heart disease: analysis of risk factors and management. J Thorac Cardiovasc Surg 1996;112(6):1600–7 [discussion: 1607–9].
20. Matsumoto M, Naitoh H, Higashi T, et al. Risk factors for pulmonary hypertensive crisis (PHC) following VSD repair in infants. Masui 1995;44:1208–12.

21. Adatia I, Beghetti M. Early postoperative care of patients with pulmonary hypertension associated with congenital cardiac disease. Cardiol Young 2009; 19:315–9.

22. Rosenzweig EB, Barst RJ. Congenital heart disease and pulmonary hypertension: pharmacology PAH and feasibility of late surgery. Prog Cardiovasc Dis 2012;55(2):128–33.

23. Beghetti M, Tissot C. Pulmonary hypertension in congenital shunts. Rev Esp Cardiol 2010;63: 1179–93.

24. Beghetti M, Galie' N, Bonnet D. Can inoperable congenital heart defects become operable in patients with pulmonary arterial hypertension? Dream or reality? Congenit Heart Dis 2012;7:3–11.

25. Lopes AA, O'Leary PW. Measurement, interpretation and use of haemodynamic parameters in pulmonary hypertension associated with congenital cardiac disease. Cardiol Young 2009;19:431–5.

26. Viswanathan S, Kumar RK. Assessment of operability of congenital cardiac shunts with increased pulmonary vascular resistance. Catheter Cardiovasc Interv 2008;71:665–70.

27. Giglia TM, Humpl T. Preoperative pulmonary hemodynamics and assessment of operability: is there a pulmonary vascular resistance that precludes cardiac operation? Pediatr Crit Care Med 2010; 11(Suppl 2):S57–69.

28. Matamis D, Pampori S, Papathanasiou A, et al. Inhaled NO and sildenafil combination in cardiac surgery patients with out-of-proportion pulmonary hypertension: acute effects on postoperative gas exchange and hemodynamics. Circ Heart Fail 2012;5:47–53.

29. Galie N, Hoeper MM, Humbert M, et al. Guidelines for the diagnosis and treatment of pulmonary hypertension: the Task Force for the Diagnosis and Treatment of Pulmonary Hypertension of the European Society of Cardiology (ESC) and the European Respiratory Society (ERS), endorsed by the International Society of Heart and Lung Transplantation (ISHLT). Eur Heart J 2009;30:2493–537.

30. Dimopoulos K, Inuzuka R, Goletto S, et al. Improved survival among patients with Eisenmenger syndrome receiving advanced therapy for pulmonary arterial hypertension. Circulation 2010; 121:20–5.

31. Galie N, Manes A, Palazzini M, et al. Management of pulmonary arterial hypertension associated with congenital systemic-to-pulmonary shunts and Eisenmenger's syndrome. Drugs 2008;68:1049–66.

32. Lopes AA, Bandeira AP, Flores PC, et al. Pulmonary hypertension in Latin America: pulmonary vascular disease: the global perspective. Chest 2010; 137(Suppl 6):78S–84S.

33. Galiè N, Humbert M, Vachiery JL, et al. 2015 ESC/ ERS guidelines for the diagnosis and treatment of pulmonary hypertension. Rev Esp Cardiol (Engl Ed) 2016;69(2):177.

34. Diller GP, Dimopoulos K, Broberg CS, et al. Presentation, survival prospects, and predictors of death in Eisenmenger syndrome: a combined retrospective and case-control study. Eur Heart J 2006;27: 1737–42.

35. Swan L, Lupton M, Anthony J, et al. Controversies in pregnancy and congenital heart disease. Congenit Heart Dis 2006;1:27–34.

36. Bedard E, Dimopoulos K, Gatzoulis MA. Has there been any progress made on pregnancy outcomes among women with pulmonary arterial hypertension? Eur Heart J 2009;30:256–65.

37. Rosenzweig EB, Kerstein D, Barst RJ. Long-term prostacyclin for pulmonary hypertension with associated congenital heart defects. Circulation 1999; 99:1858–65.

38. Barst RJ, Simonneau G, Rich S, et al, for the Uniprost PAH Study Group. Efficacy and safety of chronic subcutaneous infusion of UT-15 (Uniprost) in pulmonary arterial hypertension (PAH). Circulation 2000;102:100–1.

39. El-Kersh K, Suliman S, Smith JS. Selexipag in congenital heart disease-associated pulmonary arterial hypertension and Eisenmenger syndrome: first report. Am J Ther 2018;25(6):e714–5.

40. Galie N, Beghetti M, Gatzoulis MA, et al. Bosentan therapy in patients with Eisenmenger syndrome: a multicenter, double-blind, randomized, placebo-controlled study. Circulation 2006;114:48–54.

41. Gatzoulis MA, Beghetti M, Galie N, et al. Longer-term bosentan therapy improves functional capacity in Eisenmenger syndrome: results of the BREATHE-5 open-label extension study. Int J Cardiol 2008; 127(1):27–32.

42. Zuckerman WA, Leaderer D, Rowan CA, et al. Ambrisentan for pulmonary arterial hypertension due to congenital heart disease. Am J Cardiol 2011; 107(9):1381–5.

43. Gatzoulis MA, Landzberg M, Beghetti M, et al, MAESTRO Study Investigators. Evaluation of macitentan in patients with Eisenmenger syndrome. Circulation 2019;139(1):51–63.

44. Elshafay A, Truong DH, AboElnas MM, et al. The effect of endothelin receptor antagonists in patients with Eisenmenger syndrome: a systematic review. Am J Cardiovasc Drugs 2018;18(2):93–102.

45. Schulze-Neick I, Hartenstein P, Li J. Intravenous sildenafil is a potent pulmonary vasodilator in children with congenital heart disease. Circulation 2003;108: II167–73.

46. Sun YJ, Yang T, Zeng WJ, et al. Impact of sildenafil on survival of patients with Eisenmenger syndrome. Clin Pharmacol 2013;53(6):611–8.

47. Zhang ZN, Jiang X, Zhang R, et al. Oral sildenafil treatment for Eisenmenger syndrome: a

prospective, open-label, multicentre study. Heart 2011;97(22):1876–81.

48. Mukhopadhyay S, Nathani S, Yusuf J, et al. Clinical efficacy of phosphodiesterase-5 inhibitor tadalafil in Eisenmenger syndrome—a randomized, placebo-controlled, double-blind crossover study. Congenit Heart Dis 2011;6(5):424–31.

49. Ofori-Amanfo G, Hsu D, Lamour JM, et al. Heart transplantation in children with markedly elevated pulmonary vascular resistance: impact of right ventricular failure on outcome. J Heart Lung Transplant 2011;30(6):659–66.

50. Lang G, Taghavi S, Aigner C. Primary lung transplantation after bridge with extracorporeal membrane oxygenation: a plea for a shift in our paradigms for indications. Transplantation 2012;93: 729–36.

51. Trulock EP, Edwards LB, Taylor DO, et al. The registry of the International Society for Heart and Lung Transplantation: Twentieth Official Adult Lung and Heart-Lung Transplant Report—2003. J Heart Lung Transplant 2003;22:625–35.

52. Khambadkone S, Li J, de Leval MR, et al. Basal pulmonary vascular resistance and nitric oxide responsiveness late after Fontan-type operation. Circulation 2003;107(25):3204–8.

53. Beghetti M. Fontan and the pulmonary circulation: a potential role for new pulmonary hypertension therapies. Heart 2010;96(12):911–6.

54. Goldberg DJ, Shaddy RE, Ravishankar C, et al. The failing Fontan: etiology, diagnosis and management. Expert Rev Cardiovasc Ther 2011;9(6):785–93.

55. Ryerson L, Goldberg C, Rosenthal A, et al. Usefulness of heparin therapy in protein-losing enteropathy associated with single ventricle palliation. Am J Cardiol 2008;101:248–51.

56. Ringel RE, Peddy SB. Effect of high-dose spironolactone on protein-losing enteropathy in patients

with Fontan palliation of complex congenital heart disease. Am J Cardiol 2003;91:1031–2. A1039.

57. Yoshimura N, Yamaguchi M, Oka S, et al. Inhaled nitric oxide therapy after Fontan-type operations. Surg Today 2005;35:31–5.

58. Cai J, Su Z, Shi Z, et al. Nitric oxide and milrinone: combined effect on pulmonary circulation after Fontan-type procedure: a prospective, randomized study. Ann Thorac Surg 2008;86:882–8.

59. Miyaji K, Nagata N, Miyamoto T, et al. Combined therapy with inhaled nitric oxide and intravenous epoprostenol (prostacyclin) for critical pulmonary perfusion after the Fontan procedure. J Thorac Cardiovasc Surg 2003;125:437–9.

60. Trachte AL, Lobato EB, Urdaneta F, et al. Oral sildenafil reduces pulmonary hypertension after cardiac surgery. Ann Thorac Surg 2005;79:194–7.

61. Wang W, Hu X, Liao W, et al. The efficacy and safety of pulmonary vasodilators in patients with Fontan circulation: a meta-analysis of randomized controlled trials. Pulm Circ 2019;9(1). 2045894018790450.

62. Haseyama K, Satomi G, Yasukochi S, et al. Pulmonary vasodilation therapy with sildenafil citrate in a patient with plastic bronchitis after the Fontan procedure for hypoplastic left heart syndrome. J Thorac Cardiovasc Surg 2006;132(5):1232–3.

63. Giardini A, Balducci A, Specchia S, et al. Effect of sildenafil on haemodynamic response to exercise and exercise capacity in Fontan patients. Eur Heart J 2008;29:1681–7.

64. Apostolopoulou SC, Papagiannis J, Rammos S. Bosentan induces clinical, exercise and hemodynamic improvement in a pre-transplant patient with plastic bronchitis after Fontan operation. J Heart Lung Transplant 2005;24:1174–6.

65. Ovaert C, Thijs D, Dewolf D, et al. The effect of bosentan in patients with a failing Fontan circulation. Cardiol Young 2009;19:331–9.

Pulmonary Arterial Hypertension Secondary to Drugs and Toxins

Ramon L. Ramirez III, MD[a], Shaun M. Pienkos, MD[b],
Vinicio de Jesus Perez, MD[a,c,1], Roham T. Zamanian, MD[a,c,*]

KEYWORDS

- Drugs • Toxins • Pulmonary • Arterial • Vascular • Hypertension

KEY POINTS

- Drug- and toxin-induced pulmonary arterial hypertension is a clinically relevant subgroup of group 1 pulmonary hypertension.
- The exact mechanisms of drug- and toxin-induced pulmonary arterial hypertension vary by agent and are currently largely unknown.
- Only a small percentage of exposed patients develop clinical disease, which suggests genetic factors in the pathogenesis of drug- and toxin-induced pulmonary arterial hypertension.
- Treatments for drug- and toxin-induced pulmonary arterial hypertension include pulmonary vasodilators and removal of the offending agent.
- Pharmacovigilance and partnership with public and regulatory agencies are mandatory to prevent community outbreaks of drug- and toxin-induced pulmonary arterial hypertension.

INTRODUCTION

Since its description by Romberg in 1891,[1] pulmonary arterial hypertension (PAH) was a disease with low incidence and prevalence. However, in the 1960s a surge in PAH cases was documented in Switzerland, Germany, and Austria in association with aminorex fumarate, an amphetamine-like appetite suppressant.[2,3] Since then, other drugs and toxins have been linked to pulmonary hypertension (PH) epidemics in the United States and Europe. Based on available evidence, the current PH clinical classification recognizes the link between PH and certain drugs and toxins as either definite or possible[4] (**Table 1**). Drugs with a definite association include agents with data based on outbreaks, epidemiologic case control studies, or large multicenter series. Drugs with a possible

association are suggested by multiple case series or cases with drugs with similar mechanisms of action (**Table 2**). In this review, we cover the history and current knowledge surrounding drugs and toxins recognized to be risk factors for PAH. We also discuss the evolving evidence that links newer drugs with PAH development and the importance of pharmacovigilance, physician and public awareness, and working with regulatory agencies to prevent deadly outbreaks of PAH.

AMINOREX FUMARATE

The first agent to be implicated as a cause of PAH was aminorex fumarate. Aminorex (Menocil) was an amphetamine-like appetite suppressant that was released in Austria, Germany, and Switzerland in 1965 as a novel over-the-counter treatment for

[a] Division of Pulmonary, Allergy and Critical Care, Stanford University School of Medicine, 300 Pasteur Drive, Room S102, Stanford, CA 94305, USA; [b] Department of Medicine, Stanford University School of Medicine, 300 Pasteur Drive, Room S102, Stanford, CA 94305, USA; [c] Vera Moulton Wall Center for Pulmonary Vascular Disease, Stanford, CA, USA
[1] Present address: 300 Pasteur Drive, Grant S140 B, Stanford, CA 94305.
* Corresponding author. 300 Pasteur Drive, Room H3143, Stanford, CA 94305.
E-mail address: Zamanian@stanford.edu

Clin Chest Med 42 (2021) 19–38
https://doi.org/10.1016/j.ccm.2020.11.008

Table 1
Updated classification of drugs and toxins associated with PAH

Definite	Possible
Aminorex	Cocaine
Fenfluramine	Phenylpropanolamine
Dexfenfluramine	L-tryptophan
Benfluorex	St John's wort
Meth	Amphetamines
Dasatinib	Interferon alpha and beta
Toxic rapeseed oil	Alkylating agents
	Bosutinib
	Direct-acting antiviral agents against hepatitis C virus
	Leflunomide
	Indirubin (Chinese herb Qing-Dai)

Adapted from Simonneau G, Montani D, Celermajer DS, Denton CP, Gatzoulis MA, Krowka M, et al. Haemodynamic definitions and updated clinical classification of pulmonary hypertension. The European respiratory journal. 2019;53(1).; Reproduced with permission of the © ERS 2020.

obesity. Two years after its release, physicians began to notice a dramatic (10- to 20-fold) increase in cases of PAH in these countries.[2] The observed rate of PAH in users of aminorex was estimated at 2000 cases per million exposed, which translates to an odds ratio of more than 1000.[5] Most patients began to experience symptoms within 6 months of using aminorex.

Case series and mounting anecdotal evidence of the association between aminorex and PAH led to aminorex being withdrawn from the market in 1972.[3] Nearly 50% of patients exposed to aminorex died within 10 years of their PH diagnosis, usually owing to complications of right heart failure.[5] On autopsy, these patients were found to have precapillary PH with typical plexiform arterial lesions. Fortunately, some patients (12 of 20 in 1 series) did improve after drug withdrawal.

Aminorex fumarate produces its effects via release of catecholamines in the central nervous system.[6,7] Similar to amphetamines (**Fig. 1**), it increases basal metabolic rate and energy expenditure to induce weight loss. There is a growing body of literature linking serotonin dysregulation in the pathogenesis of drug- and toxin-induced PAH.[8] Serotonin has been demonstrated to act as a mitogen and increases pulmonary artery smooth muscle cell proliferation.[9] Occlusion of these

vessels leads to increased pulmonary pressures and the pathologic findings seen in advanced PAH. Aminorex has been shown to act as a strong substrate that interacts directly with the serotonin transporter (also called 5HTT) on pulmonary artery smooth muscle cell.[10,11] Other studies demonstrate that aminorex and similar anorexigens may also inhibit potassium channels, leading to direct vasoconstriction of pulmonary arteries owing to derangements in intracellular calcium levels.[12]

The aminorex outbreak highlighted 2 fundamental concepts in the field of PH. First, oral anorectic drugs could lead to pulmonary vascular lesions identical to those seen in other forms of PAH.[13] Second, only a very small percentage (about 2%) of patients exposed to aminorex developed clinical disease, suggesting a possible genetic predisposition.

FENFLURAMINE AND DEXFENFLURAMINE

Fenfluramine and its enantiomer, dexfenfluramine, are appetite suppressants in the phenylethylamine class, with structural and pharmacologic properties similar to amphetamine. Like aminorex, fenfluramine is also a potent serotonergic agent that interacts with the serotonin transporter.[6,11,14,15] These drugs were released in the 1970s as adjuvant therapies for obesity. In 1981, the first cases of fenfluramine-associated PAH were published.[16]

In 1993, Brenot and colleagues[17] published a retrospective study that found that 20% of patients with PAH who presented to a PH-specialized medical center reported fenfluramine use. In 67% of patients, there was a close temporal relationship between fenfluramine use and the development of PH symptoms. A handful of patients showed clinical improvement with fenfluramine withdrawal. Histologic examination of the women who had used fenfluramine showed typical advanced plexogenic pulmonary arteriopathy similar to those of primary PAH. This analysis was followed in 1996 by the International Primary Pulmonary Hypertension Study, which found that anorexic drugs such as fenfluramine and its derivatives were associated with a markedly increased risk of PAH.[18] In 2000, a prospective surveillance study of 579 patients with primary PAH and secondary PH in North America further confirmed a link between fenfluramine derivatives and PAH. The association was noted to be stronger with a longer duration of fenfluramine use.[19]

Fenfluramine was also marketed in conjunction with another amphetamine-like stimulant, phentermine, in a combination informally known as Fen/Phen. In 1997, a report identified a potential association between fenfluramine–phentermine and

Table 2
Drugs and toxins identified as risk factors for PAH, their drug or toxin class, and proposed mechanisms of PAH pathogenesis

Drug or Toxin Name	Drug or Toxin Class	Proposed Mechanism of PAH Pathogenesis
Aminorex fumarate	Amphetamine-like anorexigen	Increase in serotonin, interaction with SERT, PASMC proliferation, K+ channel inhibition mediated vasoconstriction
Fenfluramine and dexfenfluramine	Amphetamine-like anorexigen	Increase in serotonin, interaction with SERT, PASMC proliferation
Benfluorex	Amphetamine-like anorexigen	Increase in serotonin, interaction with SERT, PASMC proliferation
Methamphetamine	Amphetamine	Increase in serotonin, interaction with SERT, PASMC proliferation, Generation of ROS, Mitochondrial dysfunction
Dasatinib	Tyrosine kinase inhibitor	Generation of ROS, endothelial dysfunction, increased endothelial permeability
Toxic rapeseed oil	Oil derived from seeds of a plant, possibly contaminated with anilides	Pulmonary artery endothelial dysfunction and narrowing, intimal proliferation, fibrosis and thrombosis
Cocaine	Stimulant	Increased serotonin, interactions with SERT, increased levels of ET-1, cocaine adulterants (levamisole), decreased levels of nitric oxide and eNOS
Phenylpropanolamine	Amphetamine-like stimulant, nasal decongestant, anorexigen	Increase in serotonin, interaction with SERT, PASMC proliferation
L-Tryptophan	Essential amino acid	Adulterant, possibly 3- anilino-L-alanine, lymphocytic perivascular infiltrate, intimal thickening
St John's Wort	Over-the-counter herbal supplement	Unknown
Interferon alpha and beta	Endogenous immunomodulatory proteins	Increased ET-1 causing vasoconstriction
Mitomycin, cyclophosphamide, others	Alkylating agents	PVOD, disruption of endothelial cell repair, decrease in prostacyclin synthesis, oxidative injury
Sofosbuvir	Direct antiviral acting agents	Suppression of HCV RNA leads to rapid decrease in vasodilatory mediators via STAT-3 pathway (Renard et al 2016[94])
Leflunomide	DMARD	Inhibition of vasodilatory prostaglandin synthesis
Indirubin	Indigo plant extract, herbal medicine	Unclear, possibly impaired vasodilation owing to pulmonary artery endothelial dysfunction
Mazindol	Nonamphetamine stimulant	Possibly serotonin mediated but unclear link
MDMA	Amphetamine stimulant	Increase in serotonin, interaction with SERT, PASMC proliferation
Fluoxetine	SSRI	Serotonin dysregulation

(continued on next page)

Table 2
(continued)

Drug or Toxin Name	Drug or Toxin Class	Proposed Mechanism of PAH Pathogenesis
Diazoxide	Nondiuretic thiazide	Off target interactions with SUR2 receptor in pulmonary vasculature
Trichloroethylene	Industrial solvent	PVOD, increased vascular permeability leading to exposure of PASMCs to circulating growth factors and thus proliferation and recruitment of inflammatory cells
Anagrelide	Platelet-reducing agent	Unknown, PAH may be reversible with drug withdrawal
Carfilzomib	Proteasome inhibitor	Proteasome inhibitor mediated changes in endothelial eNOS and NO levels, leading to impaired vasodilation and endothelial dysfunction, oxidative stress, increased vascular tone

Abbreviations: DMARD, disease-modifying antirheumatic drug; eNOS, nitric oxide synthase; ET-1, endothelin-1; HCV, Hepatitis C virus; K+, potassium; MDMA, 3,4- methylenedioxymethamphetamine; PASMC, pulmonary artery smooth muscle cell; ROS, reactive oxygen species; SERT, serotonin transporter; SUR2, sulfonylurea receptor.

the development of cardiac valvular lesions,[20] potentially related to increasing levels of serotonin.[21] Interestingly, despite a case report showing a possible association between phentermine

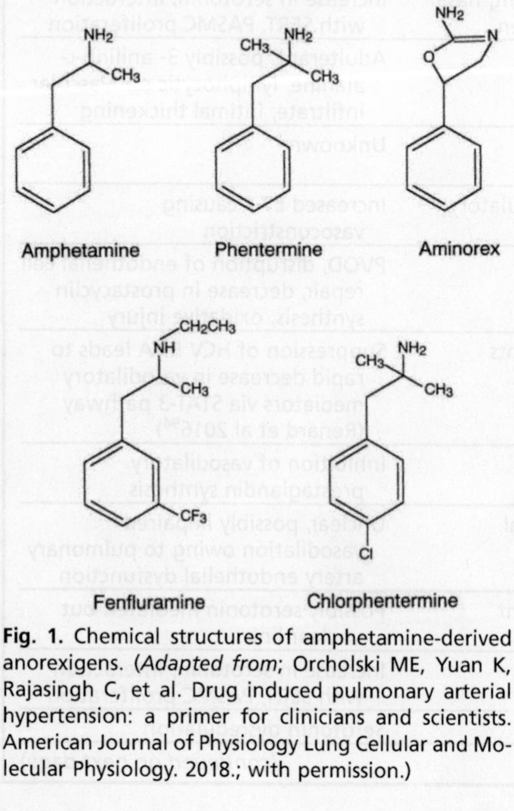

Fig. 1. Chemical structures of amphetamine-derived anorexigens. (*Adapted from;* Orcholski ME, Yuan K, Rajasingh C, et al. Drug induced pulmonary arterial hypertension: a primer for clinicians and scientists. American Journal of Physiology Lung Cellular and Molecular Physiology. 2018.; with permission.)

monotherapy and PAH[22] and the clear etiologic link between fenfluramine and PAH, phentermine monotherapy has not been conclusively shown to increase risk of PAH development.[18,19,23] This difference may be explained by phentermine's lower potency as a substrate for the serotonin transporter, because it is considerably less effective in increasing plasma 5-HT levels compared with fenfluramine and other commonly abused stimulants.[24]

Genetic susceptibility may be a factor in fenfluramine-associated PAH, because approximately 11% of patients who developed PAH secondary to fenfluramine and its derivatives carry bone morphogenetic protein receptor type 2 mutations,[25] the most common genetic cause of familial and sporadic PAH. Bone Morphogenetic protein receptor type 2 mutations could behave synergistically with fenfluramine to increase the risk of developing severe PAH.

BENFLUOREX

Benfluorex hydrochloride is an anorexigen similar in structure to the fenfluramines that was originally marketed in 1976 in France as an antidiabetic and lipid-lowering agent. The common metabolite of the fenfluramines and benfluorex is norfenfluramine, which itself has a chemical structure similar to amphetamine.[26] In 1997, benfluorex was reintroduced in France as a therapy for diabetes and the metabolic syndrome,[27] and soon afterward a report detailed 5 diabetic middle-aged women with severe PAH and 1 with valvular heart disease, all of which developed after exposure to benfluorex.[28] The French National Fund of health insurance reported that 200,000 to 300,000 patients were exposed to benfluorex, and in 2012 Savale and colleagues[29] published a study describing 85 patients with PAH associated with benfluorex. Of these 85 patients, 70 had confirmed precapillary PAH. The median duration of benfluorex exposure was 30 months. Interestingly, 33% of patients in this case series had also used other fenfluramine derivatives, and 30% of patients with precapillary PAH had other additional risk factors for PH. Owing to the increasing evidence that linked benfluorex with PAH and valvular heart disease, the drug was withdrawn in 2010.[27]

METHAMPHETAMINE

Methamphetamine (Meth) is a highly addictive and potent amphetamine-based stimulant that acts by releasing serotonin, norepinephrine, and dopamine in the central nervous system. In recent years, the distribution of Meth has expanded on a global scale, with massive increases in addiction rates.[30] There are many recognized cardiovascular complications of Meth abuse, including cardiomyopathy, increased stroke risk,[31,32] and kidney, brain, and liver injury.[33] However, it was not until recently that physicians identified an association between Meth abuse and PAH, with the first case report published in 1993.[34]

In 2006, a retrospective cohort study examined the association between stimulants (cocaine, amphetamine, or Meth) and PAH development. The authors found a history of stimulant use in 28.9% of patients with a diagnosis of idiopathic PAH (IPAH) compared with only 3.8% of patients with a diagnosis of PAH and other known risk factors, and 4.3% of patients with chronic thromboembolic PH.[35] In 2017, our research group published a prospective experience examining the association between Meth and PAH.[36] Lung biopsy samples from patients with Meth-APAH demonstrated characteristic vasculopathic changes, including plexiform angiomatoid lesions with slit-like vascular channels within the artery (**Fig. 2**), identical to those seen in patients with IPAH. Despite the similar pathologic profiles, patients with Meth-APAH presented with a more severe clinical and hemodynamic phenotype compared with patients with IPAH. A Kaplan–Meier analysis demonstrated 5-year and 10-year survival rates of 47.2% and 25.0%, respectively, in Meth-APAH versus 64.5% and 45.7% in IPAH (**Fig. 3**).

In 2018, Zhao and colleagues[37] published their experience with Meth-APAH and Meth-associated cardiomyopathy. Similar to our findings, they demonstrated that patients with Meth-APAH exhibited a higher right ventricular systolic pressure, more atrial dilation, and a greater decrease in right ventricular systolic function when compared with the Meth-induced cardiomyopathy and control cohorts. Owing to the increasing level of evidence, Meth was included as a definite risk factor in the most recent clinical classification of PH.[4]

The pathologic mechanisms of Meth-induced PAH are likely multifactorial. Meth is structurally and pharmacologically similar to anorexigens such as aminorex, the fenfluramine derivatives, and benfluorex, which are all known to be independent risk factors for PAH. These agents all have the potential to increase circulating levels of serotonin, which can act as a growth factor to stimulate pulmonary artery smooth muscle cell proliferation and obstructive vascular remodeling.[38,39] Meth has also been shown to damage pulmonary endothelial cells through the generation of harmful reactive oxygen species and the promotion of mitochondrial dysfunction.[40]

As seen with the previously mentioned anorexigens, only a small percentage of patients exposed to Meth develop PAH. This finding may indicate a complex interplay between host genetic and environmental factors, with a possible 2-hit phenomenon involved in the pathogenesis of Meth-APAH. Recent studies by our group have begun to identify potential candidate genes implicated in the pathogenesis of Meth-APAH, such as carboxylesterase 1, which is involved in the metabolism of several illicit drugs such as amphetamines, cocaine, and heroin.[41] Using immunofluorescence techniques, we found markedly decreased carboxylesterase 1 in explanted lung tissue from patients with Meth-APAH as compared with healthy controls (**Fig. 4**). Additionally, carboxylesterase 1 deficiency may result in greater Meth-induced pulmonary endothelial cell apoptosis, and ultimately lead to small vessel loss and subsequent PAH development.

The management of Meth-APAH can be challenging given the potential complications associated with easily accessible, long-term indwelling intravenous catheters for PAH-specific therapies. Our study showed that health care practitioners were more reluctant to administer intravenous or subcutaneous prostacyclin analogs to patients with Meth-APAH as compared with those with IPAH.[36] Intravenous and subcutaneous prostacyclin administration is a complex task that requires active patient engagement, adherence to the

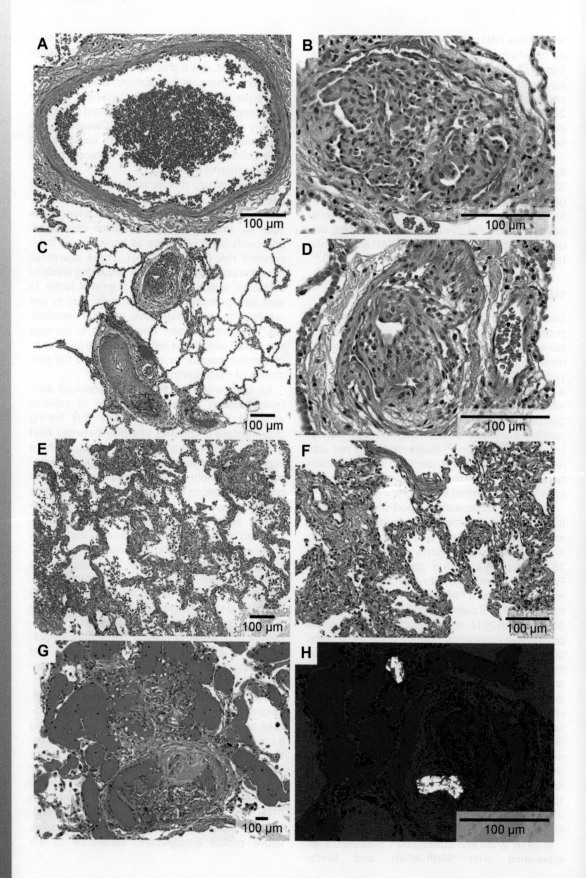

medical plan, and entrusting the patient to safely mix and self-administer these therapies.

TYROSINE KINASE INHIBITORS

Tyrosine kinase inhibitors (TKIs) with variable protein kinase affinities have been used for chronic myelogenous leukemia and other cancers. These include imatinib, dasatinib, nilotinib, bosutinib, and ponatinib, and the broader family of protein kinase inhibitors continues to expand.

Dasatinib is a second-generation tyrosine kinase inhibitor that was first linked to PAH in 2012 through a series of 9 incident cases of PAH in patients treated with the agent.[42] Eight of the 9 patients showed improvement after dasatinib discontinuation, and 2 patients died from complications apparently unrelated to PAH. Long-term follow-up of these 9 patients as well as 12 others revealed that 11 of these patients required PAH-specific therapies.[43]

An additional study describes 41 patients treated with dasatinib that developed PAH confirmed by right heart catherization.[44] Dasatinib was discontinued in 95% of cases, and in the 36 patients with follow-up data available, 34 had improvement in functional status, right heart catheterization (RHC), or echocardiographic findings. The authors of this large series noted the reversibility of dasatinib-induced PAH in most patients with treatment cessation. The histopathology of dasatinib-induced PAH was subsequently evaluated and revealed hypertrophy of the vascular media, intimal thickening, and a lack of thromboembolic disease, all of which are consistent with the vascular changes seen in IPAH.[45]

Although dasatinib has garnered the most attention for its connection with PAH, additional TKIs that have been associated in case reports include lapatinib, ponatinib, and bosutinib. Two case reports describe patients with chronic myelogenous leukemia, previously treated with other TKIs, who developed new or worsening PAH after starting bosutinib and ponatinib. Both of these patients improved after cessation of the tyrosine kinase inhibitors in question.[46,47] Lapatinib was associated with PAH in a review of 27 patients who had baseline echocardiograms before the initiation of the agent. Six patients had notable changes in pulmonary artery systolic pressures without impairment of left ventricular function, increasing from a mean of 29.0 mm Hg to 65.5 mm Hg after treatment in this subgroup.[48]

Several mechanisms have been proposed to explain dasatinib-associated PAH. One hypothesis involves the generation of reactive oxygen species by dasatinib, which disturbs the vascular endothelium and causes PAH development under specific circumstances.[43,49] Additionally, the differing off-target affinities among TKIs may determine which TKIs increase risk of PAH and which do not. Dasatinib, ponatinib, and bosutinib, for example, all affect a much wider array of tyrosine kinases than imatinib and nilotinib. Cornet and colleagues[50] showed that these 3 agents, in addition to ruxolitinib and nilotinib, were all associated with disproportionately high incidence of PAH (**Fig. 5**).

Interestingly, imatinib has been evaluated for efficacy in treating PAH before the large 2012 case series on dasatinib described elsewhere in this article. The IMPRES study, a randomized controlled trial of 202 patients, showed improvement in 6-minute walk distance and hemodynamics in the group randomized to imatinib.[51] An extension study attempted to provide long-term data on this cohort; however, a high rate of imatinib discontinuation and safety concerns led the authors to conclude that the risks likely outweigh the benefits described in the initial study.[52]

TOXIC RAPESEED OIL

In 1981, an outbreak of pulmonary disease accompanied by fever and other nonspecific symptoms arose in Spain. Exposure to rapeseed oil denatured with aniline was quickly identified as a potential cause of this mysterious epidemic. Only months after the first case, criteria for defining the toxic oil syndrome were established as (1) exposure to toxic oil, (2) diffuse pulmonary infiltrates, (3) severe myalgias, and (4) eosinophilia.[53]

Fig. 2. Histopathology of methamphetamine-associated PAH (Meth-APAH) and IPAH. (*A*) Normal muscular pulmonary artery. (*B*) Plexiform lesion in patient with IPAH who underwent lung transplantation. (*C*) Plexiform arteriopathy in Meth-APAH involving muscular artery. (*D*) High-power magnification showing proliferation of slit-like vascular channels within the artery. (*E*) Pulmonary microvasculopathy in Meth-APAH. (*F*) High-power magnification showing proliferation of capillaries within the pulmonary interstitium. (*G*) Angiomatoid lesion in Meth-APAH composed of dilated, thin-walled vascular spaces surrounding a plexiform lesion. (*H*) The patient in G also exhibited scattered intravascular collections of microcrystalline cellulose (a filler commonly used to cut amphetamines), causing an intimal proliferative response within the muscular artery. Hematoxylin and eosin stain. (*Adapted from* Zamanian, R.T., et al., Features and Outcomes of Methamphetamine Associated Pulmonary Arterial Hypertension. Am J Respir Crit Care Med, 2017. Reprinted with permission of the American Thoracic Society. Copyright © 2020 American Thoracic Society. All rights reserved.)

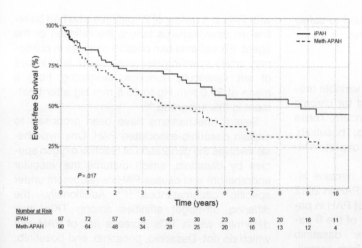

Fig. 3. Kaplan–Meier plot comparing event-free survival in patients with methamphetamine-associated PAH (Meth-APAH) versus patients with IPAH. Kaplan–Meier estimated event-free survival demonstrates worse outcomes for patients presenting with Meth-APAH (*dashed line*) as compared with those with IPAH (*solid line*). (*Adapted from* Zamanian, R.T., et al., Features and Outcomes of Methamphetamine Associated Pulmonary Arterial Hypertension. Am J Respir Crit Care Med, 2017. Reprinted with permission of the American Thoracic Society. Copyright © 2020 American Thoracic Society. All rights reserved.)

This condition typically evolved into a febrile illness with dyspnea, abdominal discomfort, nausea, vomiting, diarrhea, rash, itching, myalgias, and various neurologic complications.[54] A small portion of affected patients progressed to respiratory failure requiring mechanical ventilation, and some suffered ongoing neuropathies, contractures, and scleroderma-like skin changes. PH developed in approximately 8% of patients later in the disease course.[53] A case series of 38 such

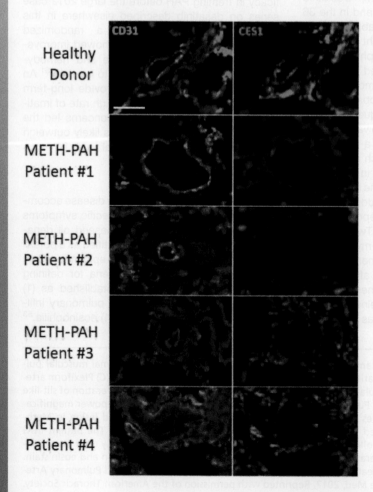

Fig. 4. Carboxylesterase 1 (CES1) expression is reduced in vascular lesions of Meth-PAH. Representative immunofluorescence studies of lung sections stained for CES1 (*red*) obtained from a healthy donor (*top*) and 4 patients with METH-PAH. CD31 (*green*) stains for endothelial cells. (*Adapted from*: Orcholski, M.E., et al., Reduced carboxylesterase 1 is associated with endothelial injury in methamphetamine-induced pulmonary arterial hypertension. Am J Physiol Lung Cell Mol Physiol, 2017. 313(2): p. L252-L266.; with permission.)

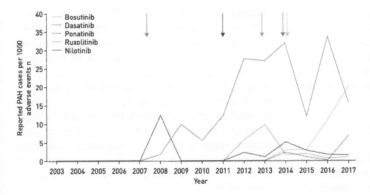

Fig. 5. Proportion of reported PAH cases per 1000 reported adverse events per year for the 5 protein kinase inhibitors with a significant disproportionality signal. The *arrows* indicate the first published case reports in MEDLINE for each drug. (*Adapted from* Cornet L, Khouri C, Roustit M, et al. Pulmonary arterial hypertension associated with protein kinase inhibitors: A pharmacovigilance-pharmacodynamic study. Eur Respir J. 2019;53(5) 1802472; DOI: 10.1183/13993003.02472-2018. Reproduced with permission of the © ERS 2020.)

patients describes echocardiographic signs of right heart failure and PH, with 11 patients going on to have RHC showing PAH. Six of these patients had follow-up catheterization 6 months later, and all of them had persistent abnormalities consistent with PAH.[55] Histopathologic studies of affected patients demonstrated a proliferative vasculopathy in multiple vascular beds.[56] More than 20 years after the exposure, additional individuals exposed to the toxic rapeseed oil were found to have elevated pulmonary artery pressures with exercise, indicating possible permanent pulmonary vascular changes.[57]

Overall, there were an estimated 20,000 cases of toxic oil syndrome reported, with a case mortality rate of 8.4%. Although the toxic oil syndrome has been difficult to reproduce experimentally, it is thought that either rapeseed oil or the anilides used for its denaturation were responsible for the Spanish epidemic. The robust epidemiologic reports from this era have been sufficient to establish toxic rapeseed oil as having a "definite" association with PAH.

COCAINE

Cocaine is a potent stimulant and one of the most commonly abused illicit substances in the United States and globally.[58,59] Cocaine produces its physiologic effects by inhibiting the reuptake of dopamine, norepinephrine, and serotonin. This inhibition results in euphoria, increased energy and libido, and decreased appetite. There are a variety of well-known cardiopulmonary toxicities associated with cocaine use, including cardiomyopathy, alveolar hemorrhage, increased stroke risk, and aortic dissection, among other multiorgan complications.

There have been reported cases of PAH developing in intravenous cocaine users, where it was postulated that embolization of adulterants could trigger a local granulomatous inflammatory response in the pulmonary circulation, with subsequent elevations in pulmonary vascular resistance.[60] However, there is also evidence that pulmonary artery pressures may increase with cocaine use despite the absence of foreign bodies.[61] This finding is supported by a histopathologic study of 20 patient deaths owing to cocaine intoxication showing pulmonary artery medial hypertrophy without foreign particle microembolization in 20% of patients.[62] Collazos and colleagues[63] reported the case of a 24-year-old intravenous cocaine user who was found to have evidence of PAH on an electrocardiogram and echocardiography that improved significantly after 5 weeks of abstinence. PH was also reported in 4 cocaine smokers with dyspnea and intermittent hemoptysis who underwent lung biopsy showing vascular remodeling.[64] More recently, a retrospective cohort study by Alzghoul and colleagues[65] used echocardiography to assess the impact of cocaine on pulmonary pressures. Cocaine users compared with the matched control group had significantly higher estimated systolic PA pressures and greater likelihood of PH.[65] Interestingly, it seems that intranasal administration of cocaine does not alter PA pressures, suggesting that the delivery route may serve as a disease modifier.[66]

The data regarding cocaine use and the risk of PAH are not uniform, however. A single blind crossover study by Kleerup and colleagues[67] demonstrated that the intravenous administration of cocaine versus placebo did not alter PA pressures or pulmonary vascular resistance in crack smoking subjects, although it did increase the heart rate and cardiac index. Additionally, a large retrospective cohort study examining the histology taken during autopsies in which the decedents had positive toxicology for cocaine demonstrated that none of the 28 patients had histopathologic evidence of PAH.[68]

Ultimately, it seems that few cocaine users develop PAH; however, there are insufficient data to identify the determinants of risk. Currently, owing to lack of large epidemiologic case control studies or large multicenter series, cocaine is listed a possible risk factor for PAH in the most recent clinical guidelines.

PHENYLPROPANOLAMINE

Phenylpropanolamine, also known as norephedrine, is a drug of the phenethylamine class with a structure similar to amphetamine. Historically, the medication has been used as a nasal decongestant, an over-the-counter anorectic, and an antiobesity agent. In 2006, a large multicenter study conducted in 13 tertiary PH centers (SOPHIA study) revealed an association between use of over-the-counter antiobesity agents, many of which contained phenylpropanolamine, and the risk of PAH.[69] In 2004, a case report surfaced of a 7-year-old boy who was heavily medicated with cold remedies containing phenylpropanolamine (Dimetapp) and subsequently died from severe PAH. On autopsy, the patient was found to have vascular changes and endarteritis consistent with severe PAH.[70]

A commonly used commercial drug Dimetapp (Pfizer, New York, NY) was removed from the market in 2000 owing to reports of an increased risk of hemorrhagic stroke.[71] The medication was then later released with phenylpropanolamine being replaced with a similar agent, pseudoephedrine. There is concern that widely available nasal decongestants containing potent vasoconstrictors similar to phenylpropanolamine (norephedrine and norpseudoephedrine) represent a risk factor for PH in the general population.[72] However, a study conducted in France in 2012 demonstrated no difference in the rate of nasal decongestant exposure among patients with PAH and controls.[73] Larger studies are needed to answer this question more definitively.

L-TRYPTOPHAN

In 1989, a syndrome of marked peripheral eosinophilia and myalgias was recognized in New Mexico in 3 patients who had been ingesting L-tryptophan–containing products. This report was followed closely by additional cases elsewhere in the United States.[74] Within 3 years, about 1512 cases had been reported and 36 deaths attributed to this exposure.[75] The condition was named eosinophilia–myalgia syndrome, and characterized by fevers, dyspnea, cough, abdominal symptoms, skin tightening, edema, pulmonary

infiltrates, and neuropathies. Three of 45 patients in 1 series[76] developed PH confirmed by RHC, but a separate series of 21 patients reported no cases of PH.[77] The syndrome was often treated with corticosteroids with overall beneficial effects.[78] The pulmonary histopathology of 5 patients with the eosinophilia–myalgia syndrome showed a lymphocyte-rich perivascular infiltrate with concomitant intimal thickening. Two of these patients were noted to have increased pulmonary artery pressures on RHC.[79] Documentation of confirmed PAH related to this syndrome is scant, however.[80]

Owing to the numerous similarities of eosinophilia–myalgia syndrome and toxic oil syndrome associated with rapeseed oil (**Table 3**), it has been suggested that a common contaminant was present in the L-tryptophan products and rapeseed oil connected to these outbreaks.[76] Toxicologic analysis of an L-tryptophan sample associated with development of the eosinophilia–myalgia syndrome revealed a possible offending agent to be 3-anilino-L-alanine,[75] which may have also been created by alanine denaturation of the rapeseed oil that caused toxic oil syndrome.[81] Despite commonalities with a toxin classified as having a definite association with PAH, L-tryptophan is currently considered to have only a possible association with PAH.

ST JOHN'S WORT

The herbal remedy *Hypericum perforatum*, colloquially referred to as St John's Wort, is commonly used as an alternative therapy for depression and other psychiatric disorders. The exact mechanism of action has remained elusive, although it has been shown to affect multiple central nervous system receptors.[82,83] In the 1990s, the data from the SOPHIA registry showed a possible association of St John's Wort with PAH. Using logistic regression to assess association of PAH with antiobesity agents, the authors found an odds ratio of 4.2 (95% confidence interval, 1.2–14.6) of PAH in those taking St John's Wort. Walker and colleagues[69] acknowledge this was an unexpected finding. No further reports of this connection have been published, and thus St John's Wort remains as a possible association with PAH.

INTERFERONS

Interferons are endogenous immunomodulatory proteins that have been used in commercial preparations since the 1990s. Interferon-α was commonly used for treatment of hepatitis C virus as well as solid and hematopoietic cancers, and

Table 3
Comparison of syndromes caused by exposure to toxic rapeseed oil and toxic L-tryptophan-containing products

	Toxic Oil Syndrome	Eosinophilia-Myalgia Syndrome
Associated toxin	Toxic rapeseed oil	L-Tryptophan–containing products
Geographic distribution	Spain	United States
No. of cases	>20,000	>1500
Common clinical features	Noncardiogenic pulmonary edema, dyspnea, myalgia, rash, neuropathy, contractures, scleroderma-like skin changes	Myalgia, weakness, arthralgias, dyspnea, cough, fever, neuropathy, rash, scleroderma-like skin changes
Laboratory findings	Eosinophilia, elevated aminotransferases	Eosinophilia, elevated aldolase, elevated aminotransferases
PAH Association	Definite	Possible

interferon-β was found to have beneficial effects in multiple sclerosis.[84] In the early 2000s, several cases were published that associated interferon-α with PAH confirmed by RHC. These cases demonstrated variable reversibility after discontinuation of the medication; however, other investigators described severe PAH with no evidence of reversal with discontinuation of interferon-α.[85] A case series of 53 individuals exposed to interferon-α who developed PAH was published from the French Registry in 2014, but an overwhelming majority of these individuals had other PAH risk factors, namely, portal hypertension (85%) and human immunodeficiency virus infection (56%).[86] Interferon-β was also implicated in a case series of 13 women undergoing treatment for multiple sclerosis, 12 of whom had no other PAH risk factors. In 2 of these interferon-β–associated PAH cases the patients died, 4 of the individuals responded to PAH therapy, and 3 had complete resolution of PAH.[84]

In vitro, interferons have been shown to increase endothelin-1 expression in pulmonary vascular smooth muscle, thereby causing vasoconstriction and increasing pulmonary vascular resistance. In a subset of human subjects, serum endothelin-1 has been demonstrated to increase with interferon exposure, supporting this mechanism and potentially explaining an association with PAH.[87] Interferon has fallen out of favor as a first-line therapy for many conditions; however, the time between interferon exposure and PAH diagnosis has been as long as 15 years.[88] Therefore, clinicians should remain aware of its possible association with PAH.

ALKYLATING AGENTS

Alkylating agents were some of the first drugs to treat solid and liquid tumors. Common alkylating agents include carmustine, bleomycin, mitomycin, and cyclophosphamide. These drugs cause numerous adverse effects owing to their nonspecific cytotoxicity, and have been categorized as possible causes of PH. In particular, these medications are linked to a postcapillary form of PH called pulmonary veno-occlusive disease (PVOD). PVOD is a rare subtype of PH characterized by the remodeling and obliteration of the pulmonary venules and veins. Case series of individuals with PVOD have notably described rapidly progressive right heart failure with higher mortality than other forms of PAH, and vasodilating agents have an unclear role in PVOD, leaving clinicians with few therapeutic options.[89]

A 2015 review of the French PH network as well as previously published cases revealed 37 cases of PVOD attributed to chemotherapies, of which 31 were associated with alkylating agents. Cyclophosphamide was the most frequent offender with 16 cases, followed by mitomycin, cisplatin, and carmustine (**Table 4**).[90] Multiple mechanisms were proposed to explain the relationship of alkylating agents and PVOD, including disruption of endothelial cell repair, a decrease in prostacyclin synthesis, and oxidative injury.[91] Despite severe PH and death in some cases associated with alkylating agents, there has also been report of reversibility and response to PAH therapies.[92]

DIRECT-ACTING ANTIVIRAL AGENTS

Direct-acting antiviral medications have revolutionized the treatment of chronic hepatitis C, leading to sustained viral response in more than 95% of patients who complete treatment.[93] These medications are, overall, well-tolerated. However, in 2016 a series reported 3 individuals who developed PAH within 2 to 6 months of initiating

Table 4
Alkylating agents associated with PVOD in a series of 37 patients

Chemotherapelitic Group	Molecule	Chemotherapy-Induced PVOD Patients, No. (%)
Alkylating or alkylating-like agents, n = 31 (83.8%)	Cyclophosphamide	16 (43.2)
	Mitomycin	9 (24.3)
	Cisplatin	8 (21.6)
	Carmustine	5 (13.5)
	Procarbazine	4 (10.8)
	Ifosfamide	2 (5.4)
	Melphalan	2 (5.4)
	Busulfan	2 (5.4)
	Mustine	1 (2.7)
	Dacarbazine	1 (2.7)

Adapted from; Ranchoux B, Günther S, Quarck R, et al. Chemotherapy-induced pulmonary hypertension: Role of alkylating agents. Am J Pathol. 2015;185(2):356-371.; with permission.

treatment with sofosbuvir, a nucleoside polymerase inhibitor that is broadly categorized as a direct-acting antiviral. All 3 patients had previous risk factors for PAH (either portal hypertension or human immunodeficiency virus infection), and 1 of them had previously been diagnosed and treated for PAH. Nevertheless, the chronologic relationship between sofosbuvir initiation and PAH diagnosis, or worsening, prompted concern.[94]

Soon afterward, a review of the French PAH Registry identified 3 additional cases of PAH in patients treated with sofosbuvir and other direct-acting antiviral agents. Two of these patients had concomitant portal hypertension, but the third had no other reported PAH risk factors. After discontinuation of the antivirals, all 3 individuals experienced hemodynamic improvement or resolution of PAH.[95] A 2019 prospective cohort study of 49 patients being treated with direct-acting antiviral agents found no evidence of increased pulmonary artery pressures as estimated by echocardiogram during treatment or after completion.[96] Given these data, as well as the uncertain connections between these therapies and PAH, this association is currently categorized as possible and certainly warrants further investigation.

LEFLUNOMIDE

Leflunomide is a DNA synthesis inhibitor that is considered disease-modifying therapy for rheumatoid and psoriatic arthritis, and has a possible association with PAH. This relationship was first proposed in a 2004 case study of a woman with rheumatoid arthritis treated with leflunomide for 13 months before a diagnosis of PH by

echocardiogram. Notably, she had a history of pulmonary embolism and left ventricular diastolic dysfunction; however, the authors report improvement in clinical status and stabilization of echocardiographic findings after leflunomide was discontinued.[97] Another case report of leflunomide-associated PH followed in 2012 in a patient with rheumatoid arthritis and no other known risk factors. This individual improved with cessation of leflunomide and the initiation of PAH therapies.[98] Finally, a case series of 4 patients with rheumatoid arthritis treated with leflunomide was published in 2018. These patients underwent RHC to confirm PAH and were ruled out for other etiologies such as thromboembolic disease. All 4 had favorable clinical and hemodynamic response to discontinuation of leflunomide, offering our most robust evidence of this relationship between leflunomide and PAH.[99]

One proposed mechanism for the association of leflunomide with PAH is the inhibition of vasodilatory prostaglandin synthesis by leflunomide[98]; however, there are few data to support this finding and further research is needed. Leflunomide remains an important treatment option for rheumatic disease, and further data regarding its possible connection to PAH are anticipated.

INDIRUBIN

Indirubin is a compound extracted from the indigo plant and has been used in herbal medicine preparations for several cancers and inflammatory conditions, such as ulcerative colitis.[100] Its first reported association with PAH was in a case report of a woman taking indigo for ulcerative colitis. She developed dyspnea after 6 months of beginning indigo therapy and was diagnosed with PAH by RHC. Repeat RHC 1 month after discontinuation showed no change in hemodynamics.[101] Misumi and colleagues[102] later reported development of PH in a patient 20 months after initiation of the indigo-containing formulation Qing-Dai, and precapillary PH was confirmed with RHC. This individual responded well to oral PAH therapies, and had resolution of PAH 3 months after discontinuing Qing-Dai.[102] Lastly, another case report describes an individual who developed PAH before the initiation of Qing-Dai, and PAH resolved after initiation of endothelin antagonist therapy but before the discontinuation of Qing-Dai,[103] therefore offering little evidence to support a causal relationship.

The mechanism of PAH development with indigo exposure is uncertain; however, pulmonary vascular reactivity testing in the presence of indigo suggested impaired vasodilation owing to pulmonary artery endothelial dysfunction.[103] More case reports will be needed to describe an association of indirubin with PAH, and this relationship is currently classified as possible.

MAZINDOL

Mazindol is a nonamphetamine central nervous system stimulant with appetite suppressant properties and is structurally related to the tricyclic antidepressants. It exerts most of its pharmacologic effects through dopamine and norepinephrine reuptake inhibition.[104] Mazindol has been used in the treatment of narcolepsy, attention deficit hyperactivity disorder, and as an antiobesity agent. A single case of PAH secondary to mazindol exposure has been reported in which a 29-year-old woman used mazindol to treat obesity. After 10 weeks of using mazindol, the patient began to notice dyspnea on exertion. Her dyspnea improved when the medication was discontinued, but unfortunately she began to experience dyspnea again 12 months later and evaluation revealed severe PAH. Although the patient was started on PAH-specific therapies, her symptoms did not resolve completely.[105] Despite this case report, there have been several studies conducted with mazindol for other therapeutic indications that have failed to document PAH as an adverse effect.[106–109]

Evidence suggests that mazindol is 2 to 4 times less potent when binding to human 5-HT2B receptors than other anorectics, which may explain why its association with PAH is not well-established. Despite there being no further case reports of PAH associated with mazindol, the drug was withdrawn from the market in several countries, but remains approved in Mexico, Argentina, and Japan.[110] Some authors recommend periodic cardiovascular examinations in patients taking mazindol given that its mechanism of action is similar to other anorectic agents, which are known risk factors for PAH.[111]

SELECTIVE SEROTONIN REUPTAKE INHIBITORS

Selective serotonin reuptake inhibitors (SSRIs) are a class of drugs used for their beneficial effects in treating depression, anxiety, and other mental health disorders. Given the role of serotonin biology in the proposed pathogenesis of many forms of drug- and toxin-induced PAH, SSRIs offered logical therapeutic potential. There have been numerous in vitro and animal model studies demonstrating the protective effects of SSRIs in PAH,[112] including the downregulation of serotonin transporter and 5HT1B receptor expression in the pulmonary arteries, attenuation of pulmonary arterial remodeling,[39] decreased right ventricular hypertrophy,[113] and decreased inflammatory responses in lung tissue.[114]

Early studies examining the role of SSRIs in humans for the treatment or prevention of PAH have yielded mixed results. A retrospective cohort study examining adult patients with who were exposed to high-affinity SSRIs found no difference in the hemodynamics or incidence of acute vasoreactivity between SSRI users and nonusers. The risk of death for high-affinity SSRI users was lower but not statistically significant.[115] A case-control study of patients enrolled in the SOPHIA registry found a protective effect of SSRIs in PH, with a decreased rate of PAH development and lower mortality once PH developed.[116] Interestingly, a population-based nested case-control study found a positive correlation between SSRI use and PAH.[117] In 2013, Sadoughi and colleagues[118] published the results of an analysis exploring SSRI use and PAH outcomes using the REVEAL registry. They found that new users of SSRIs had a higher risk of death and were less likely to be free of events indicative of clinical worsening.[118] Further data from Fox and colleagues[119] demonstrated that the use of SSRI and non-SSRI antidepressants was associated with a significantly increased risk of IPAH; however, the consistency of this risk across all antidepressant classes and the absence of a dose–response relationship suggested a noncasual association.

TRICHLOROETHYLENE

Trichloroethylene (TCE) is an occupational organic solvent used mostly for industrial purposes.

Studies have found a possible etiologic link between TCE exposure and PH, specifically PVOD. A significant exposure to TCE was found in 42% of patients with PVOD by Montani and colleagues.[120] In this study, PVOD was significantly associated with occupational exposure to organic solvents (adjusted odds ratio, 12.8) with TCE being the main culprit (adjusted odds ratio, 8.2). Additionally, histology from a PVOD patient with a positive TCE exposure history demonstrated venular, capillary, and arterial lesions typical of idiopathic or heritable PVOD (**Fig. 6**).

Although TCE is an established risk factor for PVOD, little is known about the disease mechanism. However, TCE is also a risk factor for systemic sclerosis, where TCE has been shown to cause disturbances in immune regulation and the development of autoimmunity via altered T helper 17/regulatory T cell ratios.[121] TCE has also been shown to be a source of oxidative stress and may lead to a breakdown in the endothelial barrier and increased vascular permeability.[122–124] This breakdown in the endothelial barrier may cause connective tissue and smooth muscle cells to be exposed to circulating growth factors, leading to uncontrolled proliferation and recruitment of inflammatory cells that are involved in the initial vascular remodeling observed in PAH.[125,126]

ANAGRELIDE

Anagrelide is an oral imidazoquinazoline agent used to decrease platelet levels and ameliorate

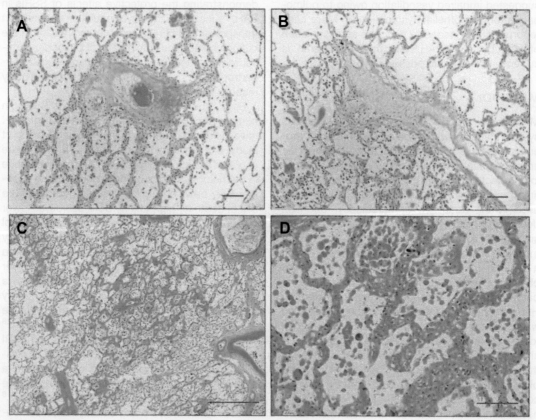

Fig. 6. Histology from the lungs of a patient with PVOD with a positive history of exposure to TCE without biallelic eukaryotic translation initiation factor 2α kinase 4 (EIF2AK4) mutations. (*A, B*) Septal veins and preseptal venules are obliterated by collagen-rich, loose fibrosis; the parenchyma is otherwise lacking important interstitial remodeling. (*C*) Patchy foci of capillary hemangiomatosis are present on most samples, frequently in association with remodeled pulmonary vessels and microvessels (*center*). (*D*) Thickening of alveolar walls is due to a multiplication of capillaries; note the abundance of pigmented macrophages (siderophages) within the alveoli. Scale bars: (*A, B, D*) 100 μm; (*C*) 1000 μm. Hematoxylin and eosin stain. (*Adapted from* Occupational exposure to organic solvents: a risk factor for pulmonary veno-occlusive disease David Montani, Edmund M. Lau, Alexis Descatha, Xavier Jaïs, Laurent Savale, Pascal Andujar, Lynda Bensefa-Colas, Barbara Girerd, Inès Zendah, Jerome Le Pavec, Andrei Seferian, Frédéric Perros, Peter Dorfmüller, Elie Fadel, Florent Soubrier, Oliver Sitbon, Gérald Simonneau, Marc Humbert. European Respiratory Journal Dec 2015, 46 (6) 1721-1731; DOI: 10.1183/13993003.00814-2015; Reproduced with permission of the © ERS 2020.)

thrombohemorrhagic events in patients with myeloproliferative disorders.[127] Sumimoto and colleagues[128] recently published a case report describing a 70-year-old female patient who developed PAH after taking anagrelide for 1 month for the treatment of polycythemia vera. Within 20 days of stopping the drug, the symptoms of PAH completely resolved. Echocardiographic and biochemical parameters also showed improvement after discontinuation of anagrelide. A prospective long-term observational cohort study of 3649 patients evaluating the efficacy and safety of anagrelide found no significant increase in PAH development.[129] The mechanisms underlying anagrelide-induced PAH remain unclear; however, given the rapid improvement in the patient described in the published case report, the toxicity fortunately may be reversible.

CARFILZOMIB

Carfilzomib is a proteasome inhibitor used in the treatment of relapsed or refractory multiple myeloma.[130] The prescribing information that accompanies Carfilzomib reports development of PAH in 1% of patients.[131] In addition, case reports have been published linking carfilzomib to PAH development.[132,133]

Several studies examining the cardiac and pulmonary safety of carfilzomib have been conducted. A retrospective study of 67 patients with relapsed and/or refractory multiple myeloma who were treated with carfilzomib revealed that 12 patients experienced cardiac or vascular adverse events. Of these events, only a small percentage were PH, and some patients had a history of PH before starting carfilzomib.[134] A study using Medicare claims data examined 635 patients with multiple myeloma who were treated with carfilzomib and revealed that 1% of patients developed PAH.[135] Furthermore, analyses of multiple phase II clinical studies with single-agent carfilzomib revealed a 2% rate of PH.[136,137] Another study evaluating the cardiac and pulmonary safety of carfilzomib reported PAH in 1 of 52 patients.[138] A prospective, observational, multi-institutional study conducted by Cornell and colleagues,[139] examining patients with relapsed multiple myeloma initiating carfilzomib or bortezomib based therapy reported a 7% rate of PH among patients taking carfilzomib. Interestingly, no patients taking bortezomib (another proteasome inhibitor) developed PH during this study.[139]

The mechanism of carfilzomib-induced PH may be due to proteasome inhibitor-mediated changes in endothelial nitric oxide synthase activity and nitric oxide levels, which can lead to impaired vasodilation

and endothelial dysfunction.[134] Other proposed mechanisms include nontargeted proteasome inhibition of the endothelium and oxidative stress playing a role in vascular dysfunction, increased vascular tone, and hypertension.[132] Several recommendations regarding monitoring patients for cardiac and pulmonary adverse events during carfilzomib therapy have been proposed, including conducting baseline and repeated echocardiograms for patients with cardiac dysfunction and monitoring brain natriuretic peptide levels.[139,140] The manufacturer of carfilzomib recommends that in instances of PH or worsening congestive heart failure, carfilzomib should be withheld until the event is resolved or the patient returns to baseline.

CLINICS CARE POINTS

- Early identification and removal of the offending agent is paramount to treatment of drug- and toxin-induced PAH.
- If additional treatment is being considered, right-heart catheterization is recommended to confirm pre-capillary pulmonary hypertension which would be amenable to pulmonary vasodilators.
- Following diagnosis of drug- and toxin-induced PAH, clinical follow up is essential to monitor for improvement or progression of disease, as there is wide variability in disease history following removal of the offending agent.

DISCLOSURE

The authors have no financial conflicts of interest to disclose.

REFERENCES

1. Romberg E. Ueber sklerose der lungen arterie. Dtsch Arch Klin Med 1891;48:197–206.
2. Gurtner HP. Pulmonary hypertension, "plexogenic pulmonary arteriopathy" and the appetite depressant drug aminorex: post or propter? Bull Eur Physiopathol Respir 1979;15(5):897–923.
3. Follath F, Burkart F, Schweizer W. Drug-induced pulmonary hypertension? Br Med J 1971;1(5743):265–6.
4. Simonneau G, Montani D, Celermajer DS, et al. Haemodynamic definitions and updated clinical classification of pulmonary hypertension. Eur Respir J 2019;53(1):1801913.
5. Gurtner HP. Aminorex and pulmonary hypertension. A Review. Cor Vasa 1985;27(2–3):160–71.
6. Rothman RB, Baumann MH. Therapeutic and adverse actions of serotonin transporter substrates. Pharmacol Ther 2002;95(1):73–88.

7. Rothman RB, Baumann MH, Dersch CM, et al. Amphetamine-type central nervous system stimulants release norepinephrine more potently than they release dopamine and serotonin. Synapse 2001;39(1):32–41.

8. Eddahibi S, Adnot S. Anorexigen-induced pulmonary hypertension and the serotonin (5-HT) hypothesis: lessons for the future in pathogenesis. Respir Res 2002;3:9.

9. Eddahibi S, Fabre V, Boni C, et al. Induction of serotonin transporter by hypoxia in pulmonary vascular smooth muscle cells. Relationship with the mitogenic action of serotonin. Circ Res 1999; 84(3):329–36.

10. Ramamoorthy S, Bauman AL, Moore KR, et al. Antidepressant- and cocaine-sensitive human serotonin transporter: molecular cloning, expression, and chromosomal localization. Proc Natl Acad Sci U S A 1993;90(6):2542–6.

11. Rothman RB, Ayestas MA, Dersch CM, et al. Aminorex, fenfluramine, and chlorphentermine are serotonin transporter substrates. Implications for primary pulmonary hypertension. Circulation 1999;100(8):869–75.

12. Weir EK, Reeve HL, Huang JM, et al. Anorexic agents aminorex, fenfluramine, and dexfenfluramine inhibit potassium current in rat pulmonary vascular smooth muscle and cause pulmonary vasoconstriction. Circulation 1996;94(9):2216–20.

13. Fishman AP. Dietary pulmonary hypertension. Circ Res 1974;35(5):657–60.

14. Rothman RB, Redmon JB, Raatz SK, et al. Chronic treatment with phentermine combined with fenfluramine lowers plasma serotonin. Am J Cardiol 2000;85(7):913–915, a910.

15. Seiler KU, Wasserman O. MAO-inhibitory properties of anorectic drugs. J Pharm Pharmacol 1973; 25(7):576–8.

16. Douglas JG, Munro JF, Kitchin AH, et al. Pulmonary hypertension and fenfluramine. Br Med J (Clin Res ed) 1981;283(6296):881–3.

17. Brenot F, Herve P, Petitpretz P, et al. Primary pulmonary hypertension and fenfluramine use. Br Heart J 1993;70(6):537–41.

18. Abenhaim L, Moride Y, Brenot F, et al. Appetite-suppressant drugs and the risk of primary pulmonary hypertension. International primary pulmonary hypertension study group. The N Engl J Med 1996; 335(9):609–16.

19. Rich S, Rubin L, Walker AM, et al. Anorexigens and pulmonary hypertension in the United States: results from the surveillance of North American pulmonary hypertension. Chest 2000;117(3): 870–4.

20. Connolly HM, Crary JL, McGoon MD, et al. Valvular heart disease associated with fenfluramine-phentermine. N Engl J Med 1997;337(9):581–8.

21. Robiolio PA, Rigolin VH, Wilson JS, et al. Carcinoid heart disease. Correlation of high serotonin levels with valvular abnormalities detected by cardiac catheterization and echocardiography. Circulation 1995;92(4):790–5.

22. Bang WD, Kim JY, Yu HT, et al. Pulmonary hypertension associated with use of phentermine. Yonsei Med J 2010;51(6):971–3.

23. Hendricks EJ, Rothman RB. RE: pulmonary hypertension associated with use of phentermine? Yonsei Med J 2011;52(5):869–70.

24. Rothman RB, Baumann MH. Methamphetamine and idiopathic pulmonary arterial hypertension: role of the serotonin transporter. Chest 2007; 132(4):1412–3.

25. Humbert M, Deng Z, Simonneau G, et al. BMPR2 germline mutations in pulmonary hypertension associated with fenfluramine derivatives. Eur Respir J 2002;20(3):518–23.

26. Frachon I, Le Gal G, Hill C, et al. Benfluorex withdrawal in France: still be hiding somewhere in the world? J Pharmacol Pharmacother 2011;2(4): 307–8.

27. Mullard A. Mediator scandal rocks French medical community. Lancet 2011;377(9769):890–2.

28. Boutet K, Frachon I, Jobic Y, et al. Fenfluramine-like cardiovascular side-effects of benfluorex. Eur Respir J 2009;33(3):684–8.

29. Savale L, Chaumais MC, Cottin V, et al. Pulmonary hypertension associated with benfluorex exposure. Eur Respir J 2012;40(5):1164–72.

30. United Nations Office on Drugs and Crime. World Drug Report 2019 (United Nations publication, Sales No. E.19.XI.8). Sales No. E. 19.XI.8 ed2019. Available at: https://wdr.unodc.org/wdr2019/prelaunch/WDR19_Booklet_4_STIMULANTS.pdf. Accessed December 3, 2020.

31. Albertson TE, Derlet RW, Van Hoozen BE. Methamphetamine and the expanding complications of amphetamines. West J Med 1999;170(4):214–9.

32. Won S, Hong RA, Shohet RV, et al. Methamphetamine-associated cardiomyopathy. Clin Cardiol 2013;36(12):737–42.

33. Gurel A. Multisystem toxicity after methamphetamine use. Clin Case Rep 2016;4(3):226–7.

34. Schaiberger PH, Kennedy TC, Miller FC, et al. Pulmonary hypertension associated with long-term inhalation of "crank" methamphetamine. Chest 1993;104(2):614–6.

35. Chin KM, Channick RN, Rubin LJ. Is methamphetamine use associated with idiopathic pulmonary arterial hypertension? Chest 2006;130(6): 1657–1663.37.

36. Zamanian RT, Hedlin H, Greuenwald P, et al. Features and outcomes of methamphetamine associated pulmonary arterial hypertension. Am J Respir Crit Care Med 2017;197(6):788–800.

37. Zhao SX, Kwong C, Swaminathan A, et al. Clinical characteristics and outcome of methamphetamine-associated pulmonary arterial hypertension and dilated cardiomyopathy. JACC Heart Fail 2018;6(3):209–18.

38. Maclean MR, Dempsie Y. The serotonin hypothesis of pulmonary hypertension revisited. Adv Exp Med Biol 2010;661:309–22.

39. Liu M, Wang Y, Wang HM, et al. Fluoxetine attenuates chronic methamphetamine-induced pulmonary arterial remodelling: possible involvement of serotonin transporter and serotonin 1B receptor. Basic Clin Pharmacol Toxicol 2013;112(2):77–82.

40. Chen PI, Cao A, Miyagawa K, et al. Amphetamines promote mitochondrial dysfunction and DNA damage in pulmonary hypertension. JCI insight 2017; 2(2):e90427.

41. Orcholski ME, Khurshudyan A, Shamskhou EA, et al. Reduced carboxylesterase 1 is associated with endothelial injury in methamphetamine-induced pulmonary arterial hypertension. Am J Physiol Lung Cell Mol Physiol 2017;313(2): L252–66.

42. Montani D, Bergot E, Günther S, et al. Pulmonary arterial hypertension in patients treated by dasatinib. Circulation 2012. https://doi.org/10.1161/CIRCULATIONAHA.111.079921.

43. Weatherald J, Chaumais MC, Savale L, et al. Long-term outcomes of dasatinib-induced pulmonary arterial hypertension: a population-based study. Eur Respir J 2017;50(1):1700217.

44. Shah NP, Wallis N, Farber HW, et al. Clinical features of pulmonary arterial hypertension in patients receiving dasatinib. Am J Hematol 2015;90(11):1060–4.

45. Daccord C, Letovanec I, Yerly P, et al. First histopathological evidence of irreversible pulmonary vascular disease in dasatinib-induced pulmonary arterial hypertension. Eur Respir J 2018;51(3): 1701694.

46. Hickey PM, Thompson AA, Charalampopoulos A, et al. Bosutinib therapy resulting in severe deterioration of pre-existing pulmonary arterial hypertension. Eur Respir J 2016;48(5):1514–6.

47. Quilot FM, Georges M, Favrolt N, et al. Pulmonary hypertension associated with ponatinib therapy. Eur Respir J 2016;47(2):676–9.

48. Alkhatib Y, Albashaireh D, Al-Aqtash T, et al. The role of tyrosine kinase inhibitor "Lapatinib" in pulmonary hypertension. Pulm Pharmacol Ther 2016;37:81–4.

49. Orlikow E, Weatherald J, Hirani N. Dasatinib-induced pulmonary arterial hypertension. Can J Cardiol 2019;35(11):1604.e1601–3.

50. Cornet L, Khouri C, Roustit M, et al. Pulmonary arterial hypertension associated with protein kinase inhibitors: a pharmacovigilance-pharmacodynamic study. Eur Respir J 2019;53(5):1802472.

51. Hoeper MM, Barst RJ, Bourge RC, et al. Imatinib mesylate as add-on therapy for pulmonary arterial hypertension: results of the randomized IMPRES study. Circulation 2013;127(10):1128–38.

52. Frost AE, Barst RJ, Hoeper MM, et al. Long-term safety and efficacy of imatinib in pulmonary arterial hypertension. J Heart Lung Transplant 2015; 34(11):1366–75.

53. Posada de la Paz M, Philen RM, Borda AI. Toxic oil syndrome: the perspective after 20 years. Epidemiol Rev 2001;23(2):231–47.

54. Tabuenca JM. Toxic-allergic syndrome caused by ingestion of rapeseed oil denatured with aniline. Lancet 1981;2(8246):567–8.

55. Garcia-Dorado D, Miller DD, Garcia EJ, et al. An epidemic of pulmonary hypertension after toxic rapeseed oil ingestion in Spain. J Am Coll Cardiol 1983;1(5):1216–22.

56. James TN. The toxic oil syndrome. Clin Cardiol 1994;17(9):463–70.

57. Tello de Meneses R, Gomez de la Camara A, Nogales-Moran MA, et al. Pulmonary hypertension during exercise in toxic oil syndrome. Med Clin (Barc) 2005;125(18):685–8.

58. United Nations Office on Drugs and Crime, World Drug Report 2017 (ISBN: 978-92-1-148291-1, eISBN: 978-92-1-060623-3, United Nations publication, Sales No. E.17.XI.6). Available at: https://www.unodc.org/wdr2017/field/Booklet_3_Plantbased_drugs.pdf. Accessed December 3. 2020.

59. Kerridge BT, Chou SP, Pickering RP, et al. Changes in the prevalence and correlates of cocaine use and cocaine use disorder in the United States, 2001-2002 and 2012-2013. Addict Behav 2019; 90:250–7.

60. Yakel DL Jr, Eisenberg MJ. Pulmonary artery hypertension in chronic intravenous cocaine users. Am Heart J 1995;130(2):398–9.

61. Lie JT, Price DD. Plexogenic pulmonary hypertension associated with intravenous cocaine abuse. Cardiovasc Pathol 1995;4(4):235–8.

62. Murray RJ, Smialek JE, Golle M, et al. Pulmonary artery medial hypertrophy in cocaine users without foreign particle microembolization. Chest 1989; 96(5):1050–3.

63. Collazos J, Martinez E, Fernandez A, et al. Acute, reversible pulmonary hypertension associated with cocaine use. Respir Med 1996;90(3):171–4.

64. Russell LAS JC, Clarke M, Lillington GA. Pulmonary hypertension in female crack users [abstr]. Am Rev Respir Dis 1992;145(A717).

65. Alzghoul BN, Abualsuod A, Alqam B, et al. Cocaine use and pulmonary hypertension. Am J Cardiol 2020;125(2):282–8.

66. Boehrer JD, Moliterno DJ, Willard JE, et al. Hemodynamic effects of intranasal cocaine in humans. J Am Coll Cardiol 1992;20(1):90–3.

67. Kleerup EC, Wong M, Marques-Magallanes JA, et al. Acute effects of intravenous cocaine on pulmonary artery pressure and cardiac index in habitual crack smokers. Chest 1997;111(1):30–5.

68. Rajab R, Stearns E, Baithun S. Autopsy pathology of cocaine users from the Eastern district of London: a retrospective cohort study. J Clin Pathol 2008;61(7):848–50.

69. Walker AM, Langleben D, Korelitz JJ, et al. Temporal trends and drug exposures in pulmonary hypertension: an American experience. Am Heart J 2006;152(3):521–6.

70. Barst RJ, Abenhaim L. Fatal pulmonary arterial hypertension associated with phenylpropanolamine exposure. Heart 2004;90(7):e42.

71. Kernan WN, Viscoli CM, Brass LM, et al. Phenylpropanolamine and the risk of hemorrhagic stroke. N Engl J Med 2000;343(25):1826–32.

72. Seferian A, Chaumais MC, Savale L, et al. Drugs induced pulmonary arterial hypertension. Presse Med 2013;42(9 Pt 2):e303–10.

73. Perrin S, Montani D, O'Connell C, et al. Nasal decongestant exposure in patients with pulmonary arterial hypertension: a pilot study. Eur Respir J 2015;46(4):1211–4.

74. Centers for Disease Control and Prevention. Eosinophilia-myalgia syndrome and L-tryptophan-containing products–New Mexico, Minnesota, Oregon, and New York, 1989. MMWR Morbidity and mortality weekly report. 1989;38(46):785–8.

75. Philen RM, Hill RH Jr. 3-(Phenylamino)alanine–a link between eosinophilia-myalgia syndrome and toxic oil syndrome? Mayo Clin Proc 1993;68(2):197–200.

76. Eidson M, Philen RM, Sewell CM, et al. L-tryptophan and eosinophilia-myalgia syndrome in New Mexico. Lancet 1990;335(8690):645–8.

77. Philen RM, Eidson M, Kilbourne EM, et al. Eosinophilia-myalgia syndrome. A clinical case series of 21 patients. New Mexico eosinophilia-myalgia syndrome study group. Arch Intern Med 1991;151(3):533–7.

78. Culpepper RC, Williams RG, Mease PJ, et al. Natural history of the eosinophilia-myalgia syndrome. Ann Intern Med 1991;115(6):437–42.

79. Tazelaar HD, Myers JL, Drage CW, et al. Pulmonary disease associated with L-tryptophan-induced eosinophilic myalgia syndrome. Clinical and pathologic features. Chest 1990;97(5):1032–6.

80. Medsger TA Jr. Tryptophan-induced eosinophilia-myalgia syndrome. N Engl J Med 1990;322(13):926–8.

81. Goda Y, Suzuki J, Maitani T, et al. 3-anilino-L-alanine, structural determination of UV-5, a contaminant in EMS-associated L-tryptophan samples. Chem Pharm Bull (Tokyo) 1992;40(8):2236–8.

82. Greeson JM, Sanford B, Monti DA. St. John's wort (Hypericum perforatum): a review of the current pharmacological, toxicological, and clinical literature. Psychopharmacology (Berl) 2001;153(4):402–14.

83. Schmidt M, Butterweck V. The mechanisms of action of St. John's wort: an update. Wien Med Wochenschr 2015;165(11–12):229–35.

84. Savale L, Chaumais MC, O'Connell C, et al. Interferon-induced pulmonary hypertension: an update. Curr Opin Pulm Med 2016;22(5):415–20.

85. Dhillon S, Kaker A, Dosanjh A, et al. Irreversible pulmonary hypertension associated with the use of interferon alpha for chronic hepatitis C. Dig Dis Sci 2010;55(6):1785–90.

86. Savale L, Sattler C, Gunther S, et al. Pulmonary arterial hypertension in patients treated with interferon. Eur Respir J 2014;44(6):1627–34.

87. George PM, Cunningham ME, Galloway-Phillipps N, et al. Endothelin-1 as a mediator and potential biomarker for interferon induced pulmonary toxicity. Pulm Circ 2012;2(4):501–4.

88. Prella M, Yerly P, Nicod LP, et al. Pulmonary arterial hypertension in patients treated with interferon. Eur Respir J 2015;46(6):1849–51.

89. Montani D, Lau EM, Dorfmüller P, et al. Pulmonary veno-occlusive disease. Eur Respir J 2016;47(5):1518–34.

90. Ranchoux B, Gunther S, Quarck R, et al. Chemotherapy-induced pulmonary hypertension: role of alkylating agents. Am J Pathol 2015;185(2):356–71.

91. Perros F, Gunther S, Ranchoux B, et al. Mitomycin-induced pulmonary veno-occlusive disease: evidence from human disease and animal models. Circulation 2015;132(9):834–47.

92. Botros L, Van Nieuw Amerongen GP, Vonk Noordegraaf A, et al. Recovery from mitomycin-induced pulmonary arterial hypertension. Ann Am Thorac Soc 2014;11(3):468–70.

93. Holmes JA, Rutledge SM, Chung RT. Direct-acting antiviral treatment for hepatitis C. Lancet 2019;393(10179):1392–4.

94. Renard S, Borentain P, Salaun E, et al. Severe pulmonary arterial hypertension in patients treated for hepatitis C with sofosbuvir. Chest 2016;149(3):e69–73.

95. Savale L, Chaumais MC, Montani D, et al. Direct-acting antiviral medications for hepatitis C virus infection and pulmonary arterial hypertension. Chest 2016;150(1):256–8.

96. Schild D, Hellige GJ, Piso RJ, et al. Pulmonary arterial hypertension in patients with direct-acting antiviral medications for hepatitis C virus infection - a prospective observational cohort study. European Heart Journal - Cardiovascular Imaging. 2020; 21(Supplement_1):834.

97. Martinez-Taboada VM, Rodriguez-Valverde V, Gonzalez-Vilchez F, et al. Pulmonary hypertension in a

patient with rheumatoid arthritis treated with leflunomide. Rheumatology (Oxford) 2004;43(11):1451–3.

98. Alvarez PA, Saad AK, Flagel S, et al. Leflunomide-induced pulmonary hypertension in a young woman with rheumatoid arthritis: a case report. Cardiovasc Toxicol 2012;12(2):180–3.

99. Coirier V, Lescoat A, Chabanne C, et al. Pulmonary arterial hypertension in four patients treated by leflunomide. Joint Bone Spine 2018;85(6):761–3.

100. Cheng X, Merz KH. The role of indirubins in inflammation and associated tumorigenesis. Adv Exp Med Biol 2016;929:269–90.

101. Nishio M, Hirooka K, Doi Y. Chinese herbal drug natural indigo may cause pulmonary artery hypertension. Eur Heart J 2016;37(25):1992.

102. Misumi K, Ogo T, Ueda J, et al. Development of pulmonary arterial hypertension in a patient treated with Qing-Dai (Chinese Herbal Medicine). Intern Med 2019;58(3):395–9.

103. Sato K, Ohira H, Horinouchi T, et al. Chinese herbal medicine Qing-Dai-induced pulmonary arterial hypertension in a patient with ulcerative colitis: a case report and experimental investigation. Respir Med Case Rep 2019;26:265–9.

104. Gonçalves CL, Scaini G, Rezin GT, et al. Effects of acute administration of mazindol on brain energy metabolism in adult mice. Acta Neuropsychiatr 2014;26(3):146–54.

105. Hagiwara M, Tsuchida A, Hyakkoku M, et al. Delayed onset of pulmonary hypertension associated with an appetite suppressant, mazindol: a case report. Jpn Circ J 2000;64(3):218–21.

106. Wigal TL, Newcorn JH, Handal N, et al. A double-blind, placebo-controlled, phase ii study to determine the efficacy, safety, tolerability and pharmacokinetics of a controlled release (CR) Formulation of mazindol in adults with DSM-5 attention-deficit/hyperactivity disorder (ADHD). CNS Drugs 2018;32(3):289–301.

107. Alvarez B, Dahlitz M, Grimshaw J, et al. Mazindol in long-term treatment of narcolepsy. Lancet 1991;337(8752):1293–4.

108. Shindler J, Schachter M, Brincat S, et al. Amphetamine, mazindol, and fencamfamin in narcolepsy. Br Med J (Clin Res ed) 1985;290(6476):1167–70.

109. Nittur N, Konofal E, Dauvilliers Y, et al. Mazindol in narcolepsy and idiopathic and symptomatic hypersomnia refractory to stimulants: a long-term chart review. Sleep Med 2013;14(1):30–6.

110. Konofal E, Benzouid C, Delclaux C, et al. Mazindol: a risk factor for pulmonary arterial hypertension? Sleep Med 2017;34:168–9.

111. Montani D, Seferian A, Savale L, et al. Drug-induced pulmonary arterial hypertension: a recent outbreak. Eur Respir Rev 2013;22(129):244–50.

112. Zhai FG, Zhang XH, Wang HL. Fluoxetine protects against monocrotaline-induced pulmonary arterial hypertension: potential roles of induction of apoptosis and upregulation of Kv1.5 channels in rats. Clin Exp Pharmacol Physiol 2009;36(8):850–6.

113. Song ZH, Wang HM, Liu M, et al. Involvement of S100A4/Mts1 and associated proteins in the protective effect of fluoxetine against MCT - induced pulmonary hypertension in rats. J Chin Med Assoc 2018;81(12):1077–87.

114. Li XQ, Wang HM, Yang CG, et al. Fluoxetine inhibited extracellular matrix of pulmonary artery and inflammation of lungs in monocrotaline-treated rats. Acta Pharmacol Sin 2011;32(2):217–22.

115. Kawut SM, Horn EM, Berekashvili KK, et al. Selective serotonin reuptake inhibitor use and outcomes in pulmonary arterial hypertension. Pulm Pharmacol Ther 2006;19(5):370–4.

116. Shah SJ, Gomberg-Maitland M, Thenappan T, et al. Selective serotonin reuptake inhibitors and the incidence and outcome of pulmonary hypertension. Chest 2009;136(3):694–700.

117. Dhalla IA, Juurlink DN, Gomes T, et al. Selective serotonin reuptake inhibitors and pulmonary arterial hypertension: a case-control study. Chest 2012;141(2):348–53.

118. Sadoughi A, Roberts KE, Preston IR, et al. Use of selective serotonin reuptake inhibitors and outcomes in pulmonary arterial hypertension. Chest 2013;144(2):531–41.

119. Fox BD, Azoulay L, Dell'Aniello S, et al. The use of antidepressants and the risk of idiopathic pulmonary arterial hypertension. Can J Cardiol 2014;30(12):1633–9.

120. Montani D, Lau EM, Descatha A, et al. Occupational exposure to organic solvents: a risk factor for pulmonary veno-occlusive disease. Eur Respir J 2015;46(6):1721–31.

121. Li SL, Yu Y, Yang P, et al. Trichloroethylene Alters Th1/Th2/Th17/Treg paradigm in mice: a novel mechanism for chemically induced autoimmunity. Int J Toxicol 2018;37(2):155–63.

122. Giovanetti A, Rossi L, Mancuso M, et al. Analysis of lung damage induced by trichloroethylene inhalation in mice fed diets with low, normal, and high copper content. Toxicol Pathol 1998;26(5):628–35.

123. Ou J, Ou Z, McCarver DG, et al. Trichloroethylene decreases heat shock protein 90 interactions with endothelial nitric oxide synthase: implications for endothelial cell proliferation. Toxicol Sci 2003;73(1):90–7.

124. Caliez J, Riou M, Manaud G, et al. EXPRESS: trichloroethylene increases pulmonary endothelial permeability: implication for pulmonary veno-

occlusive disease. Pulm Circ 2020;0(ja). 2045894020907884.

125. Burton VJ, Ciuclan LI, Holmes AM, et al. Bone morphogenetic protein receptor II regulates pulmonary artery endothelial cell barrier function. Blood 2011;117(1):333–41.

126. Huertas A, Perros F, Tu L, et al. Immune dysregulation and endothelial dysfunction in pulmonary arterial hypertension: a complex interplay. Circulation 2014;129(12):1332–40.

127. Ito T, Hashimoto Y, Tanaka Y, et al. Efficacy and safety of anagrelide as a first-line drug in cytoreductive treatment-naïve essential thrombocythemia patients in a real-world setting. Eur J Haematol 2019;103(2):116–23.

128. Sumimoto K, Taniguchi Y, Matsuoka Y, et al. "Anagrelide-induced pulmonary arterial hypertension": a rare case of drug-induced pulmonary arterial hypertension. Pulm Circ 2019;9(4). 2045894019896682.

129. Birgegård G, Besses C, Griesshammer M, et al. Treatment of essential thrombocythemia in Europe: a prospective long-term observational study of 3649 high-risk patients in the Evaluation of Anagrelide Efficacy and Long-term Safety study. Haematologica 2018;103(1):51–60.

130. Steele JM. Carfilzomib: a new proteasome inhibitor for relapsed or refractory multiple myeloma. J Oncol Pharm Pract 2013;19(4):348–54.

131. Onyx Pharmaceuticals. Kyprolis Highlights of Prescribing Information 2020. Available at: https://www.pi.amgen.com/~/media/amgen/repositorysites/pi-amgen-com/kyprolis/kyprolis_pi.pdf. Accessed December 3, 2020.

132. Hrustanovic-Kadic M, Jalil B, El-Kersh K. Carfilzomib-Induced Pulmonary Hypertension: A Rare Complication with Reversal After Discontinuation.

American Journal of Respiratory and Critical Care Medicine. 2019;199:A6790. May 17-22, 2019. Dallas, TX.

133. Krishnan U, Mark TM, Niesvizky R, et al. Pulmonary hypertension complicating multiple myeloma. Pulm Circ 2015;5(3):590–7.

134. Chari A, Hajje D. Case series discussion of cardiac and vascular events following carfilzomib treatment: possible mechanism, screening, and monitoring. BMC Cancer 2014;14:915.

135. Fakhri B, Fiala MA, Shah N, et al. Measuring cardiopulmonary complications of carfilzomib treatment and associated risk factors using the SEER-Medicare database. Cancer 2020;126(4): 808–13.

136. Wang M, Cheng J. Overview and management of cardiac and pulmonary adverse events in patients with relapsed and/or refractory multiple myeloma treated with single-agent carfilzomib. Oncology (Williston Park) 2013;27(Suppl 3):24–30.

137. Siegel D, Martin T, Nooka A, et al. Integrated safety profile of single-agent carfilzomib: experience from 526 patients enrolled in 4 phase II clinical studies. Haematologica 2013;98(11):1753–61.

138. Chen JH, Lenihan DJ, Phillips SE, et al. Cardiac events during treatment with proteasome inhibitor therapy for multiple myeloma. Cardiooncology 2017;3(1):4.

139. Cornell RF, Ky B, Weiss BM, et al. Prospective study of cardiac events during proteasome inhibitor therapy for relapsed multiple myeloma. J Clin Oncol 2019;37(22):1946–55.

140. Atrash S, Tullos A, Panozzo S, et al. Cardiac complications in relapsed and refractory multiple myeloma patients treated with carfilzomib. Blood Cancer J 2015;5(1):e272.

Pulmonary Hypertension in Left Heart Disease

Yogesh N.V. Reddy, MBBS, MSc[1], Barry A. Borlaug, MD*

KEYWORDS

• Pulmonary hypertension • Left heart disease • Heart failure

KEY POINTS

• Pulmonary hypertension (PH) is common in left heart disease and in most patients is related to passive back transmission of elevated left atrial pressure.
• Some patients with left heart disease develop a precapillary component to their PH, which worsens prognosis.
• The pathogenesis of PH varies across the different forms of left heart disease but in general is associated with impaired exercise capacity, abnormal ventilatory response with exercise, right ventricular dysfunction, and mortality.
• The objective criteria that have been used to define a precapillary component of PH in left heart disease have varied but conceptually are associated with a higher than expected PA pressure for a given left atrial pressure.
• Current therapeutic options for PH in left heart disease primarily involve treatment of the left heart component, but treatments targeting the pulmonary vasculature either directly or indirectly are being evaluated.

INTRODUCTION

Patients with heart failure (HF) secondary to left heart (LH) disease frequently present with pulmonary hypertension (PH).[1] PH in HF may be caused by 3 underlying pathophysiologic processes: (1) elevation in left atrial (LA) pressure alone, resulting in passive upstream transmission to the pulmonary circulation (isolated postcapillary [IpC] PH); (2) pathologic pulmonary vascular remodeling that coexists with LA hypertension (combined precapillary and postcapillary [CpC] PH); or (3) high flow related to a high cardiac output (CO) state (high-output heart failure), which may or may not coexist with pulmonary vascular disease (PVD) or LA hypertension (**Table 1**). This review focuses on the current state of knowledge of PH that occurs in the setting of LH disease defined by an elevation in LA or pulmonary capillary wedge pressure (PCWP).

DEFINITION OF PULMONARY HYPERTENSION

PH is defined by a pathologically elevated pressure measured in the pulmonary artery (PA). This was historically and somewhat arbitrarily defined by a mean PA pressure greater than or equal to 25 mm Hg, but it recently has been recognized that patients with a mean PA pressure between 20 mm Hg and 25 mm Hg have a higher rate of adverse outcomes, impaired exercise capacity, and progression of PH,[2] which prompted a lowering of the mean PA pressure cutpoint to define PH as greater than 20 mm Hg.[3] There is, however, a paucity of evidence to guide treatment decisions in these patients with a mean PA pressure between 20 mm Hg and 25 mm Hg, and most of the accumulated literature to date primarily has evaluated patients with a mean PA pressure greater than or equal to 25 mm Hg.

Department of Cardiovascular Medicine, Mayo Clinic, Rochester, MN 55906, USA
[1] Present address: 2391 Britwood Lane, Rochester, MN 55902.
* Corresponding author. Mayo Clinic and Foundation, 200 First Street Southwest, Rochester, MN 55905,
E-mail address: borlaug.barry@mayo.edu

Clin Chest Med 42 (2021) 39–58
https://doi.org/10.1016/j.ccm.2020.11.002

Table 1
Hemodynamic definitions of pulmonary hypertension in left heart disease

Definition	Mean Pulmonary Artery Pressure	Pulmonary Capillary Wedge Pressure	Pulmonary Vascular Resistance	Cardiac Output
IpC PH	>20 mm Hg	>15 mm Hg	<3 Wood units	<8 L/min
CpC PH	>20 mm Hg	>15 mm Hg	≥3 Wood units	<8 L/min
High-output HF	>20 mm Hg	>15 mm Hg	<3 Wood units	>8 L/min

EPIDEMIOLOGY

Regardless of underlying etiology, the presence of PH in LH disease consistently has been associated with a poor prognosis.[4–6] This in large part reflects the fact that this typically is a marker of more severe and persistent LH pathology. Once PH is established in a patient with LH disease, however, there is an elevated right ventricular (RV) afterload, which can result in progressive RV dysfunction with associated exercise intolerance, risk of hospitalization, and death.[4,7–12] Furthermore, when the PH occurs in the setting of PVD or is out of proportion to the degree of LH filling pressure elevation, outcomes are disproportionately affected.[4,6,10,13–15]

The estimated prevalence of PH in LH disease is high in general, but epidemiologic studies suffer from referral and selection biases. This is because a diagnosis of PH can be established definitively only by invasive right heart catheterization (RHC), and this test typically is performed in a more diseased cohort of patients. Echocardiography has been used for screening[5] and may provide a more valid estimate in the broader population, but this technique introduces error because of measurement inaccuracy.[16]

LH disease remains the most common cause of PH, greatly exceeding the prevalence of precapillary PA hypertension. In a cohort of 10,023 patients undergoing RHC, only 16% had precapillary PA hypertension whereas approximately 3 times as many patients (46%) had PH from LH disease.[4] In contrast, population-based echocardiography studies have identified a varying prevalence of PH in LH disease but, given the limited accuracy of echocardiography for this diagnosis, the diagnosis of PH can result in either underestimation[16] or overestimation[17] of PA pressures, depending on the specific population studied.

The prevalence of PH also differs depending on etiology of LH disease, being highest in HF with preserved ejection fraction (HFpEF) where multicomorbidity, obesity, and atrial fibrillation are common.[4,18] Although many patients with HF

with reduced ejection fraction (HFrEF) develop resting PH and high filling pressures once decompensated or with progression to end-stage HF, a substantial proportion responds well to medical therapy with normalization of filling pressures and PA pressures with preserved CO, particularly given their underlying compliant ventricles and the reversible role of extrinsic pericardial restraint that contributes to LA hypertension.[19–21] In the previously described large institutional database of 4621 patients undergoing RHC with resting PH from LH disease, only 39% of cases were a result of HFrEF, as opposed to a larger proportion (61%) from HFpEF.[4] Less common etiologies of LH disease, such as mitral or aortic valve disease and other cardiomyopathies, also are associated with a reasonably high prevalence of PH but are proportionally less common than HFpEF or HFrEF on a population level.

The frequency of precapillary PH in LH disease varies greatly in the literature, depending on definitions and cutpoints used[6,9,14,22] and different characteristics of the populations examined, including adequacy of decongestion prior to assessment,[10,23] and the rigor with which hemodynamic assessments were performed. In 1 substantial study from Vanderpool and colleagues,[4] the prevalence of CpC PH by transpulmonary gradient (TPG) (>12 mm Hg), pulmonary vascular resistance (PVR) (>3 Woods units), and diastolic pulmonary gradient (DPG) (≥7 mm Hg) criteria were 46%, 36%, and 12% respectively, in PH from LH disease. This study and most others, however, have relied on automated pressures averaged throughout respiration, which underestimates true intravascular pressure due to varying effects of pleural pressure on measured intrathoracic pressures, as opposed to the correct assessment at end expiration when pleural pressure equals atmospheric pressure.[24,25] In the same study,[4] a substantial number of patients had negative DPG gradients between the PA and PCWP, which is a physiologic impossibility at the near-zero flow state at end diastole. This violation is caused by automated pressure calculations that incorporate the PCWP V wave to create a negative DPG[26] as well as catheter ringing and whip artifact, which may cause underestimation of the nadir diastolic pressures calculated by automated analysis.[4] Finally, there also may be variations in pleural pressure during nonsimultaneous PA and PCWP assessment[25] that contribute to greater variability. There is a subset of patients with substantial obstructive lung disease where end-expiratory pressures may overestimate true intravascular pressure due to the effects of auto–positive end-expiratory pressure, and, in such cases, use of an esophageal balloon or pressures averaged throughout the respiratory cycle may be preferred.[27] Some studies also have used the left-ventricular end-diastolic pressure instead of the PCWP to calculate PVR, but this practice also introduces substantial error.[28] The PCWP better reflects the impact of the downstream pulmonary venous pressure that adds in series to pressure components related to flow, resistance, and compliance in the PA vasculature.[29] Taking all this variability into account, the prevalence of CpC PH appears to be approximately 10% to 15% of LH disease and PH.[6,9,14,22]

COMPONENTS OF MEAN PULMONARY ARTERY PRESSURE

The steady state equation of flow (ΔPressure = flow $\times$ resistance) allows understanding individual contributors to measured mean PA pressure. The mean PA pressure, which must overcome the downstream LA pressure added in series, then increases proportionally to the resistance across the pulmonary circulation through which blood must flow (PVR), and varies directly with pulmonary blood flow (CO). Expressing this in algebraic form: mean PA pressure = LA pressure + PVR * CO. Each of these 3 components (LA pressure, PVR, and CO), therefore, can contribute to measured PA pressure and PH. Primary pathology in any of the 3 components of the absolute PA pressure results in the 3 common pathophysiologic mechanisms of PH in LH disease: (1) primary LA pressure elevation (IpC PH); (2) PVR elevation (CpC PH); and (3) high-output state, resulting in high-output HF with flow-mediated PH. In reality, many patients have varying contributions from these 3 mechanisms.

ETIOLOGIC CAUSES OF PULMONARY HYPERTENSION IN LEFT HEART DISEASE

An alternative approach to classification of PH in LH disease reflects the underlying etiologic cause of LH disease. Each etiology of LH disease then can result in either pure postcapillary PH (IpC PH) or a superimposed component of PVD (CpC PH).

PULMONARY HYPERTENSION IN HEART FAILURE WITH REDUCED EJECTION FRACTION

HFrEF is characterized by LV dilatation and systolic dysfunction that leads to progressive LA hypertension, although PA pressures often improve or even normalize through use of guideline-directed medical therapy.[19,20] The presence of PH after medical therapy optimization is a poor prognostic sign reflective of a component of irreversible structural remodeling or refractory functional mitral regurgitation leading to persistent elevation in LA pressure with secondary PH. If LA pressures remain elevated for a prolonged period of time, this can result in pulmonary vascular remodeling, with an associated decrease in diffusion capacity across the lung.[30–32]

Patients may become tolerant to increased pulmonary venous hypertension over time, in part due to enhancement of pulmonary lymphatic drainage[33] and thickening of the capillary basement membrane, limiting transudation of fluid and pulmonary edema.[30,31] Although these changes may be adaptive to reduce lung congestion, there are structural changes in the pulmonary capillaries and vasculature that resembles the changes seen in precapillary PA hypertension and pulmonary veno-occlusive disease32 (Fig. 1). These substantially worsen PH to increase RV afterload at the expense of sparing the lung and LH from congestion.

The presence of CpC PH is important in the evaluation of patients for heart transplantation. Transplantation of a virgin heart (and RV) into a pulmonary vasculature with pathologic remodeling increases afterload that may lead to primary graft failure. Extensive literature has demonstrated, however, that if the PVR elevation is reversible, then transplantation can be performed successfully. This importantly indicates that not all precapillary PH in LH disease is from irreversible histologic remodeling.[34–36] In contrast, among the subset of patients whose CpC PH is not acutely reversible with short-term hemodynamic optimization, further experience with chronic LVAD support and sustained LA pressure reduction has demonstrated reversibility of the precapillary component over time, resulting in subsequent successful transplantation.[37] Why some patients with chronic LA pressure elevation are more predisposed to pulmonary vascular remodeling and development of a precapillary component compared with other HFrEF patients is unknown

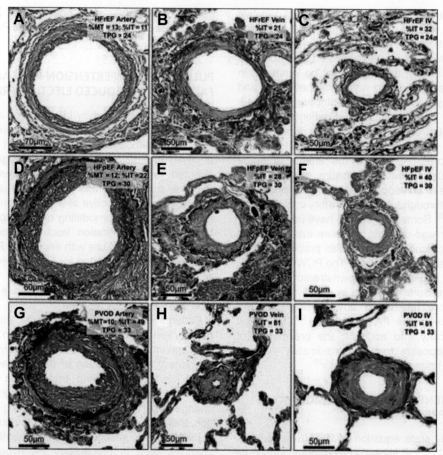

Fig. 1. Examples representative of the mean histomorphometry values for all vessels within the patient in 3 patients with approximately similar degrees of elevation in the TPG. Samples were stained with hematoxylin and eosin and Verhoeff-van Gieson, and captured with whole-field digital microscopy. Rows indicate cohort group (from top: HFrEF, HFpEF, and PVOD). Columns represent vessel type (from left: arteries, veins, and IV). Top, HFrEF: artery, ED 219 μm (*A*); vein, ED 122 μm (*B*); and IV, ED 60 μm (*C*). Middle, HFpEF: artery, ED 220 μm (*D*); vein, ED 86 μm (*E*); and IV, ED 69 μm (*F*). Bottom, PVOD: artery, ED 151 μm (*G*); vein, ED 48 μm (*H*); and IV, ED 86 μm (*I*). ED indicates external diameter; HFpEF, heart failure with preserved ejection fraction; HF-PH, heart failure–pulmonary hypertension; HFrEF, heart failure with reduced ejection fraction; IV, indeterminate vessels; PVOD, pulmonary veno-occlusive disease; TPG, transpulmonary gradient; %IT, percent intimal thickening; %MT, percent medial thickening. (*Reproduced from* Fayayz AU et al Circulation. 2018 Apr 24;137(17):1796-1810 with permission.)

but may reflect complex genetic and environmental susceptibility to development of a precapillary component in response to chronic hemodynamic stress.[22]

PULMONARY HYPERTENSION IN HEART FAILURE WITH PRESERVED EJECTION FRACTION

Although IpC PH is the most common form of PH in HFpEF,[5] pulmonary vascular reserve limitations and abnormal RV reserve is present even in the earliest stages of HFpEF, where filling pressures and pulmonary pressures may be normal at rest and abnormal only during exercise.[38,39] Even such subtle abnormal pulmonary vascular reserve

limitations may be associated with adverse outcomes,[40] limitations in exercise capacity,[39,41] and exacerbation of pulmonary edema.[42,43] Recent data have shown that the severity of LA myopathy and atrial functional mitral regurgitation play important roles and contribute to abnormal PA hemodynamics in HFpEF.[44,45] Impairments in pulmonary vascular function constrain CO reserve during exercise, even when PVR is not extremely high, and this may be treatable. Acute administration of β-adrenergic–mediated pulmonary vasodilation with dobutamine[46] or albuterol[47] improves pulmonary vascular function and CO reserve during exercise. Atrial septostomy leads to combined effects of LA pressure reduction and increases in pulmonary blood flow and O_2 content that have been found to improve pulmonary vascular function in patients with IpC PH–HFpEF.[48]

Patients with HFpEF and CpC PH may represent a unique clinical phenotype of HFpEF, with a pathophysiology that differs from HFpEF with IpC PH. Such patients with CpC PH–HFpEF have prominent abnormalities in RV-PA coupling, with disproportionate elevation in RA pressure during exercise. This increase in RA pressure then results in enhanced ventricular interdependence across the interventricular septum and pericardium during exercise and contributes to the elevation in PCWP in CpC PH.[8] Such PCWP elevation, however, is mediated by passive transmission of extrinsic pressure from the RV and pericardium from relative pericardial restraint and does not translate into a preload response or improved filling of the LV. This phenomenon also is present during exercise-induced PH in HFpEF when there is not substantial PVD present.[49] Despite a rapid rise in PCWP during exercise in CpC PH, there is an attenuated increase in LV stroke volume compared with that seen in IpC PH. This apparent uncoupling of the Frank-Starling relationship is due to the effects of ventricular interaction and relative pericardial restraint externally constraining LV filling despite a rise in measured intracavitary pressure (**Fig. 2**).[21] Therapies targeting abnormal RV-PA coupling during exercise through reduction in LA pressure and PVR or increases in PA compliance, such as albuterol[47] or inorganic nitrite therapy,[50] may hold promise in this phenotype (**Fig. 3**).

The pathogenesis of CpC PH in HFpEF remains incompletely understood because not all patients develop the precapillary component despite chronic PCWP elevation,[51] and, as discussed previously, many patients develop pulmonary vascular dysfunction relatively early in their syndrome even in the presence of normal resting PCWP.[38,39,41] As opposed to HFrEF, there may be a greater phenotypic spectrum in HFpEF, where some patients develop nonhemodynamically mediated pulmonary vascular remodeling reflective of their underlying systemic inflammatory syndrome and comorbidity burden,[5] in particular metabolic comorbidities.[52]

A large analysis demonstrated overlap in single-nucleotide polymorphisms between primary PA hypertension and CpC PH–HFpEF, suggesting that they may lie on a spectrum of disease expression[22] and their response to therapy is less than those with true primary precapillary PA hypertension.[53] The obese phenotype of HFpEF, in particular, is associated with worse RV-PA coupling and pulmonary vascular remodeling compared with nonobese HFpEF,[54] and weight loss may have a favorable impact on PA pressure,

suggesting a causal role.[55] Atrial fibrillation, weight gain, and coronary disease also appear to contribute to progressive RV dysfunction independent of the degree of PCWP elevation.[7] Further research into the mechanisms and treatment of pulmonary vascular dysfunction that develops in some patients with HFpEF is needed urgently because this now represents the most common form of PH in the modern era.[4]

PULMONARY HYPERTENSION IN VALVE DISEASE

Mitral valve stenosis (MS) represents one of the purest human disease models, allowing insight into the impact of isolated, sustained LA hypertension on pulmonary vascular remodeling and PH.[56,57] Rheumatic MS historically afflicted young patients without other comorbidities that are common in HFpEF and HFrEF, and autopsy specimens have provided insight into the pathology of pulmonary vascular remodeling from sustained LA hypertension. Multiple studies have shown that patients with severe MS and severe PVD may demonstrate acute and chronic reductions in PVR following mitral valve intervention, proving that there may be benefits to LA pressure reduction even in patients with advanced PH.[57,58]

Other left-sided valve disease, including mitral regurgitation, aortic stenosis, and regurgitation, display long asymptomatic phases, but even when LA pressure increases, CpC PH seems to develop in a minority. Even after successful valve intervention, many patients have irreversible myocardial remodeling from their original valve insult that results in persistent LA pressure elevation, pulmonary vascular remodeling, and PH, which responds poorly to PA vasodilator therapy.[59]

Severe tricuspid regurgitation (TR) frequently is observed in patients with PH due to LH disease but follows PH rather than causing it in left-sided valve disease. TR in this setting typically develops secondarily either due to RV failure from progressive PH or as a result of atrial fibrillation induced annular enlargement[60] or occult left-sided heart pathology, such as HFpEF.[7,18,61,62]

PULMONARY HYPERTENSION IN OTHER CARDIOMYOPATHIES

Hypertrophic cardiomyopathy (HCM) and amyloid heart disease are common forms of HF that frequently occur with a preserved ejection fraction and have different pathophysiology from HFpEF. The incidence of PH in HCM increases with obstruction and aging and is highest in patients with end-stage HCM with advanced HF.[63]

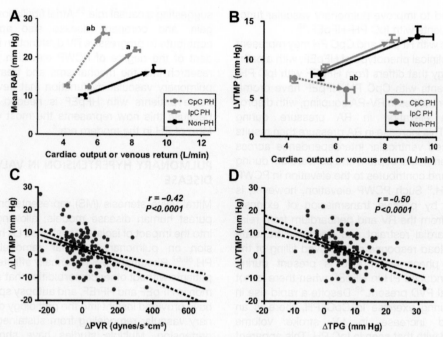

Fig. 2. Ventricular interdependence with exercise in HFpEF and PVD. (*A*) Increase in venous return during exercise was associated with more dramatic increase in right atrial pressure (RAP) in CpC PH–HFpEF compared with the other HFpEF groups. (*B*) Whereas patients with non-PH–HFpEF and IpC PH–HFpEF displayed an increase in left ventricular transmural pressure (LVTMP), CpC PH–HFpEF patients developed a paradoxic decrease in left ventricular transmural pressure as venous return to the right heart increased during exercise. The reduction in left ventricular transmural pressure was increased as exercise PVR (*C*) and TPG (*D*) increased, indicating that LH underfilling was directly related to the severity of PVD. Error bars reflect standard error of the mean. [a]P less than .05 versus non- PH–HFpEF; and [b]P less than .05 versus IpC PH–HFpEF.

Metabolic comorbidities, such as diabetes and obesity, also increase the risk for PH in HCM.[64,65] Among HCM patients with obstruction, approximately half of patients have PH, which is predominantly IpC PH. Only 11% of patients fulfilled criteria for precapillary PH, although provocative maneuvers to unmask dynamic LA pressure elevation were not performed in this subset at high risk for impaired LA compliance reserve.[65] PA pressures, however, frequently improve with septal reduction therapy in obstructive HCM.[66]

Amyloid cardiomyopathy most commonly arises from transthyretin amyloidosis, which can be either of the acquired or genetic type and is associated with higher PA pressures and PVR compared with light chain amyloidosis.[67] The genetic Val122Ile transthyretin variant of amyloidosis has the worst prognosis, quality of life, and adverse structural remodeling with highest PA pressure elevation compared with acquired wild-type transthyretin amyloidosis.[67,68]

HIGH-OUTPUT HEART FAILURE

High-output HF increasingly is recognized as a mimic of HFpEF, where patients can present with

elevated LA pressure and a high CO with associated PH in the setting of a hyperdynamic heart. The pathogenesis involves excessive increases in whole-body oxygen consumption and/or peripheral vasodilation that cause arterial underfilling, with impaired renal perfusion. This promotes salt and water retention with resultant volume overload and increase in filling pressures. Obesity, arteriovenous fistulas,[69] cirrhosis, lung disease, and myeloproliferative disorders are the most common causes in the modern era.[70] It also is important to rule out intracardiac and extracardiac shunts in suspected cases of high-output HF with PH. Regardless of etiology, a chronic high-flow state through the lungs ultimately can result in PVD analogous to the physiology of congenital left-to-right shunting.[71]

METHODS TO IDENTIFY PULMONARY HYPERTENSION AND PULMONARY VASCULAR LOAD
Echocardiography

PA pressure can be estimated using Doppler interrogation of the TR velocity jet summed with estimated RA pressure. Although this approach is

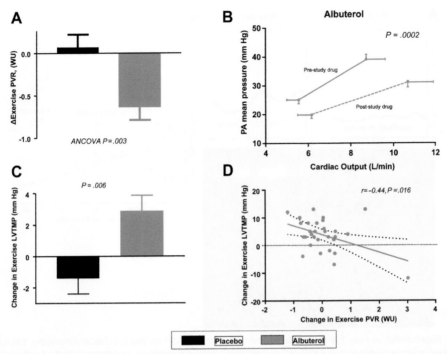

Fig. 3. (*A*) Albuterol improved the primary end point of exercise PVR compared with placebo. (*B*) Albuterol improved the PA pressure-flow relationship with a lesser increase in PA pressure relative to the increase in CO with exertion. (*C*) Left ventricular transmural pressure (LVTMP) increased in response to albuterol compared with placebo. (*D*), The degree of increase in LVTMP was correlated with the reduction in exercise PVR. ANCOVA, Analysis of Covariance; WU, Wood units.

useful for population screening and has prognostic value,[5] there are inaccuracies to this methodology, including underestimation of RA pressure by echo, particularly when assessed during exercise[16] (**Fig. 4**). There also may be greater inaccuracy with poor-quality TR tracings, and many patients do not have adequate TR velocity signals, in which case PA pressures cannot be estimated.[72] The presence or absence of TR also has an impact on this assessment and severe TR has been associated with underestimation of PA pressures.[60] Accordingly, direct measurement of PA pressures by RHC is essential in suspected cases of PH to confirm the diagnosis of PH and differentiate precapillary from postcapillary PH.

Cardiac Catheterization

The performance of a high-quality RHC is essential for PH diagnosis with assessment of severity, calculation of CO (including shunts), and discrimination of precapillary versus postcapillary components. Confirmation of PH can be made from measurement of mean PA pressures at end expiration greater than 20 mm Hg, and the presence of LH disease is inferred from an abnormal PCWP greater than or equal to 15 mm Hg,

although these resting hemodynamic cutoffs should be interpreted in the realm of a continuum of risk even at lower values[11] and poorer discriminatory performance in elderly patients with risk factors for LH disease.[73] The TPG (mean PA-PCWP) depends on the resistance (PVR) and flow rate (CO) and is higher in the presence of CpC PH. PVR is quantified as TPG/CO, with a PVR greater than 3 Wood units associated with significant precapillary component. In addition, total pulsatile load to the RV can be evaluated by PA compliance (estimated by stroke volume/PA pulse pressure) or PA elastance (PA systolic pressure/stroke volume),[74] which are more prognostic in LH disease compared with measures of steady state resistance (ie, PVR, DPG, and TPG).[74] Another formula for PA elastance that is more specific to the pulmonary vascular load recently has been proposed but has not yet been studied widely.[75]

It bears emphasis that PA compliance and PA elastance incorporate total load to the RV, including steady, pulsatile, and postcapillary load components. This contrasts with PVR, which incorporates only steady state load from the precapillary component and ignores the postcapillary and pulsatile components of load. This in part

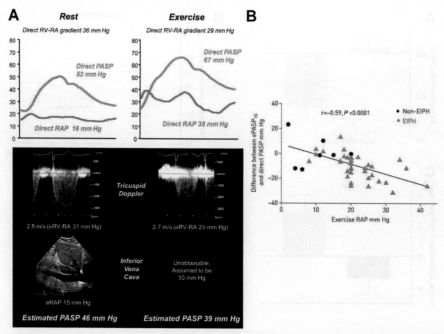

Fig. 4. (*A*) Representative case for the underestimation of true PASP by stress echocardiography. Exercise hemodynamics and echocardiography in a patient presenting exertional dyspnea and normal EF. PA (*red*) and RA (*blue*) pressures were moderately elevated at rest. Echocardiography could accurately estimate both RV-RA gradient and RAP at rest. During exercise RAP increased dramatically to 38 mm Hg, without an increase in RV-RA gradient (direct PASP 67 mm Hg). Although exercise RV-RA gradient could be estimated by echocardiography, inferior vena cava image was unobtainable during exercise. Estimated PASP (39 mm Hg) using assumed RAP of 10 mm Hg substantially underestimated direct PASP by 28 mm Hg. This underestimation even could misclassify this patient as having normal pulmonary hemodynamics response with exercise. (*B*) The magnitude of RAP rise during exercise was related to greater underestimation of PASP by echocardiogram. EIPH, Exercise Induced Pulmonary Hypertension; eRV, estimated Right Ventricular; RAP, Right Atrial Pressure; PASP, Pulmonary Artery Systolic Pressure. (*Modified from* Obokata M et al. Eur Respir J. 2020 Feb 12;55(2):1901617 with permission.)

explains the superiority of PA compliance and elastance at predicting prognosis in PH associated with LH disease.[74] This dependence of PA pulsatile loading on the degree of PCWP elevation also is reflected in a downward shift of the curvilinear PVR-PAC relationship with increasing PCWP, such that PA compliance is lower for any PVR.[15,76] This may in part reflect the retrograde transmission of reflected LA pressure V waves to the PA circulation during systole, augmenting PA systolic pressure and pulsatile RV load.[77,78] This nonlinear relationship between PCWP and PA pressure further complicates interpretation of PVD in the setting of substantial elevation in PCWP and emphasizes the need to optimize LA pressure prior to definitive diagnosis of a superimposed pulmonary vascular precapillary component to PH.[10]

Exercise Testing

In many patients with borderline or normal PCWP, exercise testing unmasks occult LH disease,

which can change an individual's classification of PH.[79] What initially was suspected to be precapillary PH based on resting hemodynamics may reflect occult LH disease or HFpEF when evaluated during the increased CO associated with exercise[80] (**Fig. 5**). The presence of obesity, atrial fibrillation, aging, hypertension, and echocardiographic signs of PH or LH filling pressure elevation can be used to estimate the probability of occult HFpEF as quantified by the H2FPEF score.[18] This can help guide the need for exercise testing in patients with normal PCWP at rest in whom it is desirable to exclude occult HFpEF. Exercise PH has prognostic significance from both the precapillary and postcapillary components, further supporting its pathophysiologic importance[11]

Right Ventricular Assessment

RV function remains a crucial determinant of prognosis in HF and, in advanced HFrEF, RV ejection fraction is more important prognostically than the LV ejection fraction.[81] RV reserve, once loading

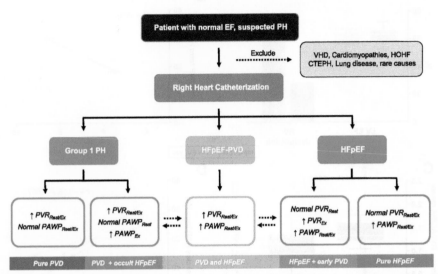

Fig. 5. The spectrum of PH in normal ejection fraction. At the ends of the spectrum there are pure PVD (group 1 PH [*green*]) and pure HFpEF with no PVD (*red*). In-between, there may be patients with PVD and some element of occult HFpEF, for example, if PCWP is normal due to diuresis or underfilling of the LA (*light green*). There also are patients with early HFpEF and abnormal pulmonary vasodilation that is restricted to exercise (*dark orange*), and others with both elevated PCWP and PVD at rest and during exercise (HFpEF-PVD [*light orange*]). In this algorithm, the presence or absence of PVD is defined by PVR, but further research is required to determine if this is the best metric to make this distinction, or alternatives, such as PA compliance and DPG, might be superior. CTEPH, chronic thromboembolic PH; EF, ejection fraction; Ex, exercise; HOHF, high-output HF; PAWP, PA wedge pressure; VHD, valvular heart disease. (*Reproduced from* Borlaug BA, Obokata M. Is it time to recognize a new phenotype? Heart failure with preserved ejection fraction with pulmonary vascular disease. Eur Heart J. 2017 Oct 7;38(38):2874–2878. doi: 10.1093/eurheartj/ehx184.)

conditions are optimized, better represents underlying RV function with improved prognostic stratification.[82] The coupling of RV function to its afterload is called RV-PA coupling, and this also has prognostic and hemodynamic importance in PH related to LH disease[83] and contributes to pulmonary edema by potentially impeding lymphatic drainage from the lung (**Fig. 6**).[42] Baseline and progressive RV function remains a crucial determinant of short-term and long-term outcomes even in HFpEF.[7,84] RV function is assessed most commonly in PH with LH disease by echocardiography, but more centers also are using magnetic resonance imaging–based assessments.

Impact of Ventricular Interaction and Pericardial Restraint

The LVEDP, PCWP, or LA pressure is used primarily clinically as a reflection of LH filling pressures. But in reality, a substantial proportion of the measured LVEDP/PCWP reflects external compressive force that is mediated across the interventricular septum and pericardium.[21] This external pericardial pressure is reflected best by the RA pressure and is elevated substantially in the presence of RV enlargement and cardiomegaly

(which are typical of CpC PH). Therefore, in the presence of substantial RV enlargement, there may be a greater portion of PCWP elevation that is not primarily due to LV disease but rather reflects enhanced diastolic ventricular interaction with relative pericardial restraint[8] (**Fig. 7**). This may result in misdiagnosis of LH disease in the setting of PH, when in fact the PCWP elevation may be driven more by the right heart as opposed to true LH pathology. This should be suspected clinically when RAP equals or even exceeds PCWP, particularly when the PA pressure is elevated greatly out of proportion to PCWP.

PATHOPHYSIOLOGIC CONTRIBUTORS TO OUT OF PROPORTION PULMONARY HYPERTENSION IN LEFT HEART DISEASE
Pulmonary Vascular Remodeling

Data from autopsy series provide insight into such pathologic vascular remodeling in LH disease, which included patients with mitral stenosis with advanced disease showing fibroelastic intimal thickening, medial hypertrophy, scarred and narrow vascular lumens, and thickening of capillary basement membranes.[57,85] In a small series of heart transplant recipients who died shortly after

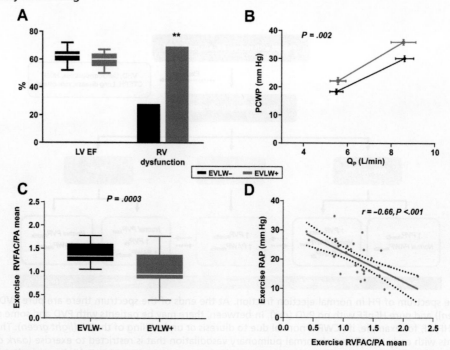

Fig. 6. The HFpEF group with extravascular lung water (EVLW+) had similar left ventricular function but worse RV function compared with the HFpEF group without extravascular lung water (EVLW−) (*A*). PCWP was higher during exercise in the EVLW + HFpEF group (*B*). RV PA uncoupling during exercise was worse in the EVLW + HFpEF group (*C*) and associated with higher right atrial pressure during exercise which potentially impacts lymphatic drainage from the lung (*D*). EF, Ejection Fraction; FAC, Fractional Area Change; LV, Left Ventricular; Qp, Pulmonary blood flow. ** p<0.05.

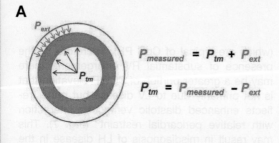

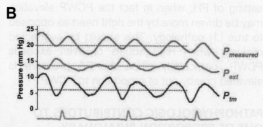

Fig. 7. (*A*) Pressure (*P*) measured is related equal to the sum of the P_{tm} and the P_{ext} applied outside. Pericardial pressure, a measure of P_{ext}, varies directly with right atrial pressure. (*B*) Example shows an estimation of LV P_{tm} as the difference between the measured PCWP (*red*) and the pericardial P_{ext}, estimated by right atrial pressure (*green*). P_{ext}, external pressure; Pra, right atrial pressure; P_{tm}, transmural pressure. Pressure (*P*) measured (Pmeasured) is related equal to the sum of the Ptm and the Pext applied outside. (*Modified from* Borlaug BA, Reddy YN. JACC Heart Fail. 2019 Jul;7(7):574-585 with permission.)

transplantation, a modest increase in TPG (>12 mm Hg) or PVR (>2.5 Wood units) was associated with an increase in muscular PA medial thickness.[86] Increased TPG and DPG have been associated with pulmonary vascular remodeling with medial hypertrophy, intimal/adventitial fibrosis, and occluded vessels.[13] This increase in small vessel disease may serve a protective purpose as a means to decrease upstream transmission of high LA pressures to the proximal PA[87] and also may serve to protect from pulmonary edema.[88] Pulmonary capillary-alveolar interface remodeling can be indirectly inferred from decrease in diffusion capacity for carbon monoxide across the lungs,[30,31] particularly when this does not improve with volume optimization[23] and in some cases even after cardiac transplantation[89] or valve intervention for mitral stenosis.[56] Recently, pan-vascular remodeling, including arterioles, intermediate vessels, and venules, was observed in HF patients regardless of EF[32] (see **Fig. 1**).

Pulmonary Vasoconstriction

Several studies have shown acute reversibility of PVR in PH from LH disease with pulmonary vasodilators.[36,90] This acute reversibility would not be possible if the PVR was driven only by structural remodeling and suggests a reversible component of autonomic, hypoxic, or neurohormonally mediated active pulmonary vasoconstriction. This may be mediated by reduced NO/adrenomedullin/angiopoietin-based signaling pathways, or increased endothelin, among other mediators, that then contribute to the precapillary component of PH.[46,91–96] Autopsy studies also have suggested disconnect between observed pulmonary vascular pathology and associated PVR, which suggests a component of functional vasoconstriction in vivo in some patients.[56,85]

Compression of Vasculature from Pulmonary Edema

Patients with overt pulmonary congestion due to LA hypertension may develop mechanical constriction of pulmonary vasculature due to vessel wall edema[97] or the mechanical effects of compressive atelectasis.[98] This is consistent with prior literature demonstrating improvement in PVR after acute decongestion.[23] One study reported that only 42% of patients initially classified as CpC PH–HF had a persistent precapillary component after decongestion.[10] Therefore, CpC PH should be diagnosed cautiously in patients who are acutely decompensated while volume overloaded and should be reassessed when euvolemic with optimized LA pressure to ensure that the PVR component is not related primarily to the acute decompensated and congested state.

Reflected V Wave and Left Atrial Compliance

In the presence of reduced LA and pulmonary venous compliance, a large V wave develops in late systole that is reflected back to the PA and augments late systolic afterload and PA pressure.[77,99] This wave reflection violates one of the fundamental assumptions involved in the PVR calculation, that the PA and PCWP measured are independent measurements without wave reflections. Therefore, for a given PCWP, the presence of a large V wave can independently contribute to PA systolic and mean pressure augmentation, potentially overestimating PVR and the precapillary component to PH. In general, the impact of wave reflections on PA afterload is not captured adequately by current hemodynamic models[100] and requires future investigation.[78]

Impact of Cardiac Output and Vascular Recruitment

Separate from the acute effect of LA pressure elevation on PA pressure and the PVR calculation, the CO also contributes to the measured PVR. The pulmonary vascular tree displays an inherent distensibility to the circulation that allows recruitment of the vascular bed in response to increased flow and elevation in LA pressures, as with exercise. This distensibility becomes impaired in HF.[12] A recent study has shown that patients with an abnormal increase in PA pressure relative to the increase in flow (PA pressure/CO relationship) display impaired exercise capacity and increased risk for adverse events, across the spectrum of resting PH, exercise-induced PH, and PH due to LH disease or other etiologies.[11] Pharmacologic augmentation of CO with albuterol in HFpEF also is associated with a decrease in PVR during exercise presumably in part from vascular recruitment[47] (see **Fig. 3**).

Thus, the normal response of the pulmonary circulation to increased flow, such as with exercise, is to decrease PVR from this vascular recruitment and distention, mitigating the increase in PA pressure, such that the normal PA pressure/CO slope is less than 3 mm Hg/L/min.[11] Conversely, in low CO states, derecruitment of the vascular tree can occur, resulting in an increase in PVR that is not due to structural remodeling but rather is due to the low flow state that improves with an increase in CO, such as with inotropes, vasodilation, or an LVAD. In addition, low CO results in a low mixed venous O_2 saturation in the PA that contributes to hypoxic vasoconstriction that can temporarily increase PVR.[101] Atrial septostomy in HFpEF to alleviate elevations in LA pressure has demonstrated favorable effects on pulmonary vascular function, presumably through increased flow-mediated recruitment and an increase in mixed venous O_2 saturation contributing to pulmonary vasodilation.[48]

TREATMENT OF PULMONARY HYPERTENSION WITH LEFT HEART DISEASE

In patients with IpC PH, normalization of LA pressure through decongestion normalizes PA pressures, because this is the primary contributor to PH. For patients with CpC PH, the evaluation of advanced HFrEF patients listed for transplantation has provided important observational evidence of the reversibility of PH, both with acute and sustained hemodynamic optimization. Patients with advanced HF demonstrate acute improvement in PVR coupled with an improvement in forward CO and PCWP, in response to the inotropic and vasodilatory effect of milrinone.[102] Similar effects on PVR also are observed in response to systemic and PA dilation with sodium nitroprusside,[35] intravenous prostaglandins,[35,36] and recently with acute neprilysin inhibition.[103] Direct pulmonary vasodilation through inhaled nitric oxide[35,90] also

Table 2
Summary of randomized trials of chronic pulmonary vasodilator therapy in left heart disease

Study	Study Population	Pulmonary Hypertension Mandated for Inclusion	Type of Pulmonary Hypertension Specified	Intervention	Results
Califf et al,[111] 1997 FIRST	HFrEF (n = 471)	No	—	Epoprostenol	Hemodynamics improved (CI, PCWP, and SVR), but there was increased mortality with epoprostenol.
Lewis et al,[104] 2007	HFrEF (n = 34)	Yes	IpC PH or Cpc PH	Sildenafil	Increased peak V_{O_2} and CO with reduced PVR. 6 min walk and QOL also improved.
Guazzi et al,[107] 2012	HFrEF (n = 32)	No	—	Sildenafil	Sildenafil improved exercise oscillatory breathing, QOL, peak V_{O_2}, mean PA pressure, wedge pressure, PVR, and CO.
Andersen et al,[110] 2013	HFpEF post-MI (n = 70)	No	—	Sildenafil	Sildenafil improved CO and SVR with an increase in LV end-diastolic volume and a trend to exercise PCWP reduction.
Redfield et al,[108] 2013 RELAX	HFpEF (n = 216)	No	—	Sildenafil	No benefit. Worsening renal function with sildenafil
Hoendermis et al,[109] 2015	HFpEF (n = 52)	HFpEF with IpC PH	IpC PH or Cpc PH	Sildenafil	No hemodynamic or clinical benefit. Higher PCWP seen with sildenafil
Guazzi et al,[43] 2011	HFpEF (n = 44)	Yes	IpC PH or Cpc PH (more patients were CpC PH)	Sildenafil	Favorable hemodynamic effects on mean PA pressure, RV function, biventricular filling pressure, cardiac index, LV diastolic function, QOL, lung diffusion, and lung water

Study	Population		IpC PH or Cpc PH	Drug	Findings
Bermejo et al,[59] 2018 SIOVAC	HFpEF 1 y after corrective valve surgery (n = 200)	Yes	IpC PH or Cpc PH	Sildenafil	Increased HF hospitalization and worsening clinical status with sildenafil
Bonderman et al,[112] 2013 LEPHT	HFrEF (n = 202)	Yes	IpC PH or Cpc PH	Riociguat	Improved cardiac index, PVR, and quality of life
Vachiery et al,[118] 2018 MELODY-1	HFpEF and HFrEF (n = 63)	Yes	CpC PH	Macitentan	No clinical or hemodynamic benefit. Worsening fluid retention with macitentan.
Anand et al,[119] 2004 EARTH	HFrEF (n = 642)	No	—	Darusentan	No benefit
Prasad et al,[120] 2006	HFrEF (n = 72)	No	—	Enrasentan	No benefit. Increase in cardiac index but worsening LV dilation, hypertrophy, NTproBNP and noradrenaline levels with more serious adverse events
Packer et al,[121] 2017 ENABLE	HFrEF (n = 1613)	No	—	Bosentan	No benefit. Worsening fluid retention with increased HF hospitalization rate. Anemia and transaminitis more common.
Zile et al,[125] 2014	HFpE (n = 192)	No	—	Sitaxsentan	Increase in treadmill time but no impact on quality of life, death, or HF hospitalization
Koller et al,[126] 2017 BADDHY	HFpEF (n = 20)	Yes	IpC PH or Cpc PH	Bosentan	Trend to worse 6-min walk distance with higher echocardiographic PA systolic and RA pressure with bosentan

Abbreviations: CI, Cardiac Index; LV, Left Ventricle; MI, Myocardial Infarction; RA, Right Atrial; QOL, Quality of Life; SVR, Systemic Vascular Resistance.

results in a reduction in PVR but at the expense of increased LA pressure. Although these effects may be demonstrated acutely, it remains unclear whether or how well they can be sustained chronically or what the effects on clinical outcomes might be.

PULMONARY VASOACTIVE THERAPIES IN PULMONARY HYPERTENSION WITH LEFT HEART DISEASE

Sildenafil is a phosphodiesterase 5 inhibitor that has demonstrated favorable effects in HFrEF patients in small single-center trials,[104–107] but a definitive trial in HFrEF patients with PH has yet to be performed (**Table 2**). Trials testing this strategy in HFpEF largely have been negative,[108–110] with the exception of 1 single-center trial, including several patients with underlying CpC PH–HFpEF and abnormal RV-PA coupling.[43] A trial testing sildenafil's efficacy in residual PH after corrective valve surgery with HFpEF-like physiology also was negative and actually showed harm with an increased risk for worsening functional status, LV dilation, and HF hospitalization with sildenafil.[59]

A trial testing intravenous epoprostenol in HFrEF was stopped prematurely due to an increased risk of death[111] despite favorable effects on hemodynamics. The β-adrenergic agonist dobutamine has been shown to elicit more substantial PVR reduction in patients with HFpEF compared with controls.[46] In an acute trial, administration of inhaled albuterol was shown to improve PVR during exercise in patients with HFpEF compared with placebo (see **Fig. 3**).[47] The participants in this study did not display evidence of CpC PH at rest, indicating that this is not necessary for a pulmonary vasoactive agent to be effective in this cohort.

Riociguat, which is a soluble guanylate cyclase stimulator, has been shown to improve various hemodynamic endpoints in HFrEF[112] and HFpEF,[113] but further study is needed. An alternative guanylate cyclase stimulator, vericiguat, demonstrated beneficial natriuretic peptide changes,[114] and a definitive outcome trial in HFrEF recently has shown reductions in HF hospitalization risk in a high-risk cohort.[115] This study included all patients with HFrEF after a recent hospitalization regardless of PH status, so the specific efficacy in HFrEF patients with CpC PH or more deranged RV-PA coupling is unknown. Favorable effects on quality of life with higher doses of vericiguat also were observed in HFpEF,[116] and a definitive outcome trial is ongoing.[117]

The endothelin antagonist macitentan was studied in CpC PH from both HFpEF and HFrEF but was associated with a tendency to fluid retention and no clear benefit despite a trend to N-terminal fragment of the prohormone brain natriuretic peptide (NTproBNP) reduction[118] (see **Table 1**). A trial targeting CpC PH–HFpEF with macitentan was undertaken but was discontinued owing to poor enrollment (NCT03153111). Clinical trials of other endothelin antagonists, including darusentan,[119] enrasentan,[120] and bosentan,[121,122] in HFrEF also have been negative, with early evidence of adverse fluid retention (see **Table 1**). This was despite studies showing elevation in endothelin levels associated with adverse outcomes and PVR[123] as well as favorable acute hemodynamic effects with endothelin antagonists in HFrEF.[92] Even though endothelin also appears to be elevated[124] and associated with abnormal pulmonary vascular reserve in HFpEF,[38] trials in unselected HFpEF populations of endothelin antagonists have to date largely been unsuccessful.[125,126] Further trials in selected subsets with prominent pulmonary vascular pathology and abnormal RV-PA coupling in HFrEF and HFpEF are required.

FUTURE DIRECTIONS

A majority of trials targeting PH in LH disease have included a mixture of patients with IpC PH, with CpC PH, and even without PH. Inclusion of such heterogeneous populations may have contributed to the failure of broadly targeting precapillary PH-directed therapies to this population. Whether there are subsets of patients with LH disease that phenotypically have disproportionate adverse pulmonary vascular physiology with resultant pericardial restraint that will benefit from PAH directed therapy is unknown. Better understanding of the hemodynamic profile of PH patients with LH disease, including exercise evaluation for occult LH or pulmonary vascular dysfunction and differentiation of the precapillary component into underlying PA structural remodeling as opposed to functional vasoconstriction, are critical for future investigation. With refinement of phenotyping and better classification of unique phenotypes with precapillary PH in LHD, future trials can better target patients who are most likely to benefit.

CLINICS CARE POINTS

- Pulmonary Hypertension is common in left heart disease and most commonly reflects the underlying left heart disease process.
- Right heart catheterization is essential to understand the mechanisms and severity of underlying pulmonary hypertension.

- Acutely decompensated heart failure patients may have a higher than expected pulmonary vascular resistance that may improve merely with optimization of their heart failure.
- Treatment in general currently is focused on treating the left heart disease.

ACKNOWLEDGMENTS

B.A. Borlaug is supported by R01 HL128526, R01 HL 126638, U01 HL125205 and U10 HL110262, all from the National Institute of Health.

DISCLOSURES

None.

REFERENCES

1. Guazzi M, Borlaug BA. Pulmonary hypertension due to left heart disease. Circulation 2012;126(8): 975–90.
2. Assad TR, Maron BA, Robbins IM, et al. Prognostic effect and longitudinal hemodynamic assessment of borderline pulmonary hypertension. JAMA Cardiol 2017;2(12):1361–8.
3. Simonneau G, Montani D, Celermajer DS, et al. Haemodynamic definitions and updated clinical classification of pulmonary hypertension. Eur Respir J 2019;53(1):1801913.
4. Vanderpool RR, Saul M, Nouraie M, et al. Association between hemodynamic markers of pulmonary hypertension and outcomes in heart failure with preserved ejection fraction. JAMA Cardiol 2018; 3(4):298–306.
5. Lam CS, Roger VL, Rodeheffer RJ, et al. Pulmonary hypertension in heart failure with preserved ejection fraction: a community-based study. J Am Coll Cardiol 2009;53(13):1119–26.
6. Miller WL, Grill DE, Borlaug BA. Clinical features, hemodynamics, and outcomes of pulmonary hypertension due to chronic heart failure with reduced ejection fraction: pulmonary hypertension and heart failure. JACC Heart Fail 2013;1(4):290–9.
7. Obokata M, Reddy YNV, Melenovsky V, et al. Deterioration in right ventricular structure and function over time in patients with heart failure and preserved ejection fraction. Eur Heart J 2019;40(8): 689–97.
8. Gorter TM, Obokata M, Reddy YNV, et al. Exercise unmasks distinct pathophysiologic features in heart failure with preserved ejection fraction and pulmonary vascular disease. Eur Heart J 2018; 39(30):2825–35.
9. Gerges M, Gerges C, Pistritto AM, et al. Pulmonary hypertension in heart failure. epidemiology, right ventricular function, and survival. Am J Respir Crit Care Med 2015;192(10):1234–46.
10. Aronson D, Eitan A, Dragu R, et al. Relationship between reactive pulmonary hypertension and mortality in patients with acute decompensated heart failure. Circ Heart Fail 2011;4(5):644–50.
11. Ho JE, Zern EK, Lau ES, et al. Exercise pulmonary hypertension predicts clinical outcomes in patients with dyspnea on effort. J Am Coll Cardiol 2020; 75(1):17–26.
12. Malhotra R, Dhakal BP, Eisman AS, et al. Pulmonary vascular distensibility predicts pulmonary hypertension severity, exercise capacity, and survival in heart failure. Circ Heart Fail 2016;9(6). https://doi.org/10.1161/CIRCHEARTFAILURE.115. 003011.
13. Gerges C, Gerges M, Lang MB, et al. Diastolic pulmonary vascular pressure gradient: a predictor of prognosis in "out-of-proportion" pulmonary hypertension. Chest 2013;143(3):758–66.
14. Palazzini M, Dardi F, Manes A, et al. Pulmonary hypertension due to left heart disease: analysis of survival according to the haemodynamic classification of the 2015 ESC/ERS guidelines and insights for future changes. Eur J Heart Fail 2018;20(2):248–55.
15. Dragu R, Rispler S, Habib M, et al. Pulmonary arterial capacitance in patients with heart failure and reactive pulmonary hypertension. Eur J Heart Fail 2015;17(1):74–80.
16. Obokata M, Kane GC, Sorimachi H, et al. Noninvasive evaluation of pulmonary artery pressure during exercise: the importance of right atrial hypertension. Eur Respir J 2020;55(2):1901617.
17. Parent F, Bachir D, Inamo J, et al. A hemodynamic study of pulmonary hypertension in sickle cell disease. N Engl J Med 2011;365(1):44–53.
18. Reddy YNV, Carter RE, Obokata M, et al. A simple, evidence-based approach to help guide diagnosis of heart failure with preserved ejection fraction. Circulation 2018;138(9):861–70.
19. Stevenson LW, Tillisch JH. Maintenance of cardiac output with normal filling pressures in patients with dilated heart failure. Circulation 1986;74(6): 1303–8.
20. Johnson W, Omland T, Hall C, et al. Neurohormonal activation rapidly decreases after intravenous therapy with diuretics and vasodilators for class IV heart failure. J Am Coll Cardiol 2002;39(10): 1623–9.
21. Borlaug BA, Reddy YNV. The role of the pericardium in heart failure: implications for pathophysiology and treatment. JACC Heart Fail 2019;7(7): 574–85.
22. Assad TR, Hemnes AR, Larkin EK, et al. Clinical and biological insights into combined post- and pre-capillary pulmonary hypertension. J Am Coll Cardiol 2016;68(23):2525–36.
23. Agostoni PG, Guazzi M, Bussotti M, et al. Lack of improvement of lung diffusing capacity following

fluid withdrawal by ultrafiltration in chronic heart failure. J Am Coll Cardiol 2000;36(5):1600–4.

24. Ryan JJ, Rich JD, Thiruvoipati T, et al. Current practice for determining pulmonary capillary wedge pressure predisposes to serious errors in the classification of patients with pulmonary hypertension. Am Heart J 2012;163(4):589–94.

25. Smiseth OA, Thompson CR, Ling H, et al. Juxtacardiac pleural pressure during positive end-expiratory pressure ventilation: an intraoperative study in patients with open pericardium. J Am Coll Cardiol 1994;23(3):753–8.

26. Nagy AI, Venkateshvaran A, Merkely B, et al. Determinants and prognostic implications of the negative diastolic pulmonary pressure gradient in patients with pulmonary hypertension due to left heart disease. Eur J Heart Fail 2017;19(1):88–97.

27. Boerrigter BG, Waxman AB, Westerhof N, et al. Measuring central pulmonary pressures during exercise in COPD: how to cope with respiratory effects. Eur Respir J 2014;43(5):1316–25.

28. Reddy YNV, El-Sabbagh A, Nishimura RA. Comparing pulmonary arterial wedge pressure and left ventricular end diastolic pressure for assessment of left-sided filling pressures. JAMA Cardiol 2018;3(6):453–4.

29. Mascherbauer J, Zotter-Tufaro C, Duca F, et al. Wedge pressure rather than left ventricular end-diastolic pressure predicts outcome in heart failure with preserved ejection fraction. JACC Heart Fail 2017;5(11):795–801.

30. Hoeper MM, Meyer K, Rademacher J, et al. Diffusion capacity and mortality in patients with pulmonary hypertension due to heart failure with preserved ejection fraction. JACC Heart Fail 2016;4(6):441–9.

31. Puri S, Baker BL, Dutka DP, et al. Reduced alveolar-capillary membrane diffusing capacity in chronic heart failure. Its pathophysiological relevance and relationship to exercise performance. Circulation 1995;91(11):2769–74.

32. Fayyaz AU, Edwards WD, Maleszewski JJ, et al. Global pulmonary vascular remodeling in pulmonary hypertension associated with heart failure and preserved or reduced ejection fraction. Circulation 2018;137(17):1796–810.

33. Uhley HN, Leeds SE, Sampson JJ, et al. Role of pulmonary lymphatics in chronic pulmonary edema. Circ Res 1962;11:966–70.

34. Costard-Jackle A, Fowler MB. Influence of preoperative pulmonary artery pressure on mortality after heart transplantation: testing of potential reversibility of pulmonary hypertension with nitroprusside is useful in defining a high risk group. J Am Coll Cardiol 1992;19(1):48–54.

35. Kieler-Jensen N, Lundin S, Ricksten SE. Vasodilator therapy after heart transplantation: effects of inhaled nitric oxide and intravenous prostacyclin, prostaglandin E1, and sodium nitroprusside. J Heart Lung Transplant 1995;14(3):436–43.

36. von Scheidt W, Costard-Jaeckle A, Stempfle HU, et al. Prostaglandin E1 testing in heart failure-associated pulmonary hypertension enables transplantation: the PROPHET study. J Heart Lung Transplant 2006;25(9):1070–6.

37. Kutty RS, Parameshwar J, Lewis C, et al. Use of centrifugal left ventricular assist device as a bridge to candidacy in severe heart failure with secondary pulmonary hypertension. Eur J Cardiothorac Surg 2013;43(6):1237–42.

38. Obokata M, Kane GC, Reddy YNV, et al. The neurohormonal basis of pulmonary hypertension in heart failure with preserved ejection fraction. Eur Heart J 2019;40(45):3707–17.

39. Borlaug BA, Kane GC, Melenovsky V, et al. Abnormal right ventricular-pulmonary artery coupling with exercise in heart failure with preserved ejection fraction. Eur Heart J 2016;37(43):3293–302.

40. Huang W, Oliveira RKF, Lei H, et al. Pulmonary vascular resistance during exercise predicts long-term outcomes in heart failure with preserved ejection fraction. J Card Fail 2018;24(3):169–76.

41. Obokata M, Olson TP, Reddy YNV, et al. Haemodynamics, dyspnoea, and pulmonary reserve in heart failure with preserved ejection fraction. Eur Heart J 2018;39(30):2810–21.

42. Reddy YNV, Obokata M, Wiley B, et al. The haemodynamic basis of lung congestion during exercise in heart failure with preserved ejection fraction. Eur Heart J 2019;40(45):3721–30.

43. Guazzi M, Vicenzi M, Arena R, et al. Pulmonary hypertension in heart failure with preserved ejection fraction: a target of phosphodiesterase-5 inhibition in a 1-year study. Circulation 2011;124(2):164–74.

44. Tamargo M, Obokata M, Reddy YNV, et al. Functional mitral regurgitation and left atrial myopathy in heart failure with preserved ejection fraction. Eur J Heart Fail 2020;22(3):489–98.

45. Reddy YNV, Obokata M, Egbe A, et al. Left atrial strain and compliance in the diagnostic evaluation of heart failure with preserved ejection fraction. Eur J Heart Fail 2019;21(7):891–900.

46. Andersen MJ, Hwang SJ, Kane GC, et al. Enhanced pulmonary vasodilator reserve and abnormal right ventricular: pulmonary artery coupling in heart failure with preserved ejection fraction. Circ Heart Fail 2015;8(3):542–50.

47. Reddy YNV, Obokata M, Koepp KE, et al. The beta-adrenergic agonist albuterol improves pulmonary vascular reserve in heart failure with preserved ejection fraction. Circ Res 2019;124(2):306–14.

48. Obokata M, Reddy YNV, Shah SJ, et al. Effects of interatrial shunt on pulmonary vascular function in

heart failure with preserved ejection fraction. J Am Coll Cardiol 2019;74(21):2539–50.

49. Parasuraman SK, Loudon BL, Lowery C, et al. Diastolic ventricular interaction in heart failure with preserved ejection fraction. J Am Heart Assoc 2019; 8(7):e010114.

50. Borlaug BA, Melenovsky V, Koepp KE. Inhaled sodium nitrite improves rest and exercise hemodynamics in heart failure with preserved ejection fraction. Circ Res 2016;119(7):880–6.

51. Thenappan T, Shah SJ, Gomberg-Maitland M, et al. Clinical characteristics of pulmonary hypertension in patients with heart failure and preserved ejection fraction. Circ Heart Fail 2011;4(3):257–65.

52. Lai YC, Tabima DM, Dube JJ, et al. SIRT3-AMP-activated protein kinase activation by nitrite and metformin improves hyperglycemia and normalizes pulmonary hypertension associated with heart failure with preserved ejection fraction. Circulation 2016;133(8):717–31.

53. Opitz CF, Hoeper MM, Gibbs JS, et al. Pre-capillary, combined, and post-capillary pulmonary hypertension: a pathophysiological continuum. J Am Coll Cardiol 2016;68(4):368–78.

54. Obokata M, Reddy YNV, Pislaru SV, et al. Evidence Supporting the existence of a distinct obese phenotype of heart failure with preserved ejection fraction. Circulation 2017;136(1):6–19.

55. Reddy YNV, Anantha-Narayanan M, Obokata M, et al. Hemodynamic effects of weight loss in obesity: a systematic review and meta-analysis. JACC Heart Fail 2019;7(8):678–87.

56. Curti PC, Cohen G, Castleman B, et al. Respiratory and circulatory studies of patients with mitral stenosis. Circulation 1953;8(6):893–904.

57. Goodale F Jr, Sanchez G, Friedlich AL, et al. Correlation of pulmonary arteriolar resistance with pulmonary vascular changes in patients with mitral stenosis before and after valvulotomy. N Engl J Med 1955;252(23):979–83.

58. Braunwald E, Braunwald NS, Ross J Jr, et al. Effects of mitral-valve replacement on the pulmonary vascular dynamics of patients with pulmonary hypertension. N Engl J Med 1965;273:509–14.

59. Bermejo J, Yotti R, Garcia-Orta R, et al. Sildenafil for improving outcomes in patients with corrected valvular heart disease and persistent pulmonary hypertension: a multicenter, double-blind, randomized clinical trial. Eur Heart J 2018;39(15):1255–64.

60. Lurz P, Orban M, Besler C, et al. Clinical characteristics, diagnosis, and risk stratification of pulmonary hypertension in severe tricuspid regurgitation and implications for transcatheter tricuspid valve repair. Eur Heart J 2020;41(29):2785–95.

61. Reddy YNV, Obokata M, Gersh BJ, et al. High prevalence of occult heart failure with preserved ejection fraction among patients with atrial fibrillation and dyspnea. Circulation 2018;137(5):534–5.

62. Andersen MJ, Nishimura RA, Borlaug BA. The hemodynamic basis of exercise intolerance in tricuspid regurgitation. Circ Heart Fail 2014;7(6):911–7.

63. Musumeci MB, Mastromarino V, Casenghi M, et al. Pulmonary hypertension and clinical correlates in hypertrophic cardiomyopathy. Int J Cardiol 2017;248:326–32.

64. Wasserstrum Y, Barriales-Villa R, Fernandez-Fernandez X, et al. The impact of diabetes mellitus on the clinical phenotype of hypertrophic cardiomyopathy. Eur Heart J 2019;40(21):1671–7.

65. Covella M, Rowin EJ, Hill NS, et al. Mechanism of progressive heart failure and significance of pulmonary hypertension in obstructive hypertrophic cardiomyopathy. Circ Heart Fail 2017;10(4):e003689.

66. Geske JB, Konecny T, Ommen SR, et al. Surgical myectomy improves pulmonary hypertension in obstructive hypertrophic cardiomyopathy. Eur Heart J 2014;35(30):2032–9.

67. Chacko L, Martone R, Bandera F, et al. Echocardiographic phenotype and prognosis in transthyretin cardiac amyloidosis. Eur Heart J 2020;41(14):1439–47.

68. Lane T, Fontana M, Martinez-Naharro A, et al. Natural history, quality of life, and outcome in cardiac transthyretin amyloidosis. Circulation 2019;140(1):16–26.

69. Reddy YNV, Obokata M, Dean PG, et al. Long-term cardiovascular changes following creation of arteriovenous fistula in patients with end stage renal disease. Eur Heart J 2017;38(24):1913–23.

70. Reddy YNV, Melenovsky V, Redfield MM, et al. High-output heart failure: a 15-year experience. J Am Coll Cardiol 2016;68(5):473–82.

71. Braunwald NS, Braunwald NS, Braunwald E, et al. The effects of surgical abolition of left-to-right shunts on the pulmonary vascular dynamics of patients with pulmonary hypertension. Circulation 1962;26:1270–8.

72. van Riel AC, Opotowsky AR, Santos M, et al. Accuracy of echocardiography to estimate pulmonary artery pressures with exercise: a simultaneous invasive-noninvasive comparison. Circ Cardiovasc Imaging 2017;10(4):e005711.

73. Maor E, Grossman Y, Balmor RG, et al. Exercise haemodynamics may unmask the diagnosis of diastolic dysfunction among patients with pulmonary hypertension. Eur J Heart Fail 2015;17(2):151–8.

74. Tampakakis E, Shah SJ, Borlaug BA, et al. Pulmonary effective arterial elastance as a measure of right ventricular afterload and its prognostic value in pulmonary hypertension due to left heart disease. Circ Heart Fail 2018;11(4):e004436.

75. Brener MI, Burkhoff D, Sunagawa K. Effective arterial elastance in the pulmonary arterial circulation: derivation, assumptions, and clinical applications. Circ Heart Fail 2020;13(3):e006591.

76. Tedford RJ, Hassoun PM, Mathai SC, et al. Pulmonary capillary wedge pressure augments right ventricular pulsatile loading. Circulation 2012;125(2):289–97.

77. Grose R, Strain J, Cohen MV. Pulmonary arterial V waves in mitral regurgitation: clinical and experimental observations. Circulation 1984;69(2):214–22.

78. Ghimire A, Andersen MJ, Burrowes LM, et al. The reservoir-wave approach to characterize pulmonary vascular-right ventricular interactions in humans. J Appl Physiol (1985) 2016;121(6):1348–53.

79. Borlaug BA, Nishimura RA, Sorajja P, et al. Exercise hemodynamics enhance diagnosis of early heart failure with preserved ejection fraction. Circ Heart Fail 2010;3(5):588–95.

80. Borlaug BA, Obokata M. Is it time to recognize a new phenotype? Heart failure with preserved ejection fraction with pulmonary vascular disease. Eur Heart J 2017;38(38):2874–8.

81. Gavazzi A, Berzuini C, Campana C, et al. Value of right ventricular ejection fraction in predicting short-term prognosis of patients with severe chronic heart failure. J Heart Lung Transplant 1997;16(7):774–85.

82. Gavazzi A, Ghio S, Scelsi L, et al. Response of the right ventricle to acute pulmonary vasodilation predicts the outcome in patients with advanced heart failure and pulmonary hypertension. Am Heart J 2003;145(2):310–6.

83. Guazzi M, Bandera F, Pelissero G, et al. Tricuspid annular plane systolic excursion and pulmonary arterial systolic pressure relationship in heart failure: an index of right ventricular contractile function and prognosis. Am J Physiol Heart Circ Physiol 2013;305(9):H1373–81.

84. Melenovsky V, Hwang SJ, Lin G, et al. Right heart dysfunction in heart failure with preserved ejection fraction. Eur Heart J 2014;35(48):3452–62.

85. Denst J, Edwards A, Neubuerger KT, et al. Biopsies of the lung and atrial appendages in mitral stenosis; correlation of data from cardiac catheterization with pulmonary vascular lesions. Am Heart J 1954;48(4):506–20.

86. Delgado JF, Conde E, Sanchez V, et al. Pulmonary vascular remodeling in pulmonary hypertension due to chronic heart failure. Eur J Heart Fail 2005;7(6):1011–6.

87. Gerges C, Gerges M, Fesler P, et al. In-depth haemodynamic phenotyping of pulmonary hypertension due to left heart disease. Eur Respir J 2018;51(5):1800067.

88. Bocchi EA, Bacal F, Auler Junior JO, et al. Inhaled nitric oxide leading to pulmonary edema in stable severe heart failure. Am J Cardiol 1994;74(1):70–2.

89. Mettauer B, Lampert E, Charloux A, et al. Lung membrane diffusing capacity, heart failure, and heart transplantation. Am J Cardiol 1999;83(1):62–7.

90. Adatia I, Perry S, Landzberg M, et al. Inhaled nitric oxide and hemodynamic evaluation of patients with pulmonary hypertension before transplantation. J Am Coll Cardiol 1995;25(7):1656–64.

91. Nishikimi T, Nagata S, Sasaki T, et al. Plasma concentrations of adrenomedullin correlate with the extent of pulmonary hypertension in patients with mitral stenosis. Heart 1997;78(4):390–5.

92. Kiowski W, Sutsch G, Hunziker P, et al. Evidence for endothelin-1-mediated vasoconstriction in severe chronic heart failure. Lancet 1995;346(8977):732–6.

93. Cooper CJ, Jevnikar FW, Walsh T, et al. The influence of basal nitric oxide activity on pulmonary vascular resistance in patients with congestive heart failure. Am J Cardiol 1998;82(5):609–14.

94. Lupi-Herrera E, Seoane M, Sandoval J, et al. Behavior of the pulmonary circulation in the grossly obese patient. Pathogenesis of pulmonary arterial hypertension at an altitude of 2,240 meters. Chest 1980;78(4):553–8.

95. Karapinar H, Esen O, Emiroglu Y, et al. Serum levels of angiopoietin-1 in patients with pulmonary hypertension due to mitral stenosis. Heart Vessels 2011;26(5):536–41.

96. Yamamoto K, Ikeda U, Shimada K. Endothelin production in mitral stenosis. N Engl J Med 1993;329(23):1740–1.

97. West JB, Dollery CT, Heard BE. Increased pulmonary vascular resistance in the dependent zone of the isolated dog lung caused by perivascular edema. Circ Res 1965;17:191–206.

98. Woodson RD, Raab DE, Ferguson DJ. Pulmonary hemodynamics following acute atelectasis. Am J Physiol 1963;205:53–6.

99. Reddy YNV, El Sabbagh A, Packer D, et al. Evaluation of shortness of breath after atrial fibrillation ablation-Is there a stiff left atrium? Heart Rhythm 2018;15(6):930–5.

100. Ting CT, Chen JW, Chang MS, et al. Pulmonary hemodynamics and wave reflections in adults with atrial septal defects. Am J Physiol Heart Circ Physiol 2020;318(4):H925–36.

101. Domino KB, Wetstein L, Glasser SA, et al. Influence of mixed venous oxygen tension (PVO2) on blood flow to atelectatic lung. Anesthesiology 1983;59(5):428–34.

102. Givertz MM, Hare JM, Loh E, et al. Effect of bolus milrinone on hemodynamic variables and

pulmonary vascular resistance in patients with severe left ventricular dysfunction: a rapid test for
reversibility of pulmonary hypertension. J Am Coll
Cardiol 1996;28(7):1775–80.

103. Zern EK, Cheng S, Wolfson AM, et al. Angiotensin
receptor-neprilysin inhibitor therapy reverses pulmonary hypertension in end-stage heart failure patients awaiting transplantation. Circ Heart Fail
2020;13(2):e006696.

104. Lewis GD, Lachmann J, Camuso J, et al. Sildenafil
improves exercise hemodynamics and oxygen uptake in patients with systolic heart failure. Circulation 2007;115(1):59–66.

105. Lepore JJ, Maroo A, Bigatello LM, et al. Hemodynamic effects of sildenafil in patients with congestive heart failure and pulmonary hypertension:
combined administration with inhaled nitric oxide.
Chest 2005;127(5):1647–53.

106. Melenovsky V, Al-Hiti H, Kazdova L, et al. Transpulmonary B-type natriuretic peptide uptake and
cyclic guanosine monophosphate release in
heart failure and pulmonary hypertension: the effects of sildenafil. J Am Coll Cardiol 2009;54(7):
595–600.

107. Guazzi M, Vicenzi M, Arena R. Phosphodiesterase
5 inhibition with sildenafil reverses exercise oscillatory breathing in chronic heart failure: a long-term
cardiopulmonary exercise testing placebo-
controlled study. Eur J Heart Fail 2012;14(1):82–90.

108. Redfield MM, Chen HH, Borlaug BA, et al. Effect of
phosphodiesterase-5 inhibition on exercise capacity and clinical status in heart failure with preserved
ejection fraction: a randomized clinical trial. JAMA
2013;309(12):1268–77.

109. Hoendermis ES, Liu LC, Hummel YM, et al. Effects
of sildenafil on invasive haemodynamics and exercise capacity in heart failure patients with preserved ejection fraction and pulmonary
hypertension: a randomized controlled trial. Eur
Heart J 2015;36(38):2565–73.

110. Andersen MJ, Ersboll M, Axelsson A, et al. Sildenafil and diastolic dysfunction after acute myocardial infarction in patients with preserved ejection
fraction: the Sildenafil and diastolic dysfunction after acute myocardial infarction (SIDAMI) trial. Circulation 2013;127(11):1200–8.

111. Califf RM, Adams KF, McKenna WJ, et al.
A randomized controlled trial of epoprostenol ther-
apy for severe congestive heart failure: the Flolan
International Randomized Survival Trial (FIRST).
Am Heart J 1997;134(1):44–54.

112. Bonderman D, Ghio S, Felix SB, et al. Riociguat for
patients with pulmonary hypertension caused by
systolic left ventricular dysfunction: a phase IIb
double-blind, randomized, placebo-controlled,
dose-ranging hemodynamic study. Circulation
2013;128(5):502–11.

113. Bonderman D, Pretsch I, Steringer-
Mascherbauer R, et al. Acute hemodynamic effects
of riociguat in patients with pulmonary hypertension associated with diastolic heart failure
(DILATE-1): a randomized, double-blind, placebo-
controlled, single-dose study. Chest 2014;146(5):
1274–85.

114. Gheorghiade M, Greene SJ, Butler J, et al. Effect of
vericiguat, a soluble guanylate cyclase stimulator,
on natriuretic peptide levels in patients with worsening chronic heart failure and reduced ejection
fraction: the SOCRATES-REDUCED randomized
trial. JAMA 2015;314(21):2251–62.

115. Armstrong PW, Pieske B, Anstrom KJ, et al. Vericiguat in patients with heart failure and reduced ejection fraction. N Engl J Med 2020;382(20):1883–93.

116. Pieske B, Maggioni AP, Lam CSP, et al. Vericiguat
in patients with worsening chronic heart failure
and preserved ejection fraction: results of the SOluble guanylate Cyclase stimulatoR in heArT failurE
patientS with PRESERVED EF (SOCRATES-PRE-
SERVED) study. Eur Heart J 2017;38(15):1119–27.

117. Butler J, Lam CSP, Anstrom KJ, et al. Rationale and
design of the VITALITY-HFpEF trial. Circ Heart Fail
2019;12(5):e005998.

118. Vachiery JL, Delcroix M, Al-Hiti H, et al. Macitentan
in pulmonary hypertension due to left ventricular
dysfunction. Eur Respir J 2018;51(2):1701886.

119. Anand I, McMurray J, Cohn JN, et al. Long-term effects of darusentan on left-ventricular remodelling
and clinical outcomes in the EndothelinA receptor
antagonist trial in heart failure (EARTH): randomised, double-blind, placebo-controlled trial. Lancet 2004;364(9431):347–54.

120. Prasad SK, Dargie HJ, Smith GC, et al. Comparison of the dual receptor endothelin antagonist enrasentan with enalapril in asymptomatic left
ventricular systolic dysfunction: a cardiovascular
magnetic resonance study. Heart 2006;92(6):
798–803.

121. Packer M, McMurray JJV, Krum H, et al. Long-term
effect of endothelin receptor antagonism with bosentan on the morbidity and mortality of patients
with severe chronic heart failure: primary results
of the ENABLE trials. JACC Heart Fail 2017;5(5):
317–26.

122. Packer M, McMurray J, Massie BM, et al. Clinical
effects of endothelin receptor antagonism with bosentan in patients with severe chronic heart failure:
results of a pilot study. J Card Fail 2005;11(1):
12–20.

123. Spieker LE, Noll G, Ruschitzka FT, et al. Endothelin
receptor antagonists in congestive heart failure: a
new therapeutic principle for the future? J Am
Coll Cardiol 2001;37(6):1493–505.

124. Valero-Munoz M, Li S, Wilson RM, et al. Dual
endothelin-a/endothelin-b receptor blockade and

cardiac remodeling in heart failure with preserved ejection fraction. Circ Heart Fail 2016;9(11): e003381.

125. Zile MR, Bourge RC, Redfield MM, et al. Randomized, double-blind, placebo-controlled study of sitaxsentan to improve impaired exercise tolerance in patients with heart failure and a

preserved ejection fraction. JACC Heart Fail 2014;2(2):123–30.

126. Koller B, Steringer-Mascherbauer R, Ebner CH, et al. Pilot study of endothelin receptor blockade in heart failure with diastolic dysfunction and pulmonary hypertension (BADDHY-Trial). Heart Lung Circ 2017;26(5):433–41.

Group 3 Pulmonary Hypertension
A Review of Diagnostics and Clinical Trials

Andrea M. Shioleno, MD[a], Nicole F. Ruopp, MD[b],*

KEYWORDS

- Pulmonary hypertension • Chronic lung disease • Group 3 PH • Interstitial lung disease
- Idiopathic pulmonary fibrosis • Chronic obstructive pulmonary disease
- Combined pulmonary fibrosis and emphysema • CLD-PH

KEY POINTS

- Pulmonary hypertension (PH) is a complication of many forms of chronic lung disease and results in increased mortality.
- Diagnosing group 3 PH can be challenging in the setting of chronic lung disease.
- Pulmonary arterial hypertension–targeted therapies in group 3 PH is controversial, and therapeutic decisions should be made at experienced PH centers where clinical trial enrollment is ongoing.
- Adjunctive therapies such as oxygen therapy when indicated, pulmonary rehabilitation, diuretics, and stabilization of the underlying lung disease remain the cornerstones of treatment.

INTRODUCTION

The World Health Organization (WHO) group 3 pulmonary hypertension (PH) is considered the ultimate sequelae of chronic respiratory disease or chronic hypoxia. Compared with group 1 PH, or pulmonary arterial hypertension (PAH), group 3 PH has a higher disease prevalence, and yet there remain no current Food and Drug Administration (FDA)-approved therapies.

CLASSIFICATION

Group 3 PH is classified as a precapillary form of PH defined on right heart catheterization (RHC) by a mean pulmonary artery pressure (mPAP) greater than 20 mm Hg, pulmonary vascular resistance (PVR) of greater than or equal to 3 Wood units (WU), and pulmonary capillary wedge pressure less than or equal to 15 mm Hg in the setting of underlying lung disease.[1] The most commonly associated lung diseases include chronic obstructive pulmonary disease (COPD), idiopathic interstitial lung diseases (ILD) including connective tissue disease–associated ILD (CTD-ILD), idiopathic pulmonary fibrosis (IPF), and other ILDs, sleep-disordered breathing (obstructive sleep apnea [OSA]), alveolar hypoventilation disorders, chronic hypoxia, and developmental abnormalities of the lung. PH is also found in other ILDs such as sarcoidosis, Langerhans cell histiocytosis, and lymphangioleiomyomatosis; however, these are placed in the WHO group 5 due to their multifactorial causes of pulmonary vascular disease.[1]

Most of the patients with group 3 PH have mild disease defined as an mPAP greater than 20 to 30 mm Hg at rest. However, there is also a subset of patients with more severe PH defined as an mPAP greater than 35 mm Hg or greater than 25 mm Hg and a low cardiac index (CI) defined as less than 2.0 L/min/m² (**Table 1**).[2] Although these represent only a minority of patients with group 3 PH, they have a statistically significant increase in their risk of mortality

a Division of Pulmonary and Critical Care Medicine, University of Miami, 1801 Northwest 9th Avenue, Miami, FL 33136, USA; b Division of Pulmonary, Critical Care, and Sleep Medicine, Tufts Medical Center, 800 Washington Street, #257 (Tupper 3), Boston, MA 02111, USA
* Corresponding author.
E-mail address: nruopp@tuftsmedicalcenter.org

Clin Chest Med 42 (2021) 59–70
https://doi.org/10.1016/j.ccm.2020.11.006
0272-5231/21/© 2020 Elsevier Inc. All rights reserved.

Table 1
Hemodynamic definitions of chronic lung disease–associated pulmonary hypertension

	Cardiopulmonary Hemodynamics (mm Hg and WU)
CLD without PH	mPAP <21 mm Hg or mPAP 21–24 mm Hg with PVR <3 WU
CLD with PH (CLD-PH)	mPAP 21–24 mm Hg with PVR ≥3 WU or mPAP 25–34 mm Hg
CLD with severe PH (CLD-severe PH)	mPAP ≥35 mm Hg or mPAP ≥25 mm Hg with low CI (<2.0 L·min^{-1}·m^{-2})

Abbreviation: CLD, chronic lung disease.

compared with those with mild-moderate disease.[3]

EPIDEMIOLOGY

Our understanding of disease prevalence in group 3 PH has been limited by insensitive screening tools, insufficient studies using RHC data, and recent changes in diagnostic thresholds. Keeping these limitations in mind, retrospective studies have demonstrated an overall 3-year survival of 44% in patients with group 3 PH, with OSA demonstrating the best survival and ILD-PH demonstrating the worst (90% vs 16%, respectively).[4]

Compared with patients with group 1 PH, patients with group 3 PH tend to be older and male predominant, have smaller right ventricles, and have a lower mPAP and PVR.[5] Despite having less severe PH, patients with group 3 PH often have worse baseline functional statuses and an increased risk of death at 3 years, especially in those with PVR greater than 7 WU.[5,6]

DIAGNOSIS

Detecting group 3 PH can be challenging and requires a high diagnostic suspicion, as the presenting symptoms for pulmonary parenchymal and vascular disease are often indistinguishable. In addition, without FDA-approved medications for this cohort of patients with PH, the recommendations for RHC have remained limited, although it is the gold standard for diagnosing group 3 PH. However, there are a variety of noninvasive tools that may point to an underlying diagnosis of PH and prompt further investigation with RHC in the appropriate population.

Standard screening studies for patients with lung diseases can assist with diagnosing underlying PH. These include a low diffusion capacity for carbon monoxide (DLCO) on pulmonary function tests (PFTs), signs of right axis deviation on electrocardiogram, and new exertional hypoxemia or a declining 6-minute walk distance (6MWD) in the setting of otherwise stable lung disease.[7,8] Detecting an enlarged pulmonary artery (PA) diameter compared with the ascending aorta diameter on a screening chest computed tomography (CT) is not only a useful indicator of PH but also predicts higher mortality in IPF and COPD.[9,10] Finally, B-type natriuretic peptide (BNP) may be elevated in group 3 PH; importantly though, it lacks sensitivity and specificity in PH and cannot rule out left-sided heart disease or detect mild PH.[11]

Transthoracic echocardiography (TTE) and cardiopulmonary exercise testing (CPET) are helpful noninvasive diagnostic tools to distinguish PH from other causes of dyspnea and help classify the severity of cardiopulmonary derangement. TTE can be limited in these patients, as poor windows due to lung artifact limit sensitivity and specificity of pulmonary artery systolic pressure measurements.[12] However, more comprehensive examinations assessing the right atrium and right ventricle (RV) as well as RV/left ventricle ratios and tricuspid annular plane systolic excursion can increase sensitivity and predict mortality, although notably do not supersede the need for diagnostic RHC.[13–15] Finally, CPET can further raise suspicion for PH with characteristic findings such as preserved breathing reserve, a reduced oxygen (O$_2$) pulse, low mixed venous O$_2$ saturation, a low CO$_2$/V$_o$2 slope, and no change or a decrease in Pa$_{co}$2 during exercise.[2] Although only available at limited centers, level 3 invasive CPET, which directly measures cardiac hemodynamics during exercise, can not only diagnose PH and discern its severity, but can also determine if a patient's dyspnea is due to a circulatory limitation from PH or a ventilatory limitation from parenchymal lung disease.[2] Level 3 CPET testing may also provide opportunities for earlier detection and treatment targets in group 3 PH in the future.[16]

RHC is required for the diagnosis of PH. Patients undergoing lung transplant evaluation are referred for RHC as standard protocol, but the guidelines for other patients with group 3 PH are less clear. The recent Sixth World Symposium on Pulmonary Hypertension (WSPH) advocates for RHC in 2 major scenarios:

1. Patients with CTD with evidence of PH but only mild lung disease as evidenced by CT chest and PFTs.
2. Patients with group 3 PH with "clinical worsening, progressive exercise limitation and/or gas exchange abnormalities that are not deemed attributable to ventilatory impairment."[2]

Patients with group 3 PH whose PH severity seems disproportionate to their degree of parenchymal or airway disease, especially those patients with CTD-ILD-PH, require careful evaluation of PFTs, RHC hemodynamics, CT imaging, and CPET results to delineate a treatment algorithm that is appropriate based on their specific PH phenotype[2] (**Fig. 1**). In general, it is recommended that these complex, individualized

decisions be made at centers with experience managing PH who are also enrolling patients in clinical trials[2] (**Fig. 2**).

TREATMENT

Treatment options for group 3 PH remain limited, and adjunctive therapies are the mainstay of treatment, including treatment and stabilization of the underlying lung disease. Although O_2 is recommended for patients who are hypoxemic at rest or with exertion, the prospective trial demonstrating the benefit of O_2 in PH are based on COPD data alone, and there are no studies addressing its use in ILD-PH.[17]

Similar to any patient with underlying lung disease, preventative measures are equally important. Pneumococcal and influenza vaccines are recommended for all these patients.[3,18] Pulmonary rehabilitation is also encouraged for those with exercise intolerance, as it improves skeletal muscle function, quality of life, and exercise capacity.[3] Despite in-situ thrombosis being seen in histopathology, anticoagulation for patients with

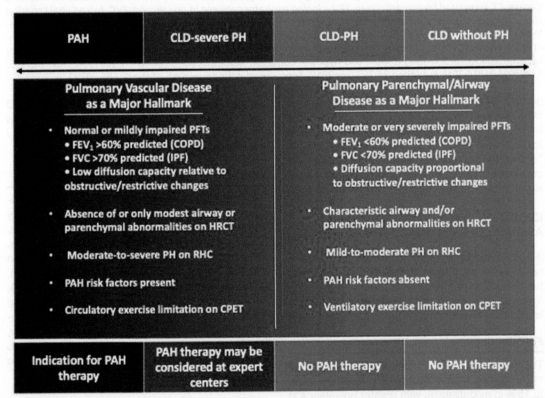

Fig. 1. Pathophysiologic continuum, diagnostic findings, and treatment algorithm of patients with PAH, patients with CLD-severe PH, patients with CLD-PH, and patients with CLD without PH. CLD, chronic lung disease; CPET, cardiopulmonary exercise test; FEV$_1$, forced expiratory volume in one second; FVC, forced vital capacity; HRCT, high-resolution computed tomography scan; PAH, pulmonary arterial hypertension; PH, pulmonary hypertension; RHC, right heart catheterization. (*From* Steven D. Nathan, Joan A. Barbera, Sean P. Gaine, Sergio Harari, Fernando J. Martinez, HorstOlschewski, Karen M. Olsson, Andrew J. Peacock, JoannaPepke-Zaba, Steeve Provencher, Norbert Weissmann, Werner-Seeger. Pulmonary hypertension in chronic lung disease and hypoxia. European Respiratory Journal 53 (1) 1801914; DOI: 10.1183/13993003.01914-2018 Published 24 January 2019; Reproduced with permission of the © ERS 2020.)

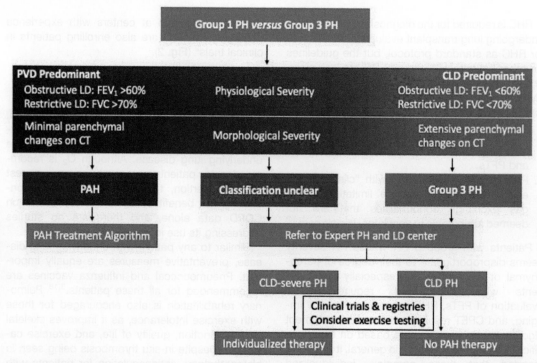

Fig. 2. Clinical classification and management algorithm of group 3 pulmonary hypertension. CLD, chronic lung disease; CT, computed tomography scan; FEV₁, forced expiratory volume in one second; FVC, forced vital capacity; LD, lung disease; PAH, pulmonary arterial hypertension; PVD, pulmonary vascular disease. (*From* Steven D. Nathan, Joan A. Barbera, Sean P. Gaine, Sergio Harari, Fernando J. Martinez, HorstOlschewski, Karen M. Olsson, Andrew J. Peacock, JoannaPepke-Zaba, Steeve Provencher, Norbert Weissmann, WernerSeeger. Pulmonary hypertension in chronic lung disease and hypoxia. European Respiratory Journal 53 (1) 1801914; DOI: 10.1183/13993003.01914-2018 Published 24 January 2019; Reproduced with permission of the © ERS 2020.)

group 3 PH is not recommended unless an alternative indication for anticoagulation exists.[3] For those with signs of RV failure, diuretics are used to maintain euvolemia. Finally, patients with "end-stage" lung disease and PH should be considered for lung transplantation referral at experienced centers.[19]

IDIOPATHIC PULMONARY FIBROSIS–ASSOCIATED PULMONARY HYPERTENSION

IPF is a progressive fibrotic disease of the lungs resulting in shortness of breath, reduced lung function, and progression to death within 3 to 5 years. PH is a frequent complication of IPF and is associated with increased mortality.[20]

Epidemiology

The prevalence of IPF-PH based on a diagnosis of mPAP greater than or equal to 25 ranges from 8% to 15% in mild disease, with greater prevalence in more advanced disease (30%–50%) and end-stage (>60%) disease.[2,20] Reassessment of patients with IPF using the new WSPH diagnostic threshold of mPAP greater than 20 with PVR greater than or equal to 3 WU found a similar

prevalence of around 51% in patients with ILD with advanced disease.[21] Ultimately, a diagnosis of PH in IPF leads to an increased 1-year mortality of 28% compared with 5.5% in IPF alone.[20]

Pathophysiology

The pathophysiology of IPF-PH remains incompletely understood. However, there are some key mediators playing a role in its pathogenesis, including vascular obliteration in areas of fibrosis, and epithelial injury ultimately leading to collagen deposition and vascular remodeling.[22] In addition, fibroblasts produce mediators, such as TGF-β, which stimulate endothelial cell apoptosis and lead to the release of vasoconstrictors (thromboxane A2, angiotensin II, and endothelin). Finally, some endothelial cells develop resistance to apoptosis and are thought to trigger the formation of plexiform lesions.[22]

Treatment

All 4 classes of PH medications have been evaluated in IPF with limited success. Indeed, the RISE IIP and ARTEMIS clinical trials, which evaluated guanylate cyclase stimulators and endothelin receptor antagonists (ERAs), were both stopped early due to a demonstration of harm including increased mortality and disease progression.[23,24] As a result, ERAs and guanylate cyclase stimulators are considered contraindicated in IPF-PH (**Table 2**).

Phosphodiesterase (PDE5) inhibitors showed initial promise with improved DLCO, oxygenation at rest, and dyspnea scores in patients with IPF.[25] However, a subsequent trial with nintedanib, an antifibrotic drug, and sildenafil (PDE5 inhibitor) in patients with IPF failed to show an improvement in dyspnea scores even in patients with RV dysfunction on TTE. Interestingly, an improvement in BNP and a lower risk of FVC decline and death were noted.[23,26] Further complicating the picture, none of these studies used RHC to accurately detect IPF-PH, and thus, PDE5 inhibitor use remains controversial in this population.

Prostacyclin therapies have had varying results in IPF depending on the mode of drug delivery. Intravenous (IV) prostacyclins have been avoided in this group due to worsening hypoxemia from ventilation-perfusion (VQ) mismatch.[27] However, some small studies showed an increase in cardiac output using iloprost or inhaled nitric oxide without exacerbating VQ mismatch.[27,28] Inhaled treprostinil was recently studied retrospectively in patients with COPD-PH and ILD-PH and demonstrated significant improvement in 6MWD and functional class.[29] This set the stage for the recently debuted INCREASE study, which is the largest and most comprehensive randomized controlled trial in group 3 PH including PH-ILD and CPFE to date.[30] This trial compared inhaled treprostinil with placebo, and the preliminary data have reported a significant improvement in 6MWD and NT-proBNP, a decreased risk of clinical worsening, and reduction in exacerbations of underlying lung disease, though more details regarding this specific cohort are pending peer-reviewed publication. Treatment with inhaled treprostinil was also well tolerated making inhaled medications a potentially promising new therapy.[30]

CONNECTIVE TISSUE DISEASE–ASSOCIATED INTERSTITIAL LUNG DISEASE AND PULMONARY HYPERTENSION

Both PH and ILD are common complications of CTD. ILD has been known to occur in rheumatoid arthritis (RA), scleroderma (SSc), systemic lupus erythematosus (SLE), inflammatory myosities, Sjogren disease, and mixed connective tissue disease (MCTD). In addition, group 1 PH can also be a sequelae of CTD, most commonly in patients with SSc. When ILD and PH coexist in this patient population, it can be difficult to ascertain how much of the disease is group 1 PH versus group 3 PH making treatment decisions challenging.

Pathophysiology

It is currently understood that immune and inflammatory mechanisms contribute to the development of pulmonary arterial hypertension (PAH) in patients with CTD.[31] The presence of inflammatory cells such as macrophages and lymphocytes inside plexiform lesions, as well as deposition of antinuclear antibodies, rheumatoid factor, immunoglobulin G, and complement inside pulmonary vessels suggest that autoimmune disease plays a major role in CTD-associated PH regardless of the WHO group classification.[32]

Epidemiology of Connective Tissue Disease–Associated Interstitial Lung Disease Pulmonary Hypertension

Although the prevalence of CTD-ILD-PH is not well characterized among all the autoimmune diseases, SSc-ILD-PH has been the most well studied. PH and ILD are the most common pulmonary manifestations in SSc and also the leading cause of death. The exact prevalence of group 3 PH in SSc is unknown, but some studies estimate 22% of patients with SSc meet criteria.[33] The presence of even mild PH in SSc-ILD results in a 5-fold increased risk of death with a 3-year survival of 39%.[33,34] Interestingly, although MCTD has some overlap with SSc and relatively high estimates of ILD (50%) and PAH (24%), there are no data regarding MCTD-ILD-PH.[35,36]

Inflammatory myosities, which include diseases such as polymyositis and antisynthetase syndrome (anti-SS), are systemic inflammatory diseases of unknown cause associated with varying degrees of muscle, skin, and joint involvement. These disorders have an ILD prevalence ranging from 20% to 78%.[37] Although limited, a screening study in patients with anti-SS found the prevalence of group 3 PH to be 7.9% based on RHC data with a 3-year survival of only 58%.[38] Accordingly, patients with SSc, inflammatory myositis, and MCTD warrant close monitoring for the development of group 3 PH, but further studies are needed to better understand these patients.

Despite the relatively high prevalence of ILD in RA, the incidence of RA-ILD-PH is not known aside from one echocardiogram-based study reporting a range of up to 6%.[39,40] The lower rates

Table 2
Randomized controlled trials of pulmonary arterial hypertension–targeted therapy in idiopathic pulmonary fibrosis–associated pulmonary hypertension

Trial Name First Author, (Reference) Year	Subject # (n)	Study Design	PH Diagnosis	Phenotype (Mean mPAP, CI and Mean FVC, DLCO)	Therapy	Duration	Primary Outcomes
STEP-IPF Zisman et al,[25] 2013	119	RCT	TTE	No RHC data FVC 57%, DLCO 26%	Sildenafil	12 wk	No improvement in 6MWD
BPHIT Corte et al,[79] 2014	60	RCT	RHC	mPAP 37 ± 9.9, CI 2.2 + 0.5%; FVC 55.7 ± 20%; DLCO 45 ± 20%	Bosentan	16 wk	No improvement PVRI
ARTEMIS Raghu et al,[24] 2015	68	RCT	RHC	mPAP 30 ± 8; FVC 67 ± 12% DLCO 39 ± 15%	Ambrisentan	Ended early	No increase in time to death *Stopped early increased harm*
RISE IIP Nathan et al,[23] 2017	147	RCT	RHC	mPAP 33.2 ± 8.2, CI 2.6 + 0.7%; FVC 76.3 ± 19%, DLCO 32 ± 12%	Riociguat	26 wk	No change in 6MWD *Stopped early increased harm*
INSTAGE Kolb et al,[26] 2018	274	RCT	TTE	Any TTE evidence of R heart dysfunction FVC 67.9 ± 19.3%, DLCO 25.8 ± 6.8%	Nintedanib Sildenafil	24 wk	No change in dyspnea score

Abbreviations: FVC, forced vital capacity; PVRI, pulmonary vascular resistance index; RCT, randomized controlled trial.

of PH and ILD in RA, SLE, and Sjogren make group 3 PH in these entities a more rare phenomenon.

Treatment

The current data in CTD-ILD-PH come predominantly from small studies in SSc-ILD-PH. To date, ERAs, PDE5 inhibitors, and prostacyclins have all been evaluated in SSc-PAH and demonstrated safety and clinical benefit ranging from early (exercise-induced) PH to severe disease. It is important to note that patients with mild lung disease were not excluded from these SSc-PAH therapeutic trials.[41–43] However, most of the CTD-ILD-PH–focused clinical trials are small and retrospective. An initial retrospective analysis of patients with SSc-ILD-PH on a variety of therapies (ERAS, PDE5 inhibitors, prostacyclins) showed no benefit and a trend toward worsening oxygenation.[44] However, a subsequent study in SSc-PAH and SSc-ILD-PH showed that an early IV prostacyclin therapy significantly improved transplant-free survival for both groups, suggesting potential benefit with initial aggressive therapy.[45] Patients with CT-ILD-PH were also included in the INCREASE trial, and initial data have demonstrated clinical improvement with inhaled treprostinil but more details regarding this specific cohort are pending peer-reviewed publication.[30]

Given the overlapping pathophysiology in CTD-ILD-PH, it is currently recommended to triage patients based on their severity of ILD and PH. (see **Fig. 1**). CTD-PH-ILD with mild lung disease and more severe PH should be treated as patients with group 1 PAH with pulmonary vasodilators.[2,19] However, patients with severe lung disease and mild PH are thought to be consistent with group 3 PH for which there is no current therapy aside from optimizing underlying ILD management.[2,19]

OTHER INTERSTITIAL LUNG DISEASES ASSOCIATED WITH PULMONARY HYPERTENSION

PH is also found in other ILDs, but our knowledge is limited due to the rarity of these diseases and sparse number of studies. In a study of PH in chronic hypersensitivity pneumonitis, 44% of patients with symptomatic dyspnea were diagnosed with precapillary PH on RHC.[46] Similarly, one study of idiopathic nonspecific interstitial pneumonia (NSIP) showed PH occurred in 31% of patients and resulted in a significantly lower transplant-free survival compared with NSIP alone (17.6 months vs 47.9 months, respectively).[47] There are no data

to support treatment with PAH-targeted therapy in these patients.

CHRONIC OBSTRUCTIVE PULMONARY DISEASE–ASSOCIATED PULMONARY HYPERTENSION

COPD is a progressive disease that comprises both chronic bronchitis and emphysema. The development of COPD-PH is associated with an increased risk of exacerbations and increased mortality.[48,49] Despite this, there exists no disease-modifying therapy and treatment options remain limited.

Epidemiology

In the ASPIRE registry from the United Kingdom and the Geissen registry from Germany, 2 of the largest registries comprising group 3 patients to date, COPD-PH accounts for 39% to 57% of all group 3 PH diagnoses, respectively.[4,50] Survival in COPD-PH is significantly better than ILD-PH (1-, 3-, and 5-year survival of 87.7%, 66.3%, and 54.0% vs 71.9%, 40.3%, and 22.5%, respectively) and seems to correlate with disease severity.[50,51] In those with severe PH (mPAP $\geq$40 mm Hg), 3-year survival was 33% compared with 55% for those with mild-moderate COPD-PH (mPAP <40 mm Hg).[51] This more severe phenotype of COPD-PH, posited to be a "pulmonary vascular phenotype," was not only associated with higher mPAPs, but also higher right atria pressures, lower CI, worsened mixed venous O_2 saturations, and worsened gas exchange despite relatively preserved spirometry and similar degrees of emphysema by imaging.[51,52]

Pathophysiology

PA remodeling has been observed in heavy smokers even in the absence of pulmonary function abnormalities.[53,54] Tobacco smoke and other noxious chemicals over time result in both epithelial and endothelial damage, resulting in vascular, airway, and lung parenchymal damage that may all contribute to elevated PAP.[55,56] Through these mechanisms, progressive airflow obstruction and emphysema ultimately lead to hypoxic pulmonary vasoconstriction and loss of vasculature. Additionally, smoke-induced endothelial damage begets vascular remodeling and decreased elasticity. These, in combination with increased intrathoracic pressure arising from air trapping, further act to raise PAP, ultimately leading to the development of COPD-PH.[52] Notably, increases in RV volume have also been associated with pulmonary arterial pruning and appear to correlate with exercise capacity and mortality in COPD.[57]

Treatment

Despite numerous clinical trials evaluating PAH-specific therapy in COPD-PH, results are largely equivocal and there remains no FDA-approved therapy. Although some therapies, such as sildenafil, have shown improvement in 6MWD and hemodynamics in clinical trials, results remain mixed for PDE5 inhibitors overall as well as ERAs[58–64] (Table 3). Overall, our clinical application of PH therapies is further complicated by the fact that RCTs pooled a wide range of COPD and PH phenotypes without distinguishing between their clinical nuances and responses to therapy. Treating mild COPD with severe PH using PAH-specific therapies is not equivalent to treating severe COPD with mild PH. Finally, the mortality benefit in COPD-PH seen in some retrospective studies has not yet been demonstrated prospectively.[51,65,66]

Importantly, although worsening V/Q mismatch with PH therapy remains a theoretic concern in COPD-PH, worsening hypoxemia has largely not been demonstrated in RCTs.[58–60,62–64] Notably, the only RCT to demonstrate worsening hypoxemia with PAH therapy was an echocardiogram-based study of bosentan (ERA), which was limited in its ability to accurately phenotype the type of PH in affected patients.[61] Of note, inhaled prostacyclins offer theoretic protection against worsening V/Q mismatch, and inhaled treprostinil has shown promise in a small, retrospective study demonstrating improved 6MWD and New York Heart Association functional class.[29]

COMBINED PULMONARY FIBROSIS AND EMPHYSEMA–ASSOCIATED PULMONARY HYPERTENSION

CPFE-PH is a syndrome characterized by upper lobe predominant emphysema and peripheral- and basilar-predominant fibrosis, subnormal spirometry, severe impairment of gas exchange, and a high incidence of PH.[67,68] As a relatively new entity, CPFE-PH is not well represented in most registries and clinical trials, thereby limiting our insight into its prognosis and treatment.

Epidemiology

PH is highly prevalent in CPFE with estimates ranging from 30% to 50% and is associated with smoking.[67,69] In addition, the hemodynamics are often severe at diagnosis with mPAP greater than 35 mm Hg in 68% and herald a significantly poorer prognosis with lower median survival times (25 vs 34 months, respectively) compared with their IPF counterparts without emphysema.[68,69]

Pathophysiology

The pathophysiology of CPFE and CPFE-PH remains largely unknown. Histopathology has noted the simultaneous presence of both emphysema and usual interstitial pneumonia.[68] Tobacco smoke is also suspected in playing a role, given its known association with emphysema and IPF.[68,70]

Treatment

Data for treatment of CPFE-PH are extremely limited, and there is no current evidence to support the use of PAH-targeted therapy in CPFE-PH.

HYPOVENTILATION AND HYPOXIA–ASSOCIATED PULMONARY HYPERTENSION

Although PH can complicate both obstructive sleep apnea (OSA) and obesity hypoventilation syndrome (OHS), the course and severity of each are distinctly unique.

Epidemiology

OSA-PH is rare and often mild.[4] In contrast, OHS-PH occurs more frequently and is associated with more severe PH as well as higher rates of RV failure.[71–74] Although mortality has not been assessed in OHS-PH specifically, patients with OHS are at increased risk of mortality and cardiovascular complications compared with their OSA counterparts.[75] Interestingly, body mass index seems to correlate with mPAP in patients with OHS-PH, whereas noninvasive ventilation (NIV) use inversely correlates with mPAP.[76]

Pathophysiology

The pathophysiology of PH in hypoventilation remains unclear. Although obesity likely plays a role given its correlation to mPAP, other factors such as hypoxic pulmonary vasoconstriction and hypercapnia in these patients may also contribute.[76–78]

Treatment

NIV remains the cornerstone of therapy for OSA-PH and OHS-PH. Indeed, the regular, sustained use of NIV is associated with improved cardiopulmonary hemodynamics and exercise capacity.[72,73] Weight loss, including via gastric bypass, has also been associated with improved cardiopulmonary hemodynamics.[74] There are no data to support the use of PAH-specific therapy in this cohort.[2]

Table 3
Randomized controlled trials of pulmonary arterial hypertension–targeted therapy in chronic pulmonary obstructive disease–associated pulmonary hypertension

Trial Name, First Author, (Reference) Year	Subjects (n)	Study Design	PH Diagnosis	Phenotype (Mean FEV$_1$ and Mean mPAP)	Therapy	Duration	Outcomes
Vonbank et al,[60] 2003	40	RCT (open label)	RHC	Severe COPD (FEV$_1$ 1.09 ± 0.4 L); mild PH (mPAP 27.6 ± 4.4 mm Hg)	"Pulsed" inhalation of nitric oxide with oxygen vs oxygen alone	3 mo	Improved mPAP and PVRI; no worsened hypoxemia
Stolz et al,[61] 2008	30	RCT (2:1)	Echo	Severe COPD (FEV$_1$ 0.92 ± 0.27 L); no PH or mild PH (median estimated sPAP at rest 32 [29–38] mm Hg)	Bosentan, 125 mg, twice daily	12 wk	No change in 6MWD; worsened hypoxemia
Valerio et al,[62] 2009	32	RCT (open label)	RHC	Moderate-severe COPD (FEV$_1$ 37 ± 18%); moderate-severe PH (mPAP 37 ± 5 mm Hg)	Bosentan, 125 mg, twice daily	18 mo	Improved mPAP, PVRI, and 6MWD; no worsened hypoxemia
Rao et al,[58] 2011	33	RCT	Echo	Severe COPD (FEV$_1$ 33 ± 11%); moderate PH (sPAP 52.7 ± 11 mm Hg)	Sildenafil, 20 mg, three times daily	12 wk	Improved 6MWD and sPAP; oxygenation not reported
Blanco et al,[63] 2013	63	RCT	RHC or ECHO	Severe COPD (FEV$_1$ 33 ± 12%); mild PH (mPAP 32 ± 6 mm Hg, n = 9; sPAP 42 ± 10 mm Hg)	Sildenafil, 20 mg, three times daily + PR	3 mo	No change in 6MWD, cycle endurance time; no worsened hypoxemia
Goudie et al,[64] 2014	120	RCT	Echo	Moderate-severe COPD (FEV$_1$ 41 ± 14%); mild PH (RVSP 42 ± 9 mm Hg)	Tadalafil 10 mg daily	12 wk	No change in 6MWD or BNP; no worsened hypoxemia
SPHERIC-1 Vitulo et al,[59] 2016	28	RCT	RHC	Mild-moderate COPD (FEV$_1$ 54 ± 22%); severe PH (mPAP 39 ± 7 mm Hg)	Sildenafil, 20 mg, three times daily	16 wk	Improved PVR, no change 6MWD; no worsened hypoxemia

Abbreviations: FEV$_1$, forced expiratory volume in 1 s; PR, pulmonary rehabilitation; PVRI, pulmonary vascular resistance index; RCT, randomized controlled trial; RVSP, right ventricular systolic pressure; sPAP, systolic pulmonary artery pressure.

SUMMARY

Group 3 PH represents the ultimate sequelae of a diversity of pulmonary diseases. The diagnosis and management of these patients remains complex and controversial owing, in part, to challenges in clinical trial design and phenotyping. As a result, the efficacy of PAH-targeted therapy in group 3 PH remains largely unknown, and thus, patients should be managed predominantly at PH centers where clinical trial enrollment is ongoing and individualized treatment approaches can be undertaken. As clinical trial design continues to evolve and new therapeutic targets emerge, there remains significant opportunity to improve our understanding of this disease.

REFERENCES

1. Simonneau G, Montani D, Celermajer DS, et al. Haemodynamic definitions and updated clinical classification of pulmonary hypertension. Eur Respir J 2019;53(1):1801913.
2. Nathan S, Bar J, Gaine S, et al. Pulmonary hypertension in chronic lung disease and hypoxia. World Symposium on Pulmonary Hypertension. Eur Respir J 2019;53:1801914.
3. Fein D, Zaidi A, Sulica R. Pulmonary hypertension due to common respiratory conditions: classifications, evaluation and management strategies. J Clin Med 2016;5:75.
4. Hurdman J, Condliffe R, Elliot CA, et al. ASPIRE registry: assessing the spectrum of pulmonary hypertension Identified at a referral centre. Eur Respir J 2012;39:945–55.
5. Awerbacha J, Stackhouseb K, Leec J, et al. Outcomes of lung disease-associated pulmonary hypertension and impact of elevated pulmonary vascular resistance. Respir Med 2019;126–30. https://doi.org/10.1016/j.rmed.2019.03.004.
6. Poms AD, Turner M, Farber HW, et al. Comorbid conditions and outcomes in patients with pulmonary arterial hypertension: a REVEAL registry analysis. Chest 2013;144:169–76.
7. Hamada K, Nagai S, Tanaka S, et al. Significance of pulmonary arterial pressure and diffusion capacity of the lung as prognosticator in patients with idiopathic pulmonary fibrosis. Chest 2007;131(3):650–6.
8. Alkukhun L, Wang XF, Ahmed MK, et al. Non-invasive screening for pulmonary hypertension in idiopathic pulmonary fibrosis. Respir Med 2016;117:65–72.
9. Yagi M, Taniguchi H, Kondoh Y, et al. CT-determined pulmonary artery to aorta ratio as a predictor of elevated pulmonary artery pressure and survival in idiopathic pulmonary fibrosis. Respirology 2017;22:1393–9.
10. Wells JM, Washko GR, Han MK, et al. Pulmonary arterial enlargement and acute exacerbations of COPD. N Engl J Med 2012;367:913–21.
11. Leuchte HH, Baumgartner RA, Nounou ME, et al. Brain natriuretic peptide is a prognostic parameter in chronic lung disease. Am J Respir Crit Care Med 2006;173:744–50.
12. Arcasoy SM, Christie JD, Ferrari VA, et al. Echocardiographic assessment of pulmonary hypertension in patients with advanced lung disease. Am J Respir Crit Care Med 2003;167:735–40.
13. Bax S, Bredy C, Kempny A, et al. A stepwise composite echocardiographic score predicts severe pulmonary hypertension in patients with interstitial lung disease. ERJ Open Res 2018;4:00124–2017.
14. Hilde JM, Skjørten I, Grøtta OJ, et al. Right ventricular dysfunction and remodeling in chronic obstructive pulmonary disease without pulmonary hypertension. J Am Collcardiol 2013;62:1103–11.
15. Rivera-Lebron BN, Forfia PR, Kreider M, et al. Echocardio- graphic and hemodynamic predictors of mortality in idio- pathic pulmonary fibrosis. Chest 2013;144:564–70.
16. Oliveira RKF, Waxman AB, Hoover PJ, et al. Pulmonary vascular and right ventricular burden during exercise in interstitial lung disease. Chest 2020;158(1):350–8.
17. Weitzenblum E, Sautegeau A, Ehrhart M, et al. Long-term oxygen therapy can reverse the progression of pulmonary hypertension in patients with chronic obstructive pulmonary disease. Am Rev Respir Dis 1985;131:493–8.
18. Galiè N, Hoeper MM, Humbert M, et al. Guidelines for the diagnosis and treatment of pulmonary hypertension: the Task Force for the diagnosis and treatment of pulmonary hypertension of the European society of cardiology (ESC) and the European respiratory society (ERS), endorsed by the International society of heart and lung transplantation (ISHLT). Eur Heart J 2009;30:2493–537.
19. Thomas C, Anderson R, Condon D. de Jesus Perez V. Diagnosis and management of pulmonary hypertension in the modern Era: Insights from the 6th World Symposium. Pulm Ther 2020 Jun;6(1):9–22.
20. Lettieri CJ, Nathan SD, Barnett SD, et al. Prevalence and outcomes of pulmonary arterial hypertension in advanced idiopathic pulmonary fibrosis. Chest 2006;129:746–52.
21. Ksovreli I, Barnett S, Shlobin O, et al. Categorization of group 3 pulmonary hypertension by the 2018 definition: who is in, who is out? Chest 2019;156(4):A872–3.
22. Farkas L, Gauldie J, Voelkel NF, et al. Pulmonary hypertension and idiopathic pulmonary fibrosis: a tale of angiogenesis, apoptosis, and growth factors. Am J Respir Cell Mol Biol 2011;45(1):1–15.

23. Nathan SD, Behr J, Collard HR, et al. Riociguat for idiopathic interstitial pneumonia-associated pulmonary hypertension (RISE-IIP): a randomised, placebo-controlled phase 2b study. Lancet Respir Med 2019;7(9):780–90.

24. Raghu G, Behr J, Brown KK, et al, ARTEMIS-IPF Investigators. Treatment of idiopathic pulmonary fibrosis with ambrisentan: a parallel, randomized trial. Ann Intern Med 2013;158(9):641–9.

25. Idiopathic Pulmonary Fibrosis Clinical Research Network, Zisman DA, Schwarz M, et al. A controlled trial of sildenafil in advanced idiopathic pulmonary fibrosis. N Engl J Med 2010;363(7):620–8.

26. Kolb M, Raghu G, Wells A, et al, INSTAGE Investigators. Nintedanib plus sildenafil in patients with idiopathic pulmonary fibrosis. N Engl J Med 2018;379:1722–31.

27. Ghofrani HA, Wiedemann R, Rose F, et al. Sildenafil for treatment of lung fibrosis and pulmonary hypertension: a randomised controlled trial. Lancet 2002;360(9337):895–900.

28. Olschewski H, Ghofrani HA, Walmrath D, et al. Inhaled prostacyclin and iloprost in severe pulmonary hypertension secondary to lung fibrosis. Am J Respir Crit Care Med 1999;160(2):600–7.

29. Faria-Urbina M, Oliveira RKF, Agarwal M, et al. Inhaled treprostinil in pulmonary hypertension associated with lung disease. Lung 2018;196(2):139–46.

30. United Therapeutics. Safety and efficacy of inhaled treprostinil in Adult PH with ILD including CPFE. (ClinicalTrials.gov Identifier: NCT02630316). 2015. Available at: https://clinicaltrials.gov/ct2/show/NCT02630316. Accessed October 5, 2020.

31. Dorfmuller P, Perros F, Balabanian K, et al. Inflammation in pulmonary arterial hypertension. Eur Respir J 2003;22:358–63.

32. Yeo PP, Sinniah R. Lupus cor pulmonale with electron microscope and immunofluorescent antibody studies. Ann Rheum Dis 1975;34:457–60.

33. Launay D, Humbert M, Berezne A, et al. Clinical characteristics and survival in systemic sclerosis-related pulmonary hypertension associated with interstitial lung disease. Chest 2011;140:1016–24.

34. Mathai S, Hummers L, Champion H, et al. Survival in pulmonary hypertension associated with the scleroderma spectrum of diseases: impact of interstitial lung disease. Arthritis Rheum 2009;60(2):569–77.

35. Mathai S, Danoff S. Management of interstitial lung disease associated with connective tissue disease. BMJ 2016;352:h6819.

36. Szodoray P, Hajas A, Kardos L, et al. Distinct phenotypes in mixed connective tissue disease: subgroups and survival. Lupus 2012;21(13):1412–22.

37. Shappley C, Paik JJ, Saketkoo LA. Myositis-related interstitial lung diseases: diagnostic features, treatment, and complications. Curr Treatm Opt Rheumatol 2019;5(1):56–83.

38. Hervier B, Meyer A, Dieval C, et al. Pulmonary hypertension in antisynthetase syndrome: prevalence, aetiology and survival. Eur Respir J 2013;42(5):1271–82.

39. Dawson JK, Goodson NG, Graham DR, et al. Raised pulmonary artery pressures measured with Doppler echocardiography in rheumatoid arthritis patients. Rheumatology 2000;39(12):1320–5.

40. Esposito A, Chu S, Madan R, et al. Thoracic manifestations of rheumatoid arthritis. Clin Chest Med 2019;3(40):545–60.

41. Coghlan JG, Galie N, Barbera JA, et al. Initial combination therapy with ambrisentan and tadalafil in connective tissue disease-associated pulmonary arterial hypertension (CTD-PAH): subgroup analysis from the AMBITION trial. Ann Rheum Dis 2017;76:1219–27.

42. Pan Z, Marra AM, Benjamin N, et al. Early treatment with ambrisentan of mildly elevated mean pulmonary arterial pressure associated with systemic sclerosis: a randomized, controlled, double-blind, parallel group study (EDITA study). Arthritis Res Ther 2019;21(1):217.

43. Badesch DB, Tapson VF, McGoon MD, et al. Continuous intravenous epoprostenol for pulmonary hypertension due to the scleroderma spectrum of disease. A randomized, controlled trial. Ann Intern Med 2000;132:425–34.

44. Le Pavec J, Girgis RE, Lechtzin N, et al. Systemic sclerosis-related pulmonary hypertension associated with interstitial lung disease: impact of pulmonary arterial hypertension therapies. Arthritis Rheum 2011;63(8):2456–64.

45. Volkmann ER, Saggar R, Khanna D, et al. Improved transplant-free survival in patients with systemic sclerosis-associated pulmonary hypertension and interstitial lung disease. Arthritis Rheumatol 2014;66:1900–8.

46. Oliveira RK, Pereira CA, Ramos RP, et al. A haemodynamic study of pulmonary hypertension in chronic hypersensitivity pneumonitis. Eur Respir J 2014;44(2):415–24.

47. King CS, Brown AW, Shlobin OA, et al. Prevalence and impact of WHO group 3 pulmonary hypertension in advanced idiopathic nonspecific interstitial pneumonia. Eur Respir J 2018;52:1800545.

48. Kessler R, Faller M, Fourgaut G, et al. Predictive factors of hospitalization for acute exacerbation in a series of 64 patients with chronic obstructive pulmonary disease. Am J Respir Crit Care Med 1999;159:158–64.

49. Oswald-Mammosser M, Weitzenblum E, Quoix E, et al. Prognostic factors in COPD patients receiving long-term oxygen therapy. Importance of pulmonary artery pressure. Chest 1995;107:1193–8.

50. Gall H, Felix JF, Schneck FK, et al. The Giessen pulmonary hypertension registry: survival in pulmonary hypertension subgroups. J Heart Lung Transplant 2017;36:957–67.

51. Hurdman J, Condliffe R, Elliot CA, et al. Pulmonary hypertension in COPD: results from the ASPIRE registry. Eur Respir J 2013;41:1292–301.

52. Kovacs G, Agusti A, Barbera' A, et al. Pulmonary vascular involvement in chronic obstructive pulmonary disease: is there a pulmonary vascular phenotype? Am J Respir Crit Care Med 2018;198:1000–11.

53. Barbera' JA. Mechanisms of development of chronic obstructive pulmonary disease-associated pulmonary hypertension. Pulm Circ 2013;3:160–4.

54. Wright JL, Petty T, Thurlbeck WM. Analysis of the structure of the muscular pulmonary arteries in patients with pulmonary hypertension and COPD: National Institutes of Health nocturnal oxygen therapy trial. Lung 1992;170:109–24.

55. Peinado VI, Barbera JA, Ramirez J, et al. Endothelial dysfunction in pulmonary arteries of patients with mild COPD. Am J Physiol 1998;274:L908–13.

56. Nyunoya T, Mebratu Y, Contreras A, et al. Molecular processes that drive cigarette smoke-induced epithelial cell fate of the lung. Am J Respir Cell Mol Biol 2014;50:471–82.

57. Washko GR, Nardelli P, Ash SY, et al. Arterial vascular pruning, right ventricular size, and clinical outcomes in chronic obstructive pulmonary disease. A longitudinal observational study. Am J Respir Crit Care Med 2019;200:454–61.

58. Rao RS, Singh S, Sharma BS, et al. Sildenafil improves six-minute walk distance in chronic obstructive pulmonary disease: a randomised, double-blind, placebo-controlled trial. Indian J Chest Dis Allied Sci 2011;53:81–5.

59. Vitulo P, Stanziola A, Confalonieri M, et al. Sildenafil in severe pulmonary hypertension associated with chronic obstructive pulmonary disease: a randomized controlled multicenter clinical trial. J Heart Lung Transplant 2017;36:166–74.

60. Vonbank K, Ziesche R, Higenbottam TW, et al. Controlled prospective randomised trial on the effects on pulmonary haemodynamics of the ambulatory long-term use of nitric oxide and oxygen in patients with severe COPD. Thorax 2003;58:289–93.

61. Stolz D, Rasch H, Linka A, et al. A randomized, controlled trial of bosentan in severe COPD. Eur Respir J 2008;32:619–28.

62. Valerio G, Bracciale P, Grazia DA. Effect of bosentan upon pulmonary hypertension in chronic obstructive pulmonary disease. Ther Adv Respir Dis 2009;3:15–21.

63. Blanco I, Santos S, Gea J, et al. Sildenafil to improve respiratory rehabilitation outcomes in COPD: a controlled trial. Eur Respir J 2013;42:982–92.

64. Goudie AR, Lipworth BJ, Hopkinson PJ, et al. Tadalafil in patients with chronic obstructive pulmonary disease: a randomised, double-blind, parallel-group, placebo-controlled trial. Lancet Respir Med 2014;2:293–300.

65. Lange TJ, Baron M, Seiler I, et al. Outcome of patients with severe PH due to lung disease with and without targeted therapy. Cardiovasc Ther 2014;32:202–8.

66. Tanabe N, Taniguchi H, Tsujino I, et al. Multi-institutional retrospective cohort study of patients with severe pulmonary hypertension associated with respiratory diseases. Respirology 2015;20:805–12.

67. Cottin V, Nunes H, Brillet P-Y, et al. Combined pulmonary fibrosis and emphysema: a distinct underrecognised entity. Eur Respir J 2005;26:586–93.

68. Cottin V, Le Pavec J, Prevot G, et al. Pulmonary hypertension in patients with combined pulmonary fibrosis and emphysema syndrome. Eur Respir J 2010;35:105–11.

69. Mejia M, Carrillo G, Rojas-Serrano J, et al. Idiopathic pulmonary fibrosis and emphysema: decreased survival associated with severe pulmonary arterial hypertension. Chest 2009;136:10–5.

70. Baumgartner KB, Samet JM, Stidley CA, et al. Cigarette smoking: a risk factor for idiopathic pulmonary fibrosis. Am J Respir Crit Care Med 1997;155:242–8.

71. Kessler R, Chaouat A, Schinkewitch P, et al. The obesity-hypoventilation syndrome revisited: a prospective study of 34 consecutive cases. Chest 2001;120:369–76.

72. Held M, Walthelm J, Baron S, et al. Functional impact of pulmonary hypertension due to hypoventilation and changes under noninvasive ventilation. Eur Respir J 2014;43:156–65.

73. Castro-Anon O, Golpe R, Perez-de-Llano LA, et al. Haemodynamic effects of non-invasive ventilation in patients with obesity–hypoventilation syndrome. Respirology 2012;17:1269–74.

74. Sugerman HJ, Baron PL, Fairman RP, et al. Hemodynamic dysfunction in obesity hypoventilation syndrome and the effects of treatment with surgically induced weight loss. Ann Surg 1988;207(5):604e13.

75. Castro-Añón O, Pérez de Llano LA, De la Fuente Sánchez S, et al. Obesity-hypoventilation syndrome: increased risk of death over sleep apnea syndrome. PLoS One 2015;10:e0117808.

76. Kauppert CA, Dvorak I, Kollert F, et al. Pulmonary hypertension in obesity- hypoventilation syndrome. Respir Med 2013;107:2061e2070.

77. Chaouat A, Weitzenblum E, Kessler R, et al. Sleep related O2 desaturation and daytime pulmonary hemodynamics in COPD patients with mild hypoxaemia. Eur Respir J 1997;10:1730–5.

78. McGuire M, Bradford A. Chronic intermittent hypercapnic hypoxia increases pulmonary arterial pressure and haematocrit in rats. Eur Respir J 2001;18:279–85.

79. Corte TJ, Keir GJ, Dimopoulos K, et al. Bosentan in pulmonary hypertension associated with fibrotic idiopathic interstitial pneumonia. Am J Respir Crit Care Med 2014;190(2):208–17.

Pulmonary Vascular Diseases Associated with Infectious Disease— Schistosomiasis and Human Immunodeficiency Viruses

Ghazwan Butrous, MB, ChB, PhD

KEYWORDS

- Schistosomiasis • HIV • Infectious diseases • Pulmonary vascular disease
- Pulmonary hypertension • Inflammation

KEY POINTS

- Infectious diseases are a leading cause of pulmo-nary hypertension worldwide.
- Many parasites, are implicated involving various pathological mechanisms.
- Schistosomiasis can induce a inflammatory reaction that contributes to the remodeling of the pulmonary vasculature.
- HIV proteins interfere with several molecular pathways that facilitate significant pulmonary vascular remodeling.

INTRODUCTION

Infection is the major cause of pulmonary hypertension globally.[1] The role of infection in pulmonary vascular diseases (PVDs) is still poorly studied except for some recent works with schistosomiasis and human immunodeficiency virus (HIV), which are discussed in this article.

A wide variety of infectious diseases contribute to the causation of PVD and, consequently, pulmonary hypertension, especially in the developing world. Schistosomiasis is the most common infection that causes pulmonary hypertension worldwide.[2–6] Other helminthic diseases have been implicated, such as *Wuchereria bancrofti* that causes elephantiasis (filariasis)[7,8] and Chinese liver fluke (*Clonorchis sinensis*) in southeast Asia.[9] Hydatid cysts also have been implicated in the development of pulmonary hypertension.[10] Viral infection, mainly HIV, can cause pulmonary hypertension (discussed later). Other viral infections, such as human herpesvirus-8, also induces PVD.[11–13] Fungal infections, like *Paracoccidioides brasiliensis,* which causes paracoccidioidomycosis in Brazil, can cause PVD in both clinical and experimental settings.[14,15] Some bacterial infections, such as *Bordetella pertussis*, may trigger pulmonary hypertension.[16] Tuberculosis has been suspected in the development of PVD but not thoroughly evaluated. Recent cases and communications from Africa and India suggest the potential role of tuberculosis in PVD.[17,18] Furthermore, coexposure and polyparasitism can be issues in developing countries because both HIV and schistosomiasis can be found in the same patients[19] (discussed later).

The study of infection enhances understanding of the complexity of PVD pathophysiology. The infection triggers complicated inflammatory and immunologic reactions. These 2 factors increasingly have been implicated in the pathophysiology of PVD in general.[20,21] Therefore, studying infection helps in understanding of the role of inflammation in PVD in other conditions like the connective tissue

Medway School of Pharmacy, The Universities of Greenwich and Kent at Medway, Anson Building, Central Avenue, Chatham Maritime, Kent ME4 4TB, UK
E-mail address: g.butrous@kent.ac.uk

Clin Chest Med 42 (2021) 71–80
https://doi.org/10.1016/j.ccm.2020.11.007

diseases that are more complex to investigate. Studying infection in PVD might help the development of new pulmonary hypertension therapies. This article concentrates on the most 2 common and most studied infectious diseases that cause PVD, schistosomiasis and HIV.

SCHISTOSOMIASIS

Schistosomiasis (bilharziasis) is caused by infection with blood flukes of the genus *Schistosoma*. It, along with malaria, is one of the most important of all human parasitic diseases. An estimated 240 million people are affected in 78 countries, and close to 800 million are at risk. Africa, in particular sub-Saharan Africa, is the main affected area, with approximately 80% of the infected global population. Eastern Mediterranean, South America, and Western Pacific regions also are affected, but not Europe or North America.[22–24] Thus, the disease is a significant public health concern in the developing world.

There are many species of schistosomiasis.[23,25] *S mansoni* and *S japonicum* primarily infect hepatic tissues. Other species, like *S haematobium*, infect the urinary system. All these species are transmitted to humans by water contact or wet soil, infested with certain freshwater snails, which act as an intermediary for the life cycle of the parasite.[23]

The Pathology of Schistosomiasis

Schistosomiasis is a chronic infection that is recognized after repeated reinfection. In general, the disease disables men and women during their most productive years. It is estimated that it can cause up to 29 million disability-adjusted life years.[26]

The adult worms produce countless eggs during their parasitic life (which can extend up to 40 years inside the human body). The eggs are highly antigenic and are the leading cause of the pathology. The immune system reacts to destroy the eggs by generating granulomatous reactions around the eggs. The granuloma eventually collapses and fibroses.[27] If there are a large number of the eggs, the fibrosis may cause functional changes in the infected organ, for example, liver fibrosis. The hepatic fibrosis in due course causes portal hypertension, which can be life-threatening, especially if esophageal varices develops.[28,29] Portal hypertension also can open collateral vessels to the lung, providing an opportunity for some eggs to find their way to the pulmonary tissues and becoming trapped in the lung's circulation. Like in the liver, the highly antigenic eggs drive an immunologic reaction that leads to the development of pulmonary granuloma[2,30,31] (**Fig. 1**).

Schistosomiasis and its Effect on Pulmonary Vasculature

The granulomas in the lung may be the main cause of subsequent remodeling of pulmonary arterioles,[32,33] which is associated with an inflammatory infiltrate, endothelial cell dysfunction, loss of endothelial barrier integrity, proliferation of endothelial cells and fibroblasts, in situ thrombi, intimal fibrosis, severe medial adventitial hypertrophy, and formation of new endothelial plexiform-like lesions.[34–36] These pathologic features are similar to the pulmonary vascular remodeling reported in pulmonary arterial hypertension.[37–39] Inflammation plays a central role in both the causes and consequences of the pathogenesis of pulmonary hypertension due to schistosomiasis. T cells, B cells, mast cells, macrophages, and dendritic cells, as well as inflammatory cytokines and chemokines, are found in the lungs of patients with pulmonary hypertension, in various parts of the remodeled small pulmonary arteries, and in plexiform lesions[5,20,32,40] (**Fig. 2**).

In the author's laboratory, mice infected with cercariae for 12 weeks showed 79% of the lungs contained evidence of granulomatous changes. Remodeled pulmonary vessels were seen in 46% of the lungs and were observed close to the granulomas, but only 15% or less showed evidence of severe right ventricular hypertrophy.[32] Thus, the more eggs trapped in the lung tissue, probably due to several reinfections, the more granulomas develop, which cause more pulmonary arterioles to be remodeled, culminating in higher pulmonary vascular resistance and eventually increasing the afterload of the right ventricle and facilitating the clinical development of pulmonary hypertension.[2,20,41]

Portal hypertension may contribute to the pathologic changes by opening the collateral vessels that help *Schistosoma* eggs to escape to the lung tissue, which increase the antigen burden in the lung and thus aggravate pulmonary hypertension.[42] Worsening pulmonary hypertension also has been described after the surgical treatment of schistosomiasis-associated portal hypertension with a shunt procedure.[28] Pulmonary hypertension has been seen in 2% to 12% of patients with portal hypertension in general[43] but in 21% of the cases with portal hypertension due to hepatosplenic *S mansoni* infection.[44]

The Prevalence of Pulmonary Hypertension Secondary to Schistosomiasis

The first report of the presence of *Schistosoma* eggs in the lungs of African natives was in 1885,[45] followed by publications from Egypt, Brazil, China, and many countries in Africa. The

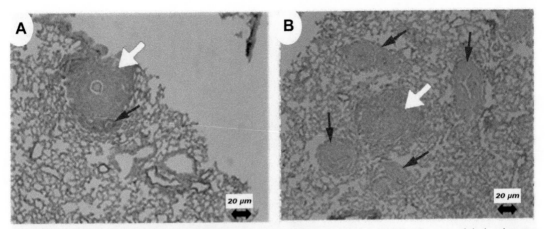

Fig. 1. *Schistosoma* eggs induced granuloma in the lung (*white arrows* in *A* and *B*). The remodeled pulmonary arterioles in the periphery or adjacent to the of the granulomas (*black arrows* in *A* and *B*).

pathologic manifestation of PVD were associated with both S mansoni and S haematobium.[46] In the review of the literature, Ward and colleagues found that the prevalence in the initial reports ranged from 7.7% to 33%.[47] There are no well-controlled epidemiologic studies on the prevalence of pulmonary hypertension secondary to schistosomiasis. Small clinical studies, however, mainly from Brazil, using more carefully controlled methodological studies in patients with hepatosplenic schistosomiasis and liver fibrosis, found that that 7.7% to 10.7% were diagnosed with pulmonary hypertension.[38] The author's experimental observation noticed that pulmonary vascular involvement is common in experimental animals,

but only a small number of animals developed significant pulmonary hypertension[32]; probably, there is a need to have a large number of remodeled vessels resulting from a large burden of eggs that clinically is achieved through continuous reinfections. Thus, PVDs are much more prevalent than clinical manifestations of pulmonary hypertension mainly in the endemic areas.

The Clinical Presentations of Pulmonary Hypertension Secondary to Schistosomiasis

The clinical presentation shows signs and symptoms that are indistinguishable from other forms of pulmonary arterial hypertension. Radiographs may reveal cardiomegaly, in particular, dilatation

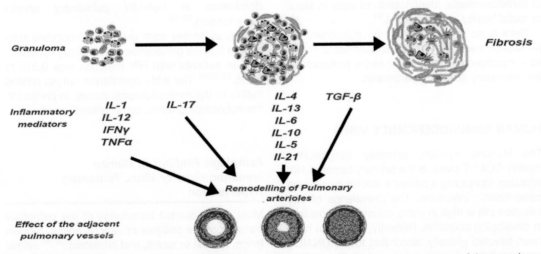

Fig. 2. The upper panel shows the stages of the development of granuloma with the resolution of the granuloma and the development of fibrosis. The inflammatory and immunologic process induced by the granuloma contributes to the remodeling process of the pulmonary arteries. The full description of these processes is beyond the scope of this article and can be found elsewhere.[6] INF, interferon gamma; TNFα, tumour necrosis factor alpha; IL, interleukin; TGFβ, transforming growth factor beta.

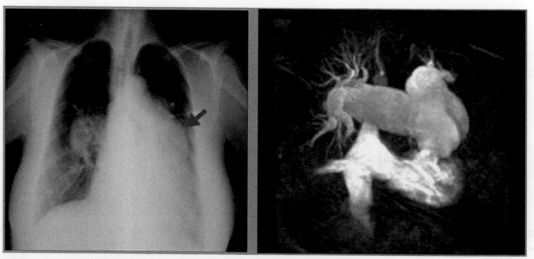

Fig. 3. .A chest radiograph of a 52-year-old man with pulmonary hypertension due to schistosomiasis. The radiographs to the left and right show the dilatation of left and right pulmonary arteries (*arrows*). The right panel shows the characteristic dilation of both main right and left pulmonary artery in patients with schistosomiasis pulmonary hypertension. (Images: courtesy of Dr Angela Bandeira.)

of the right ventricle and right atrium, and enlarged pulmonary trunk and arteries, with the pruning of the distal vasculature. Pulmonary artery enlargement, including giant pulmonary artery aneurysm and dissection, are more pronounced in schistosomiasis pulmonary hypertension than other forms of pulmonary arterial hypertension[48–50] (**Fig. 3**).

Although routine clinical investigation for pulmonary hypertension like right heart catheterization should be performed, schistosomiasis as the cause of pulmonary hypertension should be suspected in endemic areas, especially if prehepatic portal hypertension is present. Previous treatment of schistosomiasis, identification of eggs in stool, or rectal biopsy can be helpful.[51]

There is no specific therapy for pulmonary hypertension secondary to schistosomiasis; therefore, management follows the same protocols as for pulmonary arterial hypertension.

HUMAN IMMUNODEFICIENCY VIRUS

The immune system, primarily lymphocytes (mainly CD4$^+$ T cells), is the primary target of HIV infection, increasing a patient's risk for developing opportunistic infections. The prevalence of HIV infection still is high in many countries, especially in developing countries. Recently, 38 million have been infected globally, according to the UNAIDS program (https://www.unaids.org/en). The highest prevalence is in sub-Saharan Africa, contributing to 20% of the global burden of HIV-infected people.

HIV infection promotes other systemic diseases, mainly cardiovascular diseases. There is a high prevalence of pulmonary hypertension in patients with HIV, suggesting a potential relationship between HIV infection and the pathogenesis of pulmonary arterial hypertension. Kim and Factor, in 1987,[51] reported the first association of HIV with pulmonary hypertension. Many published cases followed, which showed that this association could occur in early and late stages of HIV infection, and that PAH may contribute to a rapid clinical decline in HIV. There also is 'a male predominance, in contrast to the high female predominance in non-HIV pulmonary arterial hypertension.[52–55]

Early estimates from developed countries suggested that the prevalence of pulmonary hypertension in patients with HIV infection was 0.5% to 9.9%.[53,56,57] The wide prevalence ranges related mainly to the methodological issues, in particular, the echocardiographic cutoff criteria.

Pathologic Findings in Human Immunodeficiency Virus, Pulmonary Hypertension

Most of the current knowledge of the pathology came from the analysis of various animal models (mice, rat, cat or rabbit, and primates).[58–60] Intimal and medial hyperplasia, endarteritis obliterans and plexogenic arteriopathy, thrombotic pulmonary arteriopathy, and small vessel perivascular inflammatory reaction are observed in most patients.

Furthermore, veno-occlusive disease also was observed in a few cases.[59]

There is increasing evidence that circulating HIV viral proteins are responsible for pathologic changes in the pulmonary vasculature; however, there is no evidence to date that the HIV virus is localized in lung tissue or interacts directly with the endothelium.[60,61] The main viral proteins that appear to contribute to the insult are the envelope glycoprotein 120 (gp120), transactivator of transcription (Tat) protein, and Nef and other supporting factors like CXCR4[19,62–64] (**Fig. 4**).

The gp120 protein, which is expressed on the surface of the HIV, when exposed to isolated endothelial cells results in the accumulation of hypoxia-inducible factor–1α protein and increases in platelet-derived growth factor (PDGF)-B, both of

which are known to contribute to pulmonary vascular remodeling.[62,65]

The Tat protein enhances HIV virus efficiency by promoting the transcription of all HIV genes, mainly in CD4+ T lymphocytes and macrophages. Tat interacts with the surface of endothelial cells, initiating a signaling cascade that increases the expression of hypoxia-inducible factor–1α, vascular cell adhesion molecule-1, p38 mitogen-activated protein kinase, and nuclear factor κB translocation.[66,67] It also raises the concentration of vascular endothelial growth factor and PDGF,[63] thus contributing to the remodeling of the pulmonary vascular bed.

Nef increasingly is expressed at early stages of the HIV viral life cycle.[64,68] There is increasing evidence that Nef plays a vital role in the

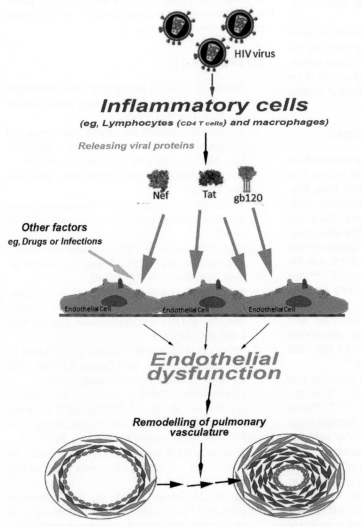

Fig. 4. Schematic presentation of the possible pathogenesis of HIV-associated pulmonary arterial hypertension. The HIV virus releases its protein after attaching the inflammatory and immune cells. These proteins cause endothelial dysfunction, which eventually causes released various mediators that enhance the remodeling of the pulmonary vasculature.

development of severe complex pulmonary vascular lesions and remodeling.[66] It induces pulmonary endothelial cell proliferation as well as apoptosis. In experimental animals infected with the HIV, Nef showed perivascular inflammatory cells, thrombosis, medial hypertrophy, and plexiform lesions.[56,67]

Furthermore, use of illicit intravenous drugs, such as opioids (heroin and morphine), may act as a disease modifier, probably enhancing the pulmonary vascular remodeling.[69–71]

Clinical Features of Human Immunodeficiency Virus–Associated Pulmonary Arterial Hypertension

Like pulmonary hypertension due to schistosomiasis, HIV-associated pulmonary hypertension shows the usual signs and symptoms of pulmonary arterial hypertension with no specific distinguishing features.[53,72] Thus, diagnosis of pulmonary hypertension associated with HIV is by exclusion.[73,74]

The impact on disease progression and outcome of pulmonary hypertension secondary to HIV by the highly effective antiretroviral therapy is still debatable. Current reports suggest opposing effects on pulmonary arterial remodeling.[75–77] Further studies are still needed in this field.

POLYPARASITISM AND COINFECTIONS

Polyparasitism and coinfections are common in many countries, mostly in tropical and subtropical regions of Africa, South America, and Asia. Diseases like HIV, tuberculosis, and schistosomiasis and other parasitic helminths coexist in the same subjects. Coinfection may change the inflammatory and immunologic milieu of the parasite-host interaction. Many patients with HIV infection in Africa had coinfection with schistosomiasis[78–83]; for example, in rural Zimbabwe, 57% of HIV patients were coinfected with S mansoni.[84] Schistosomiases influences the immunologic response and cell-to-cell transmission of HIV. The deworming of schistosomiasis reduced the rate of HIV viral replication and increased CD4+ cells.[85]

Furthermore, among HIV-infected patients, coinfection with schistosomiasis might impair the response to antiretroviral therapy.[84,86] These changes in the inflammatory and immunologic response may modify the effect of HIV or schistosomiasis on the pulmonary vasculature. This needs further investigation because of its clinical importance in the developing world, especially in Africa.[83] The recent experimental evaluation showed that the coinfection of HIV with schistosomiasis may increase the severity of pulmonary hypertension and modify the pathologic changes of pulmonary vascular remodeling.[87]

SUMMARY

Infectious diseases are a leading cause of pulmonary hypertension worldwide, especially in developing countries. Many parasites, such as worms, bacteria, viruses, and fungi, are implicated. They have not been studied thoroughly, and there has been no global epidemiologic evaluation, just estimates and speculation. There are ongoing studies, however, on schistosomiasis and HIV. Schistosomiasis can induce a critical inflammatory reaction that contributes to the remodeling of the pulmonary vasculature. HIV proteins interfere with several molecular pathways that facilitate significant pulmonary vascular remodeling. The study of infectious diseases in pulmonary hypertension helps improve understanding of the complex role of inflammation and the different molecular pathways of the various mechanisms in other etiologies of pulmonary hypertension.

REFERENCES

1. Butrous G, Ghofrani HA, Grimminger F. Pulmonary vascular disease in the developing world. Circulation 2008;118(17):1758–66.
2. Andrade ZA, Andrade SG, others. Pathogenesis of schistosomal pulmonary arteritis. Am J Trop Med Hyg 1970;19(2):305–10. Available at: http://www.cabdirect.org/abstracts/19702902421.html. Accessed July 31, 2015.
3. Butrous G. Pulmonary vascular diseases secondary to schistosomiasis. Adv Pulm Hypertens 2017;15(3):144–8.
4. Graham BB, Kumar R. Schistosomiasis and the pulmonary vasculature (2013 Grover Conference series). Pulm Circ 2014;4(3):353–62.
5. Kolosionek E, Graham BB, Tuder RM, et al. Pulmonary vascular disease associated with parasitic infection—the role of schistosomiasis. Clin Microbiol Infect 2011;17(1):15–24.
6. Butrous G. Schistosome infection and its effect on pulmonary circulation. Glob Cardiol Sci Pract 2019; 2019(1). https://doi.org/10.21542/gcsp.2019.5.
7. Obeyesekere I, Peiris D. Pulmonary hypertension and filariasis. Br Heart J 1974;36(7):676–81. Available at: https://www.ncbi.nlm.nih.gov/pmc/articles/PMC458879/. Accessed November 3, 2018.
8. Walloopillai NJ. Primary pulmonary hypertension, an unexplained epidemic in Sri Lanka. Pathobiology 1975;43(2–3):248–50.
9. Lai KS, McFadzean AJ, Yeung R. Microembolic pulmonary hypertension in pyogenic cholangitis. Br Med J 1968;1(5583):22–4. Available at: https://www.

ncbi.nlm.nih.gov/pmc/articles/PMC1984939/. Accessed November 3, 2018.

10. Buz S, Knosalla C, Mulahasanovic S, et al. Severe chronic pulmonary hypertension caused by pulmonary embolism of hydatid cysts. Ann Thorac Surg 2007;84(6):2108–10.

11. Cool CD, Rai PR, Yeager ME, et al. Expression of human herpesvirus 8 in primary pulmonary hypertension. N Engl J Med 2003;349(12):1113–22.

12. Hsue PY, Deeks SG, Farah HH, et al. Role of HIV and human herpesvirus-8 infection in pulmonary arterial hypertension. AIDS 2008;22(7):825–33.

13. Katano H, Hogaboam CM. Herpesvirus-associated pulmonary hypertension? Am J Respir Crit Care Med 2005;172(12):1485–6.

14. Batah S, dos Santos Leao P, Veronez J, et al. Pulmonary hypertension due to the human paracoccidioidomycosis. In: B108. Pulmonary hypertension: the latest findings. American thoracic society international conference abstracts. American Thoracic Society, San Diego, CA, 2018. p. A4378. https://doi.org/10.1164/ajrccm-conference.2018.197.1_MeetingAbstracts.A4378.

15. Leao P, Setembre Batah S, dos Santos A L, et al. Paracoccidioidomycosis-induced pulmonary hypertension. In: B108. Pulmonary hypertension: the latest findings. American thoracic society international conference abstracts. American Thoracic Society, San Diego, CA, 2018. p. A4376. https://doi.org/10.1164/ajrccm-conference.2018.197.1_MeetingAbstracts.A4376.

16. Peters MJ, Pierce CM, Klein NJ. Mechanisms of pulmonary hypertension in Bordetella pertussis. Arch Dis Child 2003;88(1):92–3.

17. Ahmed AEH, Ibrahim AS, Elshafie SM. Pulmonary hypertension in patients with treated pulmonary tuberculosis: analysis of 14 consecutive cases. Clin Med Insights Circ Respir Pulm Med 2011;5:1. Available at: http://www.ncbi.nlm.nih.gov/pmc/articles/PMC3040077/. Accessed July 6, 2012.

18. Bhattacharyya P, Saha D, Bhattacherjee PD, et al. Tuberculosis associated pulmonary hypertension: the revelation of a clinical observation. Lung India 2016;33(2):135–9.

19. Butrous G. Human immunodeficiency virus–associated pulmonary arterial hypertension considerations for pulmonary vascular diseases in the developing world. Circulation 2015;131(15):1361–70.

20. Kumar R, Graham B. How does inflammation contribute to pulmonary hypertension? Eur Respir J 2018;51(1):1702403.

21. Rabinovitch M, Guignabert C, Humbert M, et al. Inflammation and immunity in the pathogenesis of pulmonary arterial hypertension. Circ Res 2014;115(1):165–75.

22. Ciddio M, Mari L, Gatto M, et al. The temporal patterns of disease severity and prevalence in schistosomiasis. Chaos 2015;25(3):036405.

23. Colley DG, Bustinduy AL, Secor WE, et al. Human schistosomiasis. Lancet 2014;383(9936):2253–64.

24. Chitsulo L, Engels D, Montresor A, et al. The global status of schistosomiasis and its control. Acta Trop 2000;77(1):41–51.

25. Barsoum RS, Esmat G, El-Baz T. Human schistosomiasis: clinical perspective. J Adv Res 2013. https://doi.org/10.1016/j.jare.2013.01.005.

26. van der Werf MJ, de Vlas SJ, Brooker S, et al. Quantification of clinical morbidity associated with schistosome infection in sub-Saharan Africa. Acta Trop 2003; 86(2):125–39. Available at: http://www.sciencedirect.com/science/article/pii/S0001706X03000299.

27. Andrade Cheever AW, Cheever AW, Cheever AW. Characterization of the murine model of schistosomal hepatic periportal fibrosis. Int J Exp Pathol 1993;74(2):195–202.

28. De Cleva R, Pugliese V, Zilberstein B, et al. Systemic hemodynamic changes in mansonic schistosomiasis with portal hypertension treated by azygoportal disconnection and splenectomy. Am J Gastroenterol 1999;94(6):1632–7. Available at: http://www.nature.com/ajg/journal/v94/n6/abs/ajg1999380a.html. Accessed June 21, 2017.

29. Lichtenberg F von. Portal hypertension and schistosomiasis*. Ann N Y Acad Sci 1970;170(1):100–14.

30. Doenhoff MJ, Hassounah O, Murare H, et al. The schistosome egg granuloma: immunopathology in the cause of host protection or parasite survival? Trans R Soc Trop Med Hyg 1986;80(4):503–14.

31. Hams E, Aviello G, Fallon PG. The schistosoma granuloma: friend or foe? Front Immunol 2013;4. https://doi.org/10.3389/fimmu.2013.00089.

32. Kolosionek E, King J, Rollinson D, et al. Schistosomiasis causes remodeling of pulmonary vessels in the lung in a heterogeneous localized manner: detailed study. Pulm Circ 2013;3(2):356–62.

33. Kolosionek EJ, King J, Rollinson D, et al. Vascular changes in the schistosoma mansoni model of pulmonary vascular diseases. In: B61. Pulmonary hypertension: experimental models I. Denver, Colorado: American Thoracic Society; 2011. p. A3405.

34. Almeida AZA, Andrade ZA, Andrade ZA. Effect of chemotherapy on experimental pulmonary schistosomiasis. Am J Trop Med Hyg 1983;32(5):1049–54.

35. Warren. Experimental pulmonary schistosomiasis. Trans R Soc Trop Med Hyg 1964;58:228–33.

36. Crosby A, Jones FM, Kolosionek E, et al. Praziquantel reverses pulmonary hypertension and vascular remodeling in murine schistosomiasis. Am J Respir Crit Care Med 2011;184(4):467–73. Available at: http://

cat.inist.fr/?aModele=afficheN&cpsidt=24441614. Accessed April 15, 2013.

37. Lapa M, Dias B, Jardim C, et al. Cardiopulmonary manifestations of hepatosplenic schistosomiasis. Circulation 2009;119(11):1518–23.

38. Lapa MS, Ferreira EVM, Jardim C, et al. Clinical characteristics of pulmonary hypertension patients in two reference centers in the city of Sao Paulo. Rev Assoc Med Bras 2006;52(3):139–43. Available at: http://www.scielo.br/scielo.php?pid=S0104-42302006000300012&script=sci_arttext&tlng=es. Accessed January 15, 2017.

39. Graham B, Bandeira A, Butrous G, et al. Significant intrapulmonary Schistosoma egg antigens are not present in schistosomiasis-associated pulmonary hypertension. Pulm Circ 2011;1(4):456.

40. Ali Z, Kosanovic D, Kolosionek E, et al. Enhanced inflammatory cell profiles in schistosomiasis-induced pulmonary vascular remodeling. Pulm Circ 2017; 7(1):244–52.

41. Cheever Andrade ZA, Andrade ZA, Andrade ZA. Pathological lesions associated with Schistosoma mansoni infection in man. Trans R Soc Trop Med Hyg 1967;61(5):626–39.

42. Lambertucci JR, Serufo JC, Gerspacher-Lara R, et al. Schistosoma mansoni: assessment of morbidity before and after control. Acta Trop 2000; 77(1):101–9.

43. Donovan CL, Marcovitz PA, Punch JD, et al. Two-dimensional and dobutamine stress echocardiography in the preoperative assessment of patients with end-stage liver disease prior to orthotopic liver transplantation. Transplantation 1996;61(8):1180–8. Available at: http://journals.lww.com/transplantjournal/Abstract/1996/04270/TWO_DIMENSIONAL_AND_DOBUTAMINE_STRESS.11.aspx.

44. de Cleva R, Herman P, Pugliese V, et al. Prevalence of pulmonary hypertension in patients with hepatosplenic Mansonic schistosomiasis–prospective study. Hepatogastroenterology 2002;50(54): 2028–30. Available at: http://europepmc.org/abstract/med/14696458.

45. Belleli V. Les oeufs de Bilharzia haematobia dans les poumons. Unione Á Med Áegiz Á1 1885;22–3.

46. Shaw A, Ghareeb AA, et al, Ghareeb AA. The pathogenesis of pulmonary schistosomiasis in Egypt with special reference to Ayerza's dis-ease. J Pathol Bacteriol 1938;46(3):401–24.

47. Ward T, Fenwick A, Butrous G. The prevalence of pulmonary hypertension in schistosomiasis: A systematic review. PVRI Review; Mumbai 2011;3(1): 12–21.

48. Santarém OL de A, Cleva R de, Sasaya FM, et al. Left ventricular dilation and pulmonary vasodilation after surgical shunt for treatment of presinusoidal portal hypertension. PLoS One 2016; 11(4):e0154011.

49. Gavilanes F, Piloto B, Fernandes CJC. Giant pulmonary artery aneurysm in a patient with schistosomiasis-associated pulmonary arterial hypertension. J Bras Pneumol 2018;44(2):167.

50. Corrêa R de A, Silva LC, dos S, et al. Pulmonary hypertension and pulmonary artery dissection. J Bras Pneumol 2013;39(2):238–41.

51. Kim KK, Factor SM. Membranoproliferative glomerulonephritis and plexogenic pulmonary arteriopathy in a homosexual man with acquired immunodeficiency syndrome. Hum Pathol 1987; 18(12):1293–6.

52. Himelman RB, Dohrmann M, Goodman P, et al. Severe pulmonary hypertension and cor pulmonale in the acquired immunodeficiency syndrome. Am J Cardiol 1989;64(19):1396–9.

53. Speich R, Jenni R, Opravil M, et al. Primary pulmonary hypertension in HIV infection. Chest 1991; 100(5):1268–71.

54. Duchesne N, Gagnon JA, Fouquette B, et al. Primary pulmonary hypertension associated with HIV infection. Can Assoc Radiol J 1993;44(1):39–41.

55. Krishnan U, Horn EM. Pulmonary arterial hypertension in HIV. In: Myerson M, Glesby MJ, editors. Cardiovascular care in patients with HIV. Springer International Publishing; 2019. p. 159–70. https://doi.org/10.1007/978-3-030-10451-1_12.

56. Mette SA, Palevsky HI, Pietra GG, et al. Primary pulmonary hypertension in association with human immunodeficiency virus infection: a possible viral etiology for some forms of hypertensive pulmonary arteriopathy. Am Rev Respir Dis 1992;145(5): 1196–200.

57. Sitbon O, Lascoux-Combe C, Delfraissy J-F, et al. Prevalence of HIV-related pulmonary arterial hypertension in the current antiretroviral therapy era. Am J Respir Crit Care Med 2008;177(1):108–13.

58. Hatziioannou T, Evans DT. Animal models for HIV/AIDS research. Nat Rev Microbiol 2012;10(12): 852–67.

59. Ruchelli E, Nojadera G, Rutstein R, et al. Pulmonary veno-occlusive disease. Another vascular disorder associated with human immunodeficiency virus infection? Arch Pathol Lab Med 1994;118(6):664–6. Available at: http://europepmc.org/abstract/MED/8204018/reload=0. Accessed April 23, 2014.

60. Letvin NL, King NW. Immunologic and pathologic manifestations of the infection of rhesus monkeys with simian immunodeficiency virus of macaques. J Acquir Immune Defic Syndr 1990;3:1023–40.

61. Chalifoux L, Simon M, Pauley D, et al. Arteriopathy in macaques infected with simian immunodeficiency virus. Lab Invest 1992;67(3):338–49. Available at: http://europepmc.org/abstract/MED/1405492. Accessed April 23, 2014.

62. O'Brien-Ladner A, Dhillon NK, Mermis J. HIV-associated viral proteins induce parallel hypoxia-

inducible factor-1Alpha and platelet derived growth factor accumulation. Am J Respir Crit Care Med 2011;183:A5014. Available at: http://www.atsjournals.org/doi/pdf/10.1164/ajrccm-conference.2011.183.1_MeetingAbstracts.A5014. Accessed May 11, 2014.

63. Humbert M, Monti G, Fartoukh M, et al. Platelet-derived growth factor expression in primary pulmonary hypertension: comparison of HIV seropositive and HIV seronegative patients. Eur Respir J 1998; 11(3):554–9. Available at: http://erj.ersjournals.com/content/11/3/554. Accessed April 26, 2014.

64. Foster JL, Garcia JV. HIV-1 Nef: at the crossroads. Retrovirology 2008;5(1):84. Available at: http://www.biomedcentral.com/1742-4690/5/84. Accessed May 8, 2014.

65. Porter KM, Walp ER, Elms SC, et al. Human immunodeficiency virus-1 transgene expression increases pulmonary vascular resistance and exacerbates hypoxia-induced pulmonary hypertension development. Pulm Circ 2013;3(1):58–67.

66. Almodovar S, Knight R, Allshouse AA, et al. Human immunodeficiency virus *nef* signature sequences are associated with pulmonary hypertension. AIDS Res Hum Retroviruses 2012;28(6):607–18.

67. Marecki JC, Cool CD, Parr JE, et al. HIV-1 Nef is associated with complex pulmonary vascular lesions in SHIV- nef –infected macaques. Am J Respir Crit Care Med 2006;174(4):437–45.

68. O'Neill E, Kuo LS, Krisko JF, et al. Dynamic evolution of the human immunodeficiency virus type 1 pathogenic factor, Nef. J Virol 2006;80(3):1311–20. Available at: http://jvi.asm.org/content/80/3/1311.short. Accessed May 8, 2014.

69. Dhillon NK, Li F, Xue B, et al. Effect of cocaine on human immunodeficiency virus–mediated pulmonary endothelial and smooth muscle dysfunction. Am J Respir Cell Mol Biol 2011;45(1):40–52.

70. Spikes L, Dalvi P, Tawfik O, et al. Enhanced pulmonary arteriopathy in simian immunodeficiency virus–infected macaques exposed to morphine. Am J Respir Crit Care Med 2012;185(11):1235–43.

71. Spikes L, Gu H, Dalvi P, et al. Alterations in apoptosis and proliferation of endothelial cells on exposure to HIV-tat and morphine: implications for HIV-PAH. Am J Respir Crit Care Med 305:A3408. Available at: http://www.atsjournals.org/doi/abs/10.1164/ajrccm-conference.2012.185.1_MeetingAbstracts.A3408. Accessed May 12, 2014.

72. Coplan NL, Shimony RY, Ioachim HL, et al. Primary pulmonary hypertension associated with human immunodeficiency viral infection. Am J Med 1990; 89(1):96–9.

73. Vazquez ZGS, Klinger JR. Guidelines for the treatment of pulmonary arterial hypertension. Lung 2020;198(4):581–96.

74. Galiè N, Humbert M, Vachiery J-L, et al. 2015 ESC/ERS Guidelines for the diagnosis and treatment of pulmonary hypertension: the joint task force for the diagnosis and treatment of pulmonary hypertension of the European society of cardiology (ESC) and the European respiratory society (ERS)Endorsed by: association for European Paediatric and Congenital Cardiology (AEPC), international society for heart and lung transplantation (ISHLT). Eur Respir J 2015;46(4):903–75.

75. Opravil M, Sereni D. Natural history of HIV-associated pulmonary arterial hypertension: trends in the HAART era. AIDS 2008;22:S35–40. Available at: http://journals.lww.com/aidsonline/Abstract/2008/09003/Natural_history_of_HIV_associated_pulmonary.6.aspx. Accessed May 16, 2014.

76. Mondy KE, Gottdiener J, Overton ET, et al. High prevalence of echocardiographic abnormalities among HIV-infected persons in the era of highly active antiretroviral therapy. Clin Infect Dis 2011; 52(3):378–86.

77. Pugliese A, Isnardi D, Saini A, et al. Impact of highly active antiretroviral therapy in HIV-positive patients with cardiac involvement. J Infect 2000;40(3):282–4.

78. Hotez PJ, Harrison W, Fenwick A, et al. Female genital schistosomiasis and HIV/AIDS: reversing the neglect of girls and women. PLoS Negl Trop Dis 2019;13(4):e0007025.

79. Mbabazi PS, Andan O, Fitzgerald DW, et al. Examining the relationship between urogenital schistosomiasis and HIV infection. PLoS Negl Trop Dis 2011; 5(12):e1396.

80. Downs JA, Dupnik KM, Dam GJ van, et al. Effects of schistosomiasis on susceptibility to HIV-1 infection and HIV-1 viral load at HIV-1 seroconversion: a nested case-control study. PLoS Negl Trop Dis 2017;11(9):e0005968.

81. Masikini P, Colombe S, Marti A, et al. Schistosomiasis and HIV-1 viral load in HIV-infected outpatients with immunological failure in Tanzania: a case-control study. BMC Infect Dis 2019;19(1):249.

82. Colombe S, Machemba R, Mtenga B, et al. Impact of schistosome infection on long-term HIV/AIDS outcomes. PLoS Negl Trop Dis 2018;12(7):e0006613.

83. Bustinduy A, King C, Scott J, et al. HIV and schistosomiasis co-infection in African children. Lancet Infect Dis 2014. https://doi.org/10.1016/S1473-3099(14)70001-5.

84. Mazigo HD, Nuwaha F, Wilson S, et al. Epidemiology and interactions of human immunodeficiency virus-1 and schistosoma mansoni in sub-saharan Africa. Infect Dis Poverty 2013;2(1):2–11. Available at: http://www.biomedcentral.com/content/pdf/2049-9957-2-2.pdf. Accessed May 19, 2014.

85. Kallestrup P, Zinyama R, Gomo E, et al. Schistosomiasis and HIV-1 infection in rural Zimbabwe: effect of treatment of schistosomiasis on CD4 Cell Count and

Plasma HIV-1 RNA Load. J Infect Dis 2005;192(11):1956–61.

86. Efraim L, Peck RN, Kalluvya SE, et al. Schistosomiasis and impaired response to antiretroviral therapy among HIV-infected patients in Tanzania. J Acquir Immune Defic Syndr 2013;62(5):e153–6.

87. Morales Cano D, Mondejar Parreño G, Medrano Garcia S, et al. Effects of schistosoma mansoni and HIV-1 co-exposure on pulmonary vascular pathology. In: B108. Under pressure: the role of cellular stress in pulmonary vascular remodeling. American Thoracic Society International Conference Abstracts. American Thoracic Society; Dallas, TX, 2019. p. A4204. https://doi.org/10.1164/ajrccm-conference.2019.199.1_MeetingAbstracts.A4204.

Chronic Thromboembolic Disease and Chronic Thromboembolic Pulmonary Hypertension

Irene M. Lang, MD*, Ioana A. Campean, MD, Roela Sadushi-Kolici, MD,
Roza Badr-Eslam, MD, Christian Gerges, MD, PhD, Nika Skoro-Sajer, MD

KEYWORDS

- Chronic thromboembolic pulmonary hypertension
- Chronic thromboembolic pulmonary vascular disease • Venous thromboembolism
- Acute pulmonary embolism

KEY POINTS

- Chronic thromboembolic pulmonary hypertension (CTEPH) occurs in roughly 50 patients per million.
- CTEPH is a manifestation of inflammatory thrombosis.
- CTEPH/CTED are likely to be the consequence of failure to resolve thrombotic vascular obstruction in the pulmonary arteries.
- Treatments of CTEPH/CTED are based on mechanical interventions (PEA and BPA) and are assisted by drugs that are approved for PAH.
- Patients who are suitable for mechanical treatments have a far better outcome compared with those on medical treatments.

INTRODUCTION AND DEFINITIONS

Chronic thromboembolic pulmonary hypertension (CTEPH) is a progressive pulmonary vascular disease characterized by chronic obstruction of major pulmonary arteries with flow-limiting organized thrombi. In the clinical classification of the 6th World Symposium on Pulmonary Hypertension, CTEPH/ chronic thromboembolic pulmonary disease (CTED) are in group 4, labeled as *PH due to pulmonary artery obstruction* (**Table 1**).[1]

The diagnosis of CTEPH is based on findings obtained after at least 3 months of effective anticoagulation to discriminate this condition from "subacute" pulmonary embolism (PE). These findings are a mean pulmonary artery pressure (mPAP) $\geq$25 mm Hg, with pulmonary artery wedge pressure $\leq$15 mm Hg; and specific vascular lesions

by multidetector computed tomography (CT) angiography, MRI, or conventional pulmonary cineangiography, such as ringlike stenoses, webs/slits, and chronic total occlusions (pouch lesions, or tapered lesions) leading to segmental perfusion defects. CTED carries vascular lesions identical to CTEPH[2] (**Fig. 1**), but lacks pulmonary hypertensive hemodynamics at rest (**Table 2**). The 6th World Symposium on Pulmonary Hypertension Task Force on pulmonary hypertension (PH) diagnosis and classification[1] has put forward a new threshold for PH (mPAP >20 mm Hg) and for precapillary PH (combination of mPAP >20 mm Hg, pulmonary arterial wedge pressure $\leq$15 mm Hg, and pulmonary vascular resistance [PVR] $\geq$3 Wood Units). Potential consequences of these new thresholds for the management of CTEPH and CTED, respectively, are not yet established;

Department of Internal Medicine II, Division of Cardiology, Medical University of Vienna, Währinger Gürtel 18-20, Vienna 1090, Austria
* Corresponding author.
E-mail address: irene.lang@meduniwien.ac.at

Clin Chest Med 42 (2021) 81–90
https://doi.org/10.1016/j.ccm.2020.11.014
0272-5231/21/© 2020 The Authors. Published by Elsevier Inc. This is an open access article under the CC BY-NC-ND license (http://creativecommons.org/licenses/by-nc-nd/4.0/).

chestmed.theclinics.com

Table 1
World Health Organization group 4: pulmonary hypertension due to pulmonary artery obstructions

Group	Description
Group 4	Pulmonary hypertension due to pulmonary artery obstructions
	4.1. Chronic thromboembolic pulmonary hypertension (CTEPH)
	4.2. Other pulmonary artery obstructions
	4.2.1. Sarcoma or angiosarcoma
	4.2.2. Other malignant tumors Renal, uterine, germ cell tumors of the testis, others
	4.2.3. Nonmalignant tumors Uterine leiomyoma
	4.2.4. Arteritis without connective tissue disease
	4.2.5. Congenital pulmonary artery stenoses
	4.2.6. Parasites Hydatidosis

however, it has been demonstrated that elevated mPAP is correlated with poorer survival in thromboembolic disease,[3] and that borderline PAP is associated with increased mortality compared with normal PAP.[4,5]

EPIDEMIOLOGY AND NATURAL HISTORY

Single case reports and epidemiologic observations[6] suggest that CTEPH/CTED are consequences of venous thromboembolism. CTEPH has been reported with a cumulative incidence between 0.1% and 9.1% within the first 2 years after a symptomatic PE event,[6] with a recent meta-analysis suggesting that the incidence of CTEPH in survivors of acute pulmonary embolism is approximately 3%.[7] The large margin of error is due to referral bias, paucity of early symptoms, and the difficulty to differentiate acute PE from symptoms of preexisting CTEPH. Although the exact prevalence and annual incidence of CTEPH are unknown, some data suggest that this condition may occur in approximately 5 individuals per million population per year,[8] and may affect 43 to 50 cases per million people in Europe.[9]

It remains unclear whether CTEPH/CTED is the direct sequelae of acute PE because data suggest that CTEPH cases diagnosed early after symptomatic acute PE appear to be preexisting CTEPH cases that were misdiagnosed as acute PE.[10] Furthermore, a proportion of 40% to 60% of CTEPH cases lack an acute PE history.[11] In the new guidelines on the diagnosis and management of acute PE,[12] a separate chapter is dedicated to long-term sequelae of PE. Recent research has identified recurrent venous thromboembolism (VTE), post-thrombotic syndrome, bleeding, and functional limitations as important outcome measures of acute PE treatment.[13–18] Dyspnea, anxiety, chest pain, post-thrombotic panic syndrome, and depression[18–21] that lead to persistent functional limitations and/or decreased quality of life have been labeled as post-PE syndrome (PPS).[15] PPS includes

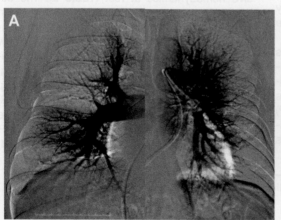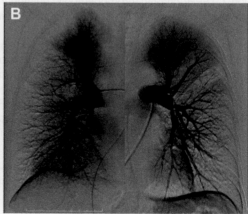

Fig. 1. Case examples of pulmonary angiograms (*A* and *B*) of patients with CTEPH and CTED. (*A*) A 74-year old male patient with CTEPH; mPAP was 38 mm Hg. (*B*) A 54-year-old female patient with CTED; mPAP was 21 mm Hg.

Table 2
CTEPH and CTED clinical characteristics

Diagnostic Criteria	CTEPH	CTED
Symptoms	Exercise and resting dyspnea	Exercise dyspnea, or no symptoms
RHC	mPAP ≥25 mm Hg, PAWP ≤15	mPAP <25 mm Hg (usually 21–24), PAWP ≤15
RHC at exercise	—	Pressure-flow slope >3 mm Hg/L/min
V/Q scan	Mismatched perfusion defects	Mismatched perfusion defects
Angiography (CTPA or DSA)	Ringlike stenoses, webs/slits, and chronic total occlusions (pouch lesions, or tapered lesions)	Ringlike stenoses, webs/slits, and chronic total occlusions (pouch lesions, or tapered lesions)
CPET	—	mPAP/CO slope >1 (correlated with dead-space ventilation) and ventilatory equivalents for carbon dioxide slope >20[75]
TTE	Normal or enlarged RV and RA	Usually normal RV and (mildly enlarged) RA
Anticoagulation before diagnosis	At least 3 mo	At least 3 mo

Abbreviations: CO, cardiac output; CPET, cardio pulmonary exercise test; CTED, chronic thromboembolic pulmonary disease; CTEPH, chronic thromboembolic pulmonary hypertension; CTPA, computed tomography pulmonary angiography; DSA, digital subtraction angiography; mPAP, mean pulmonary artery pressure; PAWP, pulmonary artery wedge pressure; RA, right atrium; RHC, right heart catherization; RV, right ventricle; TTE, transthoracic echocardiography; V/Q, ventilation/perfusion.

CTEPH/CTED, deconditioning, and all other functional limitations after acute PE.[15,22] PPS is common and is observed in up to 40% to 60% of PE survivors, whereas CTEPH remains rare with an incidence of 2% to 3% in PE survivors.[23] A similar proportion of CTEPH (4%) presents as CTED.[2]

PATHOPHYSIOLOGY

One of the limitations of CTEPH research is the difficulty to reproduce the disease in animal models.[24] Repeated thrombo-emboli resolve quickly,[25] both in the canine[26] and in the porcine models,[24,27] without leading to chronic PH. In humans, imaging data suggest that in contrast to animal models, resolution takes at least 3 months and remains incomplete in many patients (**Table 3**). These data suggest that there may be a spectrum of thromboembolic disease, including CTEPH and CTED, representing different magnitudes of thromboembolic obstructions that are based on the same basic pathophysiological mechanisms. Unilateral pulmonary artery obstruction represents a particular subset of CTEPH/CTED.

The hallmark of CTEPH/CTED is fibrotic transformation of pulmonary arterial thrombus, leading to mechanical obstruction of pulmonary arteries.[11] Unlike in acute PE, there is no linear correlation between the degree of mechanical obstruction and hemodynamics,[28] presumably because of a concomitant small vessel pulmonary arteriopathy

that is seen in approximately 40% of cases.[29] There is also no correlation between perfusion defects and oxygen consumption at peak exercise ($V_{O_{2max}}$).[21]

No pulmonary arterial hypertension (PAH)-specific mutations have been identified in CTEPH,[30] but associations with blood group non-O[31] and ADAMTS13.[32] Previous splenectomy, a history of infected ventriculo-atrial shunts for the treatment of hydrocephalus, and indwelling catheters and leads,[33] thyroid replacement therapy, cancer, and chronic inflammatory disorders, such as osteomyelitis and inflammatory bowel diseases are significantly associated with CTEPH[34,35] and have a negative impact on survival.[36]

Endothelial dysfunction,[37] unbalanced fibrinolysis,[38–41] dysfunctional angiogenesis,[42] and immunologic mechanisms[43] have been associated with disease mechanisms underlying CTEPH. Despite some evidence that thrombophilia, particularly antiphospholipid antibodies and elevated factor VIII, may be risk factors for CTEPH,[35] thrombolytic treatment did not affect long-term mortality rates, and it did not appear to reduce the occurrence of CTEPH within 2 years of follow-up.[44]

CLINICAL PRESENTATION AND DIAGNOSIS

Algorithms for predicting CTEPH at the time of PE,[45] and ruling out CTEPH,[46] have been limited by a lack of specificity, and CTEPH has remained largely underdiagnosed.

Table 3
Residual perfusion defects after acute PE

Study	Number of Patients	Follow-up after Diagnosis	Imaging Technique	Perfusion Defects (% Patients)
Lim et al,[76] 2020	190	3–6 mo	V/Q-scan	VKA: 38.9 Rivaroxaban: 23.2
Pesavento et al,[77] 2017	647	6 mo	V/Q-scan	50
Meysman et al,[78] 2017	46	6 mo	Q-SPECT	52
den Exter et al,[79] 2015	157	6 mo	MDCT	16
Pesavento et al,[80] 2014	113	6 mo	MDCT	15
Poli et al,[81] 2013	235	Median 11 mo	Q-scan	26
Alonso-Martínez et al,[82] 2012	120	Mean 5 mo	MDCT	26
Cosmi et al,[83] 2011	173	Mean 9 mo	MDCT/Q-scan	15 MDCT 28 Q scan
Sanchez et al,[84] 2010	254	Median 12 mo	V/Q-scan	29
Nijkeuter et al,[85] 2006	268	8 d–11 mo	V/Q-scan CT	50

Abbreviations: CT, computed tomography; DSA, digital subtraction angiography; MDCT, multidetector computed tomography; PE, pulmonary embolism; VKA, vitamin K antagonists; V/Q, ventilation/perfusion.

CTEPH/CTED equally affect both genders, median age of patients at diagnosis is 63 years.[11] Clinically, CTEPH symptoms and signs are nonspecific and may resemble those of acute PE. In Europe, a median of 14 months is counted between symptom onset and diagnosis in expert centers.[8]

Patients with complete unilateral obstruction may present with normal pulmonary hemodynamics at rest despite symptomatic disease. These patients are classified as having CTED.

Although CT pulmonary angiography is the investigation of choice for the diagnosis of acute PE, planar V/Q lung scan is a suitable first-line screening modality for CTEPH, as it carries a 96% to 97% sensitivity and 90% to 95% specificity for the diagnosis[47] (**Fig. 2**). By contrast, in idiopathic PAH and pulmonary veno-occlusive disease, perfusion scans typically show nonsegmental defects or are normal. Both V/Q scanning and modern CT pulmonary angiography may be accurate methods for the detection of CTEPH with excellent diagnostic efficacy in expert hands (100%, 93.7%, and 96.5% sensitivity, specificity, and accuracy for V/Q, and 96.1%, 95.2%, and 95.6% for CT pulmonary angiography).[48]

Multi detector (MD) CT pulmonary angiography has become an established imaging modality for confirming CTEPH[49]; however, this investigation alone cannot exclude the disease.[47] CT pulmonary angiography may help to identify complications of the disease such as pulmonary artery (PA) dilatation resulting in left main coronary artery compression, and hypertrophied bronchial arterial collaterals, which may lead to hemoptysis.

A high-resolution CT scan of the chest delivers images of the lung parenchyma, and identifies emphysema, bronchial disease, or interstitial lung disease, as well as infarcts, vascular and pericardial malformations, and thoracic wall deformities. Perfusion inequalities manifest as a mosaic parenchymal pattern with dark areas corresponding to

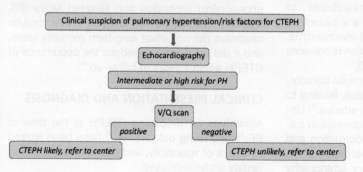

Fig. 2. Diagnostic algorithm for CTEPH/CTED.

relatively decreased perfusion. Although a mosaic pattern is frequent in CTEPH, it also can be observed in up to 12% of patients with PAH. MRI of the pulmonary vasculature is still considered inferior to CT,[50,51] but this modality, as well as cone beam CT,[52] angioscopy,[53] intravascular ultrasound, optical coherence tomography, and pressure wire[54] may be complementary, and may be used according to local experience and practice.

Final diagnosis and operability assessment are achieved by right heart catheterization (RHC) and selective pulmonary angiography in the anterior-posterior and lateral projections illustrating ringlike stenosis, webs ("slits"), pouches, wall irregularities, and complete vascular obstructions, as well as bronchial collaterals, supporting the assessment of technical operability or suitability for balloon pulmonary angioplasty (BPA). The diagnosis of CTED cannot be made without an RHC, and may be supplemented by an invasive or noninvasive exercise study to demonstrate inappropriate rise of PAP under exercise[55,56] (see **Table 2**). In the differential diagnosis of CTEPH, PA sarcoma, tumor cell embolism, parasites (hydatid cyst), foreign body embolism, tumor embolism, and congenital or acquired PA stenoses have to be considered (see **Table 1**). In addition, mediastinal fibrosis may appear like CTEPH on V/Q scanning, but leads to characteristic lesions on pulmonary angiography.

TREATMENTS

CTEPH/CTED are potentially curable by pulmonary endarterectomy (PEA); however, more than half of patients are not eligible for surgery,[8,57] or experience persistent or recurrent PH after PEA.[8,58–60] These previous no-option patients are treated medically today, and/or percutaneously by BPA, or still remain untreated.

Although PEA is formally the gold standard of CTEPH treatments, current registries illustrate that at least 40% of patients are poor surgical candidates, and remain unoperated.[8] Suitability of patients for PEA, BPA, medical therapy, or any combination of these treatments in any sequence is determined by multiple factors that cannot yet be standardized; these are related to patient factors, the expertise of the surgical and percutaneous multidisciplinary teams (**Fig. 3**), and available resources. General criteria include preoperative New York Heart Association functional classes and surgical accessibility of thrombi in the main, lobar, or segmental pulmonary arteries. Advanced age per se is no contraindication for surgery. There is no PVR threshold or measure of

right ventricular (RV) dysfunction that can be considered to preclude PEA or BPA.

Surgical Treatment

PEA is the treatment of choice for CTEPH. In Europe, in-hospital mortality is currently as low as 4.7%[61] or even lower in high-volume single centers.[62] Most patients experience substantial relief from symptoms and near-normalization of hemodynamics.[61,63,64] In contrast to surgical embolectomy for acute PE, treatment of CTEPH necessitates a true bilateral endarterectomy through the medial layer of the pulmonary arteries, which is performed under deep hypothermia and circulatory arrest,[64] without the need for cerebral perfusion.[65]

Postoperative extracorporeal membrane oxygenation (ECMO) is recommended as a standard of care in PEA centers for severe cases.[64] Early postoperative reperfusion edema may require veno-arterial ECMO, and severe persistent PH may be bridged to emergency lung transplantation with veno-venous ECMO.

Patients who do not undergo PEA or suffer from untreated persistent or recurrent PH after PEA face a poor prognosis,[57] unless they are considered for BPA.[66]

In CTED, PEA resulted in significant improvement in symptoms and quality of life.[2] Although there was no in-hospital mortality, complications occurred in 40% of patients.

Percutaneous Catheter-Directed Treatment

In 2001, Feinstein and Landzberg published a series of 18 patients with nonoperable CTEPH who they subjected to balloon dilatation of the pulmonary arteries. Despite a significant decrease of mPAP, 11 patients developed reperfusion pulmonary edema and 3 required mechanical ventilation.[67] Over the past 10 years, Japanese investigators have refined BPA by titration of balloon size and number of treated lesions to the level of mPAP. On average, 5 sessions are needed per patient to improve parameters of RV function.[68] Although BPA is not extensively used, it is rapidly gaining attention worldwide. One of the largest Japanese registries has reported results similar to those derived from PEA both on short-term and long-term clinical follow-up.[69] In CTED, BPA is safe, with few complications (2.9% of the interventions, 10% of patients). After the procedures, World Health Organization functional class, 6-minute walking distance, PVR, and pulmonary arterial compliance improved, and N-terminal pro-brain natriuretic peptide concentrations declined.[70]

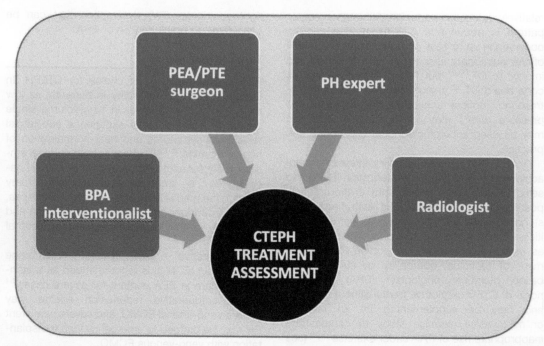

Fig. 3. Key players of the CTEPH team.

Pharmacologic Treatment

Optimal medical treatment for CTEPH/CTED consists of anticoagulants and diuretics, and oxygen in cases of heart failure or hypoxemia. Lifelong anticoagulation is recommended, even after PEA, although no comparative data exist on the efficacy and safety of new oral anticoagulants.[71] Although there is no consensus, routine inferior vena cava filter placement is not justified by the available evidence. Pulmonary microvascular disease in CTEPH has provided the rationale for off-label use of drugs approved for PAH. Whether these drugs work in CTED is unknown. Medical treatment of CTEPH with targeted therapy may be justified in technically nonoperable patients or in the presence of an unacceptable surgical risk-benefit ratio. However, the precise position of medical treatment of CTEPH in relation to interventional techniques is uncertain. The only data derive from the randomized RACE trial testing the efficacy and safety of medical therapy with riociguat against BPA (NCT02634203). By week 26, geometric mean PVR decreased to 41% of baseline value in 52 patients of the BPA group, compared with 68% of baseline value in 53 patients of the riociguat group. Although these data suggest greater efficacy of BPA, complication rates were higher in patients undergoing BPA.

Patients with persistent or recurrent PH after PEA may be candidates for targeted medical therapy. The use of targeted therapy in operable patients with severe hemodynamic compromise as bridge to PEA has not yet been supported by scientific evidence.

An enteral stimulator of soluble guanylate cyclase, riociguat led to a mean increase of 39 m in the 6-minute walk distance of patients with nonoperable CTEPH, or persistent/recurrent PH after PEA after 16 weeks, with a least-squares mean difference of 246 dyn cm·s^{-5} in PVR ($P<.001$, secondary end-point); the time to clinical worsening remained unchanged.[72] Riociguat received approval by both the Food and Drug Administration and European Medicines Agency for the treatment of adults with persistent or recurrent CTEPH after surgical treatment, or inoperable CTEPH, to improve exercise capacity and World Health Organization Functional Classification. Recently, the dual endothelin receptor blocker macitentan significantly improved PVR in patients with inoperable CTEPH and was well tolerated.[73] Furthermore, a recent multicenter randomized controlled trial demonstrated that treatment with subcutaneous treprostinil was safe, and improved exercise capacity in patients with severe CTEPH.[74] Subcutaneous treprostinil was approved for the treatment of inoperable CTEPH and persistent/recurrent PH after PEA in the beginning of 2020.

Prospective randomized controlled trials comparing different treatment modalities, and sequences of treatment, are needed in patients with potential treatment benefit for example, in patients with high PVR and technically challenging anatomy. Furthermore, medical treatments before mechanical treatments, that is, PEA and BPA, have not been systematically studied.

SOURCES OF FUNDING

This research was funded by the Austrian Science Fund F54.

CLINICS CARE POINTS

- Severe acute PE and a history of acute pulmonary embolism should make you think of CTEPH.
- Symptomatic patients 3-6 months after acute PE should have an echocardiogram.
- Ascertain that patients were on 3 months of anticoagulation before they are seen for tests to diagnose CTEPH
- Patients with CTEPH should be managed at a CTEPH center.

DISCLOSURES

I.M. Lang has relationships with drug companies including AOPOrphan Pharmaceuticals AG, Actelion-Janssen, MSD, United Therapeutics, Medtronic, and Ferrer. In addition to being investigator in trials involving these companies, relationships include consultancy service, research grants, and membership of scientific advisory boards. I.A. Campean has nothing to disclose. R. Sadushi-Kolici has relationships with drug companies including Actelion, AOP Orphan Pharmaceuticals, Bayer-Schering, GlaxoSmithKline, and SciPharm Sàrl. In addition, Roela Sadushi-Kolici is an investigator in trials involving these companies, relationships include consultancy service, and research grants. R. Badr-Eslam has received compensation for scientific symposia from Actelion-Janssen, AOPOrphan Pharmaceuticals, AstraZeneca, and GlaxoSmithKline. C. Gerges has received compensation for scientific symposia from Actelion-Janssen, AOPOrphan Pharmaceuticals, AstraZeneca, and GlaxoSmithKline. N. Skoro-Sajer has relationships with drug companies, including Actelion, AOP Orphan Pharmaceuticals, Bayer AG, GlaxoSmithKline, Pfizer, and United Therapeutics. In addition, Nika Skoro-Sajer is an investigator in trials involving these companies, relationships include consultancy service, and research grants.

REFERENCES

1. Simonneau G, Montani D, Celermajer DS, et al. Haemodynamic definitions and updated clinical classification of pulmonary hypertension. Eur Respir J 2019;53(1):1801913.
2. Taboada D, Pepke-Zaba J, Jenkins DP, et al. Outcome of pulmonary endarterectomy in symptomatic chronic thromboembolic disease. Eur Respir J 2014;44(6):1635–45.
3. Riedel M, Stanek V, Widimsky J, et al. Longterm follow-up of patients with pulmonary thromboembolism. Late prognosis and evolution of hemodynamic and respiratory data. Chest 1982;81(2):151–8.
4. Heresi GA, Minai OA, Tonelli AR, et al. Clinical characterization and survival of patients with borderline elevation in pulmonary artery pressure. Pulm Circ 2013;3(4):916–25.
5. Maron BA, Hess E, Maddox TM, et al. Association of borderline pulmonary hypertension with mortality and hospitalization in a large patient cohort: insights from the veterans affairs clinical assessment, reporting, and tracking program. Circulation 2016; 133(13):1240–8.
6. Lang IM, Simonneau G, Pepke-Zaba JW, et al. Factors associated with diagnosis and operability of chronic thromboembolic pulmonary hypertension. A case-control study. Thromb Haemost 2013; 110(1):83–91.
7. Ende-Verhaar YM, Cannegieter SC, Vonk Noordegraaf A, et al. Incidence of chronic thromboembolic pulmonary hypertension after acute pulmonary embolism: a contemporary view of the published literature. Eur Respir J 2017;49(2):1601792.
8. Pepke-Zaba J, Delcroix M, Lang I, et al. Chronic thromboembolic pulmonary hypertension (CTEPH): results from an international prospective registry. Circulation 2011;124(18):1973–81.
9. Cottin V, Avot D, Levy-Bachelot L, et al. Identifying chronic thromboembolic pulmonary hypertension through the French national hospital discharge database. PLoS One 2019;14(4):e0214649.
10. Guérin L, Couturaud F, Parent F, et al. Prevalence of chronic thromboembolic pulmonary hypertension after acute pulmonary embolism. Prevalence of CTEPH after pulmonary embolism. Thromb Haemost 2014;112(3):598–605.
11. Lang IM, Madani M. Update on chronic thromboembolic pulmonary hypertension. Circulation 2014; 130(6):508–18.
12. Konstantinides SV, Meyer G, Becattini C, et al. 2019 ESC guidelines for the diagnosis and management of acute pulmonary embolism developed in collaboration with the European Respiratory Society (ERS): the Task Force for the diagnosis and management of acute pulmonary embolism of the European Society of Cardiology (ESC). Eur Respir J 2019;54(3):1901647.
13. Klok FA, Zondag W, van Kralingen KW, et al. Patient outcomes after acute pulmonary embolism. A pooled survival analysis of different adverse events. Am J Respir Crit Care Med 2010;181(5):501–6.

14. Sista AK, Klok FA. Late outcomes of pulmonary embolism: the post-PE syndrome. Thromb Res 2018; 164:157–62.

15. Klok FA, van der Hulle T, den Exter PL, et al. The post-PE syndrome: a new concept for chronic complications of pulmonary embolism. Blood Rev 2014; 28(6):221–6.

16. Kahn SR, Ducruet T, Lamping DL, et al. Prospective evaluation of health-related quality of life in patients with deep venous thrombosis. Arch Intern Med 2005;165(10):1173–8.

17. Klok FA, van Kralingen KW, van Dijk AP, et al. Prevalence and potential determinants of exertional dyspnea after acute pulmonary embolism. Respir Med 2010;104(11):1744–9.

18. Hunter R, Noble S, Lewis S, et al. Long-term psychosocial impact of venous thromboembolism: a qualitative study in the community. BMJ Open 2019; 9(2):e024805.

19. Lukas PS, Krummenacher R, Biasiutti FD, et al. Association of fatigue and psychological distress with quality of life in patients with a previous venous thromboembolic event. Thromb Haemost 2009;102(6):1219–26.

20. Keller K, Tesche C, Gerhold-Ay A, et al. Quality of life and functional limitations after pulmonary embolism and its prognostic relevance. J Thromb Haemost 2019;17(11):1923–34.

21. Kahn SR, Hirsch AM, Akaberi A, et al. Functional and exercise limitations after a first episode of pulmonary embolism: results of the ELOPE prospective cohort study. Chest 2017;151(5):1058–68.

22. Klok FA, Barco S. Follow-up after acute pulmonary embolism. Hamostaseologie 2018;38(1):22–32.

23. Ende-Verhaar YM, Meijboom LJ, Kroft LJM, et al. Usefulness of standard computed tomography pulmonary angiography performed for acute pulmonary embolism for identification of chronic thromboembolic pulmonary hypertension: results of the InShape III study. J Heart Lung Transplant 2019;38(7):731–8.

24. Mercier O, Fadel E. Chronic thromboembolic pulmonary hypertension: animal models. Eur Respir J 2013;41(5):1200–6.

25. Lang IM, Marsh JJ, Konopka RG, et al. Factors contributing to increased vascular fibrinolytic activity in mongrel dogs. Circulation 1993;87(6):1990–2000.

26. Marsh JJ, Konopka RG, Lang IM, et al. Suppression of thrombolysis in a canine model of pulmonary embolism. Circulation 1994;90(6):3091–7.

27. Schultz J, Andersen A, Gade IL, et al. Riociguat, sildenafil and inhaled nitric oxide reduces pulmonary vascular resistance and improves right ventricular function in a porcine model of acute pulmonary embolism. Eur Heart J Acute Cardiovasc Care 2020; 9(4):293–301.

28. Azarian R, Wartski M, Collignon MA, et al. Lung perfusion scans and hemodynamics in acute and chronic pulmonary embolism. J Nucl Med 1997; 38(6):980–3.

29. Gerges C, Gerges M, Friewald R, et al. Microvascular disease in chronic thromboembolic pulmonary hypertension: hemodynamic phenotyping and histomorphometric assessment. Circulation 2020;141(5):376–86.

30. Suntharalingam J, Machado RD, Sharples LD, et al. Demographic features, BMPR2 status and outcomes in distal chronic thromboembolic pulmonary hypertension. Thorax 2007;62(7):617–22.

31. Bonderman D, Turecek PL, Jakowitsch J, et al. High prevalence of elevated clotting factor VIII in chronic thromboembolic pulmonary hypertension. Thromb Haemost 2003;90(3):372–6.

32. Newnham M, South K, Bleda M, et al. The ADAMTS13-VWF axis is dysregulated in chronic thromboembolic pulmonary hypertension. Eur Respir J 2019;53(3):1801805.

33. Natali D, Jais X, Abraham M, et al. Chronic thromboembolic pulmonary hypertension associated with indwelling Port-A-Cath® central venous access systems. Am J Respir Crit Care Med 2011;183:A2409.

34. Bonderman D, Jakowitsch J, Adlbrecht C, et al. Medical conditions increasing the risk of chronic thromboembolic pulmonary hypertension. Thromb Haemost 2005;93(3):512–6.

35. Bonderman D, Wilkens H, Wakounig S, et al. Risk factors for chronic thromboembolic pulmonary hypertension. Eur Respir J 2009;33(2):325–31.

36. Bonderman D, Skoro-Sajer N, Jakowitsch J, et al. Predictors of outcome in chronic thromboembolic pulmonary hypertension. Circulation 2007;115(16): 2153–8.

37. Chibana H, Tahara N, Itaya N, et al. Pulmonary artery dysfunction in chronic thromboembolic pulmonary hypertension. Int J Cardiol Heart Vasc 2017; 17:30–2.

38. Lang IM, Marsh JJ, Olman MA, et al. Expression of type 1 plasminogen activator inhibitor in chronic pulmonary thromboemboli. Circulation 1994;89(6): 2715–21.

39. Lang IM, Marsh JJ, Olman MA, et al. Parallel analysis of tissue-type plasminogen activator and type 1 plasminogen activator inhibitor in plasma and endothelial cells derived from patients with chronic pulmonary thromboemboli. Circulation 1994;90(2): 706–12.

40. Lang IM, Moser KM, Schleef RR. Expression of Kunitz protease inhibitor–containing forms of amyloid beta-protein precursor within vascular thrombi. Circulation 1996;94(11):2728–34.

41. Satoh T, Satoh K, Yaoita N, et al. Activated TAFI promotes the development of chronic thromboembolic pulmonary hypertension: a possible novel therapeutic target. Circ Res 2017;120(8):1246–62.

42. Alias S, Redwan B, Panzenboeck A, et al. Defective angiogenesis delays thrombus resolution: a

potential pathogenetic mechanism underlying chronic thromboembolic pulmonary hypertension. Arterioscler Thromb Vasc Biol 2014;34(4):810–9.

43. Frey MK, Alias S, Winter MP, et al. Splenectomy is modifying the vascular remodeling of thrombosis. J Am Heart Assoc 2014;3(1):e000772.

44. Konstantinides SV, Vicaut E, Danays T, et al. Impact of thrombolytic therapy on the long-term outcome of intermediate-risk pulmonary embolism. J Am Coll Cardiol 2017;69(12):1536–44.

45. Klok FA, Dzikowska-Diduch O, Kostrubiec M, et al. Derivation of a clinical prediction score for chronic thromboembolic pulmonary hypertension after acute pulmonary embolism. J Thromb Haemost 2016; 14(1):121–8.

46. Klok FA, Surie S, Kempf T, et al. A simple non-invasive diagnostic algorithm for ruling out chronic thromboembolic pulmonary hypertension in patients after acute pulmonary embolism. Thromb Res 2011; 128(1):21–6.

47. Tunariu N, Gibbs SJ, Win Z, et al. Ventilation-perfusion scintigraphy is more sensitive than multidetector CTPA in detecting chronic thromboembolic pulmonary disease as a treatable cause of pulmonary hypertension. J Nucl Med 2007;48(5):680–4.

48. Lang IM, Plank C, Sadushi-Kolici R, et al. Imaging in pulmonary hypertension. JACC Cardiovasc Imaging 2010;3(12):1287–95.

49. He J, Fang W, Lv B, et al. Diagnosis of chronic thromboembolic pulmonary hypertension: comparison of ventilation/perfusion scanning and multidetector computed tomography pulmonary angiography with pulmonary angiography. Nucl Med Commun 2012;33(5):459–63.

50. Ley S, Ley-Zaporozhan J, Pitton MsB, et al. Diagnostic performance of state-of-the-art imaging techniques for morphological assessment of vascular abnormalities in patients with chronic thromboembolic pulmonary hypertension (CTEPH). Eur Radiol 2012;22(3):607–16.

51. Renapurkar RD, Shrikanthan S, Heresi GA, et al. Imaging in chronic thromboembolic pulmonary hypertension. J Thorac Imaging 2017;32(2):71–88.

52. Fukuda T, Ogo T, Nakanishi N, et al. Evaluation of organized thrombus in distal pulmonary arteries in patients with chronic thromboembolic pulmonary hypertension using cone-beam computed tomography. Jpn J Radiol 2016;34(6):423–31.

53. Shure D, Gregoratos G, Moser KM. Fiberoptic angioscopy: role in the diagnosis of chronic pulmonary arterial obstruction. Ann Intern Med 1985;103(6 Pt 1):844–50.

54. Ishiguro H, Kataoka M, Inami T, et al. Diversity of lesion morphology in CTEPH analyzed by OCT, pressure wire, and angiography. JACC Cardiovasc Imaging 2016;9(3):324–5.

55. Guth S, Wiedenroth CB, Rieth A, et al. Exercise right heart catheterisation before and after pulmonary endarterectomy in patients with chronic thromboembolic disease. Eur Respir J 2018;52(3):1800458.

56. Held M, Grün M, Holl R, et al. Cardiopulmonary exercise testing to detect chronic thromboembolic pulmonary hypertension in patients with normal echocardiography. Respiration 2014;87(5):379–87.

57. Delcroix M, Lang I, Pepke-Zaba J, et al. Long-term outcome of patients with chronic thromboembolic pulmonary hypertension: results from an international prospective registry. Circulation 2016;133(9): 859–71.

58. Archibald CJ, Auger WR, Fedullo PF, et al. Long-term outcome after pulmonary thromboendarterectomy. Am J Respir Crit Care Med 1999;160(2): 523–8.

59. Skoro-Sajer N, Marta G, Gerges C, et al. Surgical specimens, haemodynamics and long-term outcomes after pulmonary endarterectomy. Thorax 2014;69(2):116–22.

60. Cannon JE, Su L, Kiely DG, et al. Dynamic risk stratification of patient long-term outcome after pulmonary endarterectomy: results from the United Kingdom National cohort. Circulation 2016;133(18): 1761–71.

61. Mayer E, Jenkins D, Lindner J, et al. Surgical management and outcome of patients with chronic thromboembolic pulmonary hypertension: results from an international prospective registry. J Thorac Cardiovasc Surg 2011;141(3):702–10.

62. Mahmud E, Madani MM, Kim NH, et al. Chronic thromboembolic pulmonary hypertension: evolving therapeutic approaches for operable and inoperable disease. J Am Coll Cardiol 2018;71(21): 2468–86.

63. Madani MM, Auger WR, Pretorius V, et al. Pulmonary endarterectomy: recent changes in a single institution's experience of more than 2,700 patients. Ann Thorac Surg 2012;94(1):97–103 [discussion: 103].

64. Jenkins D, Madani M, Fadel E, et al. Pulmonary endarterectomy in the management of chronic thromboembolic pulmonary hypertension. Eur Respir Rev 2017;26(143):160111.

65. Vuylsteke A, Sharples L, Charman G, et al. Circulatory arrest versus cerebral perfusion during pulmonary endarterectomy surgery (PEACOG): a randomised controlled trial. Lancet 2011;378(9800):1379–87.

66. Araszkiewicz A, Darocha S, Pietrasik A, et al. Balloon pulmonary angioplasty for the treatment of residual or recurrent pulmonary hypertension after pulmonary endarterectomy. Int J Cardiol 2019;278: 232–7.

67. Feinstein JA, Goldhaber SZ, Lock JE, et al. Balloon pulmonary angioplasty for treatment of chronic thromboembolic pulmonary hypertension. Circulation 2001;103(1):10–3.

68. Lang I, Meyer BC, Ogo T, et al. Balloon pulmonary angioplasty in chronic thromboembolic pulmonary hypertension. Eur Respir Rev 2017;26(143):160119.

69. Ogawa A, Satoh T, Fukuda T, et al. Balloon pulmonary angioplasty for chronic thromboembolic pulmonary hypertension: results of a multicenter registry. Circ Cardiovasc Qual Outcomes 2017; 10(11):e004029.

70. Wiedenroth CB, Olsson KM, Guth S, et al. Balloon pulmonary angioplasty for inoperable patients with chronic thromboembolic disease. Pulm Circ 2018; 8(1). 2045893217753122.

71. Bunclark K, Newnham M, Chiu YD, et al. A multicenter study of anticoagulation in operable chronic thromboembolic pulmonary hypertension. J Thromb Haemost 2020;18(1):114–22.

72. Ghofrani HA, D'Armini AM, Grimminger F, et al. Riociguat for the treatment of chronic thromboembolic pulmonary hypertension. N Engl J Med 2013; 369(4):319–29.

73. Ghofrani HA, Simonneau G, D'Armini AM, et al. Macitentan for the treatment of inoperable chronic thromboembolic pulmonary hypertension (MERIT-1): results from the multicentre, phase 2, randomised, double-blind, placebo-controlled study. Lancet Respir Med 2017;5(10):785–94.

74. Sadushi-Kolici R, Jansa P, Kopec G, et al. Subcutaneous treprostinil for the treatment of severe non-operable chronic thromboembolic pulmonary hypertension (CTREPH): a double-blind, phase 3, randomised controlled trial. Lancet Respir Med 2019;7(3):239–48.

75. van Kan C, van der Plas MN, Reesink HJ, et al. Hemodynamic and ventilatory responses during exercise in chronic thromboembolic disease. J Thorac Cardiovasc Surg 2016;152(3):763–71.

76. Lim MS, Nandurkar D, Jong I, et al. Incidence of residual perfusion defects by lung scintigraphy in patients treated with rivaroxaban compared with warfarin for acute pulmonary embolism. J Thromb Thrombolysis 2020;49(2):220–7.

77. Pesavento R, Filippi L, Palla A, et al. Impact of residual pulmonary obstruction on the long-term outcome of patients with pulmonary embolism. Eur Respir J 2017;49(5):1601980.

78. Meysman M, Everaert H, Vincken W. Factors determining altered perfusion after acute pulmonary embolism assessed by quantified single-photon emission computed tomography-perfusion scan. Ann Thorac Med 2017;12(1):30–5.

79. den Exter PL, van Es J, Kroft LJ, et al. Thromboembolic resolution assessed by CT pulmonary angiography after treatment for acute pulmonary embolism. Thromb Haemost 2015;114(1):26–34.

80. Pesavento R, Filippi L, Pagnan A, et al. Unexpectedly high recanalization rate in patients with pulmonary embolism treated with anticoagulants alone. Am J Respir Crit Care Med 2014;189(10):1277–9.

81. Poli D, Cenci C, Antonucci E, et al. Risk of recurrence in patients with pulmonary embolism: predictive role of D-dimer and of residual perfusion defects on lung scintigraphy. Thromb Haemost 2013;109(2):181–6.

82. Alonso-Martínez JL, Anniccherico-Sánchez FJ, Urbieta-Echezarreta MA, et al. Residual pulmonary thromboemboli after acute pulmonary embolism. Eur J Intern Med 2012;23(4):379–83.

83. Cosmi B, Nijkeuter M, Valentino M, et al. Residual emboli on lung perfusion scan or multidetector computed tomography after a first episode of acute pulmonary embolism. Intern Emerg Med 2011;6(6): 521–8.

84. Sanchez O, Helley D, Couchon S, et al. Perfusion defects after pulmonary embolism: risk factors and clinical significance. J Thromb Haemost 2010;8(6): 1248–55.

85. Nijkeuter M, Hovens MM, Davidson BL, et al. Resolution of thromboemboli in patients with acute pulmonary embolism: a systematic review. Chest 2006;129(1):192–7.

Pulmonary Hypertension in Pregnancy

Inderjit Singh, MD, FRCP[a],*, Evelyn Horn, MD[b], Jennifer Haythe, MD[c]

KEYWORDS

- Pulmonary hypertension • PAH • Pregnancy • Pregnancy management
- Physiologic changes of pregnancy

KEY POINTS

- Pregnancy in patients with any form of pulmonary hypertension (PH) is associated with significant maternal-fetal morbidity and mortality.
- The adaptive and expectant mechanical and hormonal changes of pregnancy have deleterious consequences on the cardiopulmonary circulation of the pregnant PH patient.
- Management of pregnancy in PH involves a multispecialty care approach preferably in a pulmonary arterial hypertension referral center.

INTRODUCTION

The anatomic and physiologic changes that occur during pregnancy involve multiple organs that facilitate fetal development. It is important that pulmonary hypertension (PH) providers recognize these expectant changes, as it will help them anticipate and manage the consequences of these adaptive in the pregnant PH patient. Pulmonary arterial hypertension (PAH) is a disease characterized by obliterative vasculopathy of the pulmonary circulation that eventually culminates in right ventricle (RV) failure and death. PAH most commonly occurs in women of child-bearing age, and women are 3 to 4 times more likely to develop PAH compared with men.[1,2] The expectant physiologic and anatomic burden during pregnancy further compromises the RV-pulmonary circulatory function in PH patients and contributes to the high maternal and fetal mortality seen.[3]

This article focuses on the normal expectant physiologic changes encountered during pregnancy and the effects of these changes on the cardiopulmonary circulation in patients with PH to help inform appropriate management of the PH patient during pregnancy.

NORMAL PHYSIOLOGIC CHANGES OF PREGNANCY
Mechanical and Hormonal Changes

Mechanical changes during pregnancy relate to the effects of gravid uterus and hormonal-mediated changes to maternal chest wall compliance (discussed later). With regards to the former, the gravid uterus can compromise venous return by compressing the inferior cava particularly in the supine position. Turning from lateral to supine position can result in 25% reduction in venous return with resulting decrease in stroke volume.[4] Deep vein thrombosis of the lower extremities typically has a left-sided predilection during pregnancy. This left-sided predilection is thought to be related to mechanical compression of the left iliac vein by the gravid uterus (at the point where it crosses the right iliac artery).[5]

The first hormone to peak during pregnancy is plasma human choriogonadotropin; this occurs

[a] Yale School of Medicine, Yale New Haven Health, LCI-106, 20 York Street, New Haven, CT 06519, USA; [b] Weill Cornell Medical College, New York Presbyterian-Weill Cornell Medical Center, Starr Pavilion, 520 East 70th Street, 4th Floor, New York City, NY 10021, USA; [c] Columbia University Vagelos College of Physicians and Surgeons, New York Presbyterian-Columbia University Hospital, CUMC/Vivian & Seymour Milstein Family, 173 Fort Washington Avenue, New York City, NY 10032, USA
* Corresponding author.
E-mail address: Inderjit.singh@yale.edu

Clin Chest Med 42 (2021) 91–99
https://doi.org/10.1016/j.ccm.2020.10.006
0272-5231/21/© 2020 Elsevier Inc. All rights reserved.

around the 10th week of pregnancy, and its production stimulates relaxin, which in turn promotes systemic vasodilation.[6] Progesterone and estrogen are the main sex hormones that predominate for the remainder of pregnancy, and their trajectory along with their systemic and pulmonary vascular effects is depicted in **Fig. 1**.

Changes to the Cardiovascular System

Hematological changes

Plasma volume progressively increases throughout pregnancy and peaks just before delivery at values 50% to 70% greater than prepregnancy values.[6] This expansile increase in volume is related to sex hormone–mediated systemic vasodilatation. The resulting reduced systemic vascular filling and diminished atrial stretch activate the renin-angiotensin-aldosterone system and decrease the release of natriuretic peptides, respectively, allowing for significant fluid and sodium retention.[7–9] Although there is a commensurate increase in red cell mass during pregnancy from increased erythropoietin production, there is a decrease in hemoglobin and hematocrit concentrations because the expansion in plasma volume is greater than the increase in red cell mass.[4] The resulting decrease in blood viscosity reduces the systemic and pulmonary vascular resistance (PVR) and helps augment the cardiac output. During pregnancy, there is an increased risk of thrombophilia. All 3 elements of Virchow's triad are present, including venous stasis, venous trauma,

and hypercoagulability. Venous stasis is the consequence of (a) venodilation possibly mediated by nitric oxide and (b) mechanical compression of the pelvic veins by the gravid uterus.[5] Venous trauma of the pelvic veins commonly occurs during both cesarean and vaginal deliveries. The pulsatile compression of the pelvic veins from uterine contraction is thought to contribute to vascular endothelial damage and therefore thrombus formation.[2] Finally, during gestation, alterations to the fibrinolytic system that enhances thrombosis and impairs clot lysis are encountered. The alteration of the fibrinolytic system include an increase in coagulation factors V, XI, X, VIII and fibrinogen levels along with concomitant decrease in protein S levels.[10,11] In addition, there is also an increase in activated protein C resistance, plasminogen-activator inhibitor-1 (PAI-1) and PAI-2, and thrombin-activatable fibrinolysis factor.[5]

Changes in cardiac anatomy

The increase in plasma volume culminates in cardiac chamber dilatation as well as mild tricuspid regurgitation.[12,13] Although the RV and left ventricle (LV) masses increase,[12,14] the ratio of wall thickness to ventricular radius does not change akin to the eccentric hypertrophy that is encountered in athletes.[15] Pregnancy-induced cardiac eccentric hypertrophy is reversible and regresses following delivery.[6] Increase in plasma volume and resulting atrial stretch likely account for increases in heart rate seen with pregnancy.[16]

Changes in cardiac performance

Cardiac output increases abruptly in the first trimester before it gradually peaks to about 40% to 50% of prepregnancy values (see **Fig. 1**). The increase in cardiac output is related to a 35% increase in stroke volume and increase in heart rate.[6] Augmentation in stroke volume in pregnancy can be attributed to increased plasma volume, decreased RV and systemic afterload, increased contractility, as well as eccentric hypertrophy with resulting increased LV compliance.[15,17] Although transient reduction in LV contractility has been described,[18] myocardial contractility typically increases during pregnancy. The increase in myocardial contractility results from the combination of plasma volume expansion–mediated heterometric adaptation (ie, Frank-Starling mechanism) and from direct inotropic effects of sex hormones (eg, estrogen and prolactin).[6]

Changes in systemic vascular resistance

Systemic vascular resistance (SVR) decreases by about 40% during the course of pregnancy and accounts for the low diastolic blood pressure

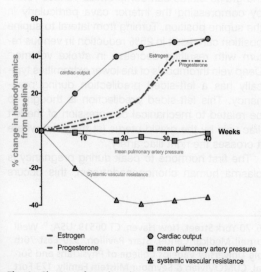

Fig. 1. Changes from baseline in cardiac output, mean pulmonary artery pressure (mPAP), and systemic vascular resistance (CO) relative to changes in sex hormone (estrogen and progesterone) from baseline levels during pregnancy.

seen with pregnancy (see **Fig. 1**).[19] This decrease in SVR is the result of progesterone and estrogen–mediated vasodilation and the low SVR state generated by the extensive network of capillaries of the uteroplacental circulation.[20] The mechanism of sex hormone–mediated vasodilation is thought to be related to increased endotheial nitric oxide and prostacyclin synthesis along with blunted responsiveness to angiotensin II and norepineph-rine.[6] The opposing effects of pregnancy on the SVR (ie, decrease in SVR) and cardiac output (ie, increase in CO) allow for the mean systemic arte-rial pressure to decrease slightly during the initial course of pregnancy before returning to prepreg-nancy levels in the third trimester.[21]

Changes in pulmonary vascular resistance
The increase in cardiac output reduces the PVR by initially recruiting and later distending under perfused pulmonary capillaries.[22,23] Similar to the systemic circulation, the opposing effects on PVR (ie, decreases) and cardiac output (ie, in-crease in CO) allow for preservation of mean pul-monary artery pressure (mPAP) values throughout pregnancy (see **Fig. 1**).

Changes to the Respiratory System

Changes to airway anatomy, lung mechanics, and gas exchange during pregnancy have important implications particularly pertaining to airway and anesthesia management.

Chest wall anatomy
The relaxing effects of the hormone relaxin on the ligamentous attachment of the lower rib cage in-crease the circumference of the lower chest, allowing for an increase in the subcostal angle.[6] Consequently, the thorax now assumes a barrel chest appearance which allows for accommoda-tion of the enlarging uterus. The cephalad displacement of the gravid uterus and therefore diaphragm results in approximately 20% reduction in the functional residual capacity (FRC).[6] During endotracheal intubation, cephalad displacement of diaphragm from supine positioning and admin-istration of neuromuscular blockade further reduce the FRC, hastening the onset of oxygen desaturation.[24]

Upper airway anatomy
Pregnancy-induced fluid retention contributes to upper airway oropharyngeal edema. The combina-tion of oropharyngeal edema and reduced FRC highlights the precarious scenario of endotracheal intubation in pregnant PH patients with an already compromised RV-pulmonary circulation.

Gas exchange
Because pregnancy is a hypermetabolic state, the oxygen consumption (Vo_2) is increased by approximately 20%.[25] This increase in Vo_2 coin-cides with an increase in minute ventilation driven primarily by progesterone-mediated increase in tidal volume. The resulting increase in minute ventilation by approximately 50% results in a res-piratory alkalosis, a compensatory metabolic acidosis, and an increase in arterial oxygen ten-sion.[6] This increase in minute ventilation also contributes to sensation of dyspnea seen in pregnancy.

EFFECTS OF PREGNANCY ON CARDIOPULMONARY CIRCULATION IN PULMONARY HYPERTENSION

The increased cardiac output throughout preg-nancy and fluid shifts following delivery pose a grave threat to maternal mortality and morbidity in PH patients with their fixed and elevated PVR. Increased maternal-fetal morbidity and mortality are commonly observed between weeks 20 and 24 (ie, second trimester), during labor and delivery, and up to 2 months in postpartum period.[6] Deteri-oration during the second trimester reflects the inability of the RV-pulmonary circulation to accom-modate the major volume expansion encountered during this period. Deterioration during labor and delivery or the postpartum period is triggered by large-volume shifts, alteration in RV preload generated by intrathoracic pressure swings from pain and Valsalva maneuvers, negative effects of hypoxemia and acidosis on pulmonary vascula-ture and RV function, and increased predisposition to venous thromboembolism.

The obliterative pulmonary vasculopathy seen in PAH prevents the normal physiologic pulmonary vasodilatory response leading to increases in mPAP and PVR (**Fig. 2**). Failure of the pulmonary vasculature to accommodate increases in cardiac output culminates in RV pressure/volume over-load. The enlarging RV begins to compromise LV filling by 2 mechanisms: (a) parallel interventricular dependence, whereby the RV end-diastolic pres-sure exceeds LV end-diastolic pressure shifting the interventricular septum toward the LV and therefore reducing the LV end-diastolic volume and filling; and (b) serial interventricular depen-dence, whereby the reduction in RV stroke volume results in impaired LV filling.[20] In addition, the compensatory tachycardia seen during preg-nancy, which helps augment cardiac output, is likely compromised because of beta-adrenergic receptor desensitization commonly encountered in PH.[26] Systemic hypotension will subsequently

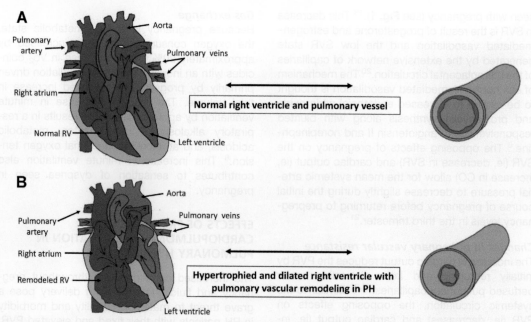

Fig. 2. (*A*) The normal pulmonary vasculature is a high capacitance and low resistance circuit. (*B*) With pulmonary hypertension, the associated pulmonary vasculopathy results in progressive remodeling and narrowing of the pulmonary vasculature leading to elevated right ventricular (RV) afterload and eventually RV remodeling.

ensue, increasing the PVR-to-SVR ratio, causing RV ischemia and the subsequent downward spiral of RV failure. The increased PVR-to-SVR ratio may also precipitate refractory hypoxemia from the increased right-to-left shunt via patent foramen ovale (PFO).

MANAGEMENT OF THE PREGNANT PULMONARY HYPERTENSION PATIENT
General Measures

The care of a pregnant PH patient requires a multi-disciplinary approach, involving obstetricians, anesthesiologists, neonatologists, PH specialists, and intensivists specialized in managing high-risk pregnancies. Additionally, the availability of the mechanical circulatory support team for the provision of extra corporeal membrane oxygenation (ECMO) support for the critically ill pregnant PH should also be a part of the multi-disciplinary team planning.

Because of the increased maternal morbidity and mortality associated with PH, pregnancy in PH is strongly discouraged and termination of pregnancy should be offered regardless of functional class or other favorable prognostic outcomes.[6] Some patients may even present with an initial diagnosis of PH during their pregnancy. However, despite appropriate counseling, some pregnant PH patients may decide to proceed with their pregnancy. In this setting, the pregnant PH patient should

receive her care at a PH referral center. PH referral center such as a pulmonary hypertension association accredited care center (PHCC) with expertise in both pulmonary hypertension and maternal fetal medicine. Patients should be monitored closely, and their visit frequency tailored to the individual patient and their risks.

Hypoxemia may complicate PH as a result of right-to-left shunt via PFO or low cardiac output with resulting low mixed venous oxygen saturation (Mvo$_2$). Hypoxia, if present, should be corrected with supplemental oxygenation to mitigate the effects of reflexive hypoxic vasoconstriction[27,28] on the already elevated PVR and to prevent intrauterine growth restriction and prematurity.[29] A Pao$_2$ greater than 70 mm Hg is recommended in pregnant PH patients.[30]

Because of the thrombotic tendency associated with pregnancy, prophylactic anticoagulation is recommended for all PAH patients in the peripartum period.[21] For patients already on therapeutic anticoagulation therapy (eg, CTEPH [chronic thromboembolic pulmonary hypertension] patients), low-molecular-weight heparin (LMWH) is favored over coumadin because of the teratogenic effects associated with the latter. LMWH can be transitioned to unfractionated heparin in preparation for delivery. Unfractionated heparin is readily reversible with protamin and has a shorter half-life, making it ideal if patients experience significant bleeding during delivery. The newer direct oral anticoagulants (eg, rivaroxaban, dabigatran, and apixaban) have not been studied in patients' PAH and are therefore not recommended.[6]

Diuretic therapy during pregnancy helps reduce intravascular volume and therefore the RV end-diastolic pressure. Diuretics are particularly important during the second trimester of pregnancy during which time volume expansion is a major physiologic occurrence. Furosemide is preferred, whereas spironolactone is avoided because of its teratogenic effects.[6] Maternal administration of diuretic therapy promotes fetal diuresis and typically causes a small increase in amniotic fluid volume. However, prolonged use of high-dose diuretic therapy can result in transient oligohydramnios from maternal intravascular volume contraction.[31] In addition to judicious diuretic use, a low-salt diet and fluid restriction (1.5–2.0 L) are recommended to prevent volume overload. Patients should nurse in the lateral position to avoid compression of their inferior vena cava by the gravid uterus, which can impede venous return.

Therapeutic abortion is commonly performed in the first trimester but can also be considered in the second trimester up to the point of fetal viability. Beyond which point, early delivery may be performed if clinically indicated.[6] Uterine dilatation and evacuation are safer compared with medical abortion.[32] The drugs used to facilitate medical abortion, including prostaglandin E_1 or E_2 and misoprostol, have vasodilatory properties. They can be absorbed into the systemic circulation and lower the SVR/blood pressure, therefore reducing the systemic to RV perfusion gradient with resulting RV ischemia. This systemic vasodilatory effect is more pronounced with prostaglandin E_2 compared with E_1.[32]

For patients who decide to pursue their pregnancy, comprehensive evaluation that encompasses history and physical examination, 6-minute walk testing, serum brain natriuretic peptide, and frequent echocardiographic assessment is essential. Echocardiography frequency can be increased to every 2 weeks during the second and third trimester to allow for close monitoring of RV function and adjustment of PAH-specific medications if necessary.[6] For pregnant patients with a suspected diagnosis of PH on presentation, a right heart study is required to establish the diagnosis. Patients should be advised and counseled on the initiation of PAH-specific therapy during pregnancy, delivery, and the postpartum period.

Delivery

During labor and delivery, continuous monitoring with electrocardiogram, pulse oximetry, central venous pressure, and invasive systemic arterial monitoring should be the standard of care.[33] Real-time echocardiography allowing for close monitoring of RV function is also recommended. Routine use of a pulmonary artery catheter is not necessary[34] and may even increase the risk of hemodynamic-relevant arrhythmias.[35] Vasopressors, inotropes, and inhaled pulmonary vasodilator therapy (eg, inhaled nitric oxide or prostacyclin) should be readily available to provide hemodynamic support. It is prudent to avoid and correct factors that could worsen the PVR, including hypoxia, iron deficiency, acidosis, and anxiety, and pain-induced catecholamine release.[36,37]

The ideal anesthetic care for these patients involves maintenance of normoxia, normotension, and euvolemia while minimizing surges in catecholamine-mediated increase in PVR with adequate analgesia and mitigating increase in RV preload during and in the immediate postpartum period. If intubation is necessary, nasotracheal intubation is best avoided given the capillary engorgement of the nasopharynx frequently observed in the pregnant population increases the risk for epistaxis.[38] The reduced FRC during pregnancy is further compounded when these patients are positioned supine for intubation and subjected to neuromuscular blockade. Optimum preoxygenation or apneic oxygenation is therefore important during this period to prevent oxygen desaturation with consequent hypoxic pulmonary vasoconstriction. Following intubation, general anesthetic use, in particular, volatile anesthetics, can depress cardiac contractility.[39,40] General anesthesia is also associated with increased RV afterload during laryngeal intubation or with positive pressure ventilation. The latter effect can be mitigated by low tidal volume/lung protective ventilatory strategy; however, care must be taken to avoid hypercapnic acidosis.[6] Spinal anesthesia alone should be avoided in these patients because of the risk of marked sympathetic blockade with systemic hypotension causing hemodynamic instability.[6] Low-dose combined spinal-epidural anesthesia is a preferable option because it provides denser perineal sensory block compared with epidural anesthesia alone, with limited risk of systemic hypotension.[41]

The optimum timing and mode of delivery (vaginal vs cesarean section) need to be carefully evaluated in particular to ensure the best support staff is available (e.g. avoid planning for elective delivery in the middle of the night). In stable pregnant PH patients, planned delivery around 34 to 36 weeks' gestation is recommended. Delivery before this is indicated if there is evidence of worsening cardiopulmonary status.[6] Although among healthy population, vaginal delivery is associated with fewer infections and reduced blood loss,[42] a protracted and difficult labor can have detrimental effects on right heart hemodynamics. Vaginal delivery is associated with repeated Valsalva maneuvers generating positive intrathoracic pressures and causing impediment of venous return. In patients with PH, a higher right-sided filling pressure is required to sustain an adequate RV stroke volume; consequently, the Valsalva maneuver can precipitate hemodynamic collapse through reduction in RV preload. In addition, the pain that frequently accompanies childbirth is associated with sympathetic nervous stimulation, increasing the heart rate, and therefore, RV afterload.[43] Oxytocin, commonly used to induce labor, has unwanted hemodynamic effects, including systemic vasodilatation, and can also increase the PVR.[44]

In the hours and days following childbirth, maternal blood volume is augmented by autotransfusion of blood from the contracting uterus and from relief of inferior cava compression by the gravid uterus. In the setting of a fixed and elevated RV afterload, hemodynamic collapse and poor outcome are common.[3,34] This immediate postpartum period is therefore recognized as a critical period for acute decompensation in PH patients. Following delivery, the hyperdynamic circulation ceases and the PVR returns to prepregnancy levels (Fig. 3). In patients with PH, in the setting of a fixed and elevated PVR, augmentation of venous return to the right heart can precipitate acute RV failure. Because of the increased risk of hemodynamic compromise and mortality, PH physicians should be vigilant to detect the onset of RV failure heralded by a low cardiac output and rising central venous pressure. Patients are recommended to be closely monitored in the intensive care unit for several days postpartum.[6] Prophylactic anticoagulation is important during this period as well.

ROLE OF PULMONARY ARTERIAL HYPERTENSION–SPECIFIC THERAPIES DURING PREGNANCY AND DELIVERY

PAH can present for the first time during pregnancy, or PAH patients may elect to become pregnant despite appropriate counseling against pregnancy. If there is a suspicion of possible PH, a right heart study is indicated and can be safely conducted, as this would help dictate management. PH providers may diagnose previously undiagnosed congenital heart defects (eg, atrial septal defect) or connective tissue disease–associated PAH. The latter may warrant concomitant immunotherapy along with PAH-targeted therapy. In a normal cardiopulmonary circulation, an elevated CO reduces the PVR because incremental recruitment and distension of the pulmonary vasculature. PH providers should therefore account for the hyperdynamic circulation of pregnancy when determining the presence of an abnormal PVR. Recently, it was shown that patients with a "borderline" PVR of 2.2 woods unit (WU) (interquartile range 1.9–2.7 WU) have significant functional limitation at baseline with increased 5-year mortality. Treatment with PAH-specific therapies in this patient population resulted in improvement in walk distance and functional class.[45]

Of course, there is also the scenario where PAH patients accidentally become pregnant. If the patient decides to pursue her pregnancy, there are several case studies describing the successful use of PAH-specific therapies in pregnancy.

Calcium Channel Blockers

Calcium channel blockers, nifedipine and diltiazem, are safe in pregnancy.[46,47] In those patients who are vasoresponsive to pulmonary vasodilators, such as inhaled nitric oxide (defined by a drop in mPAP by 10 mm Hg to 40 mm Hg or less with or without an increase in CO), high-dose calcium channel blockers are recommended.[6] Pregnant PAH patients who are not vasoresponsive are not candidates for calcium channel blocker therapy because its use can precipitate further reduction in SVR through its systemic vasodilatory effects.

Prostaglandins

Current available prostacyclin therapies, including epoprostenol, treprostinil, and iloprost, are not

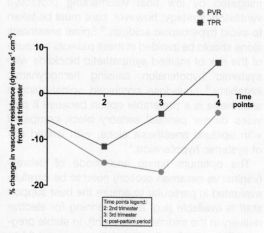

Fig. 3. Changes in pulmonary vascular resistance (PVR) and total peripheral resistance (TPR) during the second and third trimester and post-partum periods compared to the first trimester.[19,23]

known to be teratogenic.[6] Reproductive studies involving rats and rabbits showed no impaired fertility or fetal harm with epoprostenol at 2.5 to 4.8 times the recommended human dose.[48] Systemic prostacyclins are indicated in patients with World Health Organization functional class III or IV symptoms and reduced function. In addition, systemic prostacyclin is also indicated in patients who have progressive worsening of symptoms or deteriorating RV function despite being on established phosphodiesterase-5 inhibitors (PDE-5 inhibitors) and nonparental prostaglandins.[6] Inhaled treprostinil and iloprost are options for those with less severe symptoms. In addition, inhaled pulmonary vasodilators, such as inhaled treprostinil, iloprost, and nitric oxide, can be administered continuously in the acutely ill patient as a bridge to systemic or parenteral prostaglandin therapy.[6] The use of continuously inhaled prostacyclin and/or inhaled nitric oxide therapy during delivery is recommended.

Phosphodiesterase-5 Inhibitors

There have been numerous case studies demonstrating PDE-5 inhibitors' successful use in pregnant patients with PAH.[6] There are no data on the safety and efficacy of tadalafil in pregnant patients with PAH. Because of this, sildenafil is the preferred PDE-5 inhibitor for use in pregnancy. Sildenafil should be reserved in pregnant PAH patients in combination with prostaglandin therapy. If sildenafil is used as monotherapy, it should be reserved for patients with mild PAH with preserved RV function or as an alternative to patients who decline parenteral therapy.

Other Oral Pulmonary Arterial Hypertension Therapies

Endothelin receptor antagonists (macitentan, ambrisentan, bosentan, and sitaxentan) and the soluble guanylate cyclase stimulator, riociguat, are pregnancy category X and therefore should not be prescribed in pregnant PAH patients or should be discontinued when pregnancy is discovered.[6]

USE OF ASSISTED REPRODUCTIVE STRATEGY IN PATIENTS WITH PULMONARY HYPERTENSION

The use of assisted reproductive technologies with a gestational carrier offers a viable option for women with PAH who desire children. Successful ovarian stimulation and egg retrieval in a PAH patient followed by successful gestational carrier pregnancy have been reported.[49] The management of patients with PAH for assisted reproductive technology requires multidisciplinary care consisting of PH provider, reproductive endocrinologist, and cardiac or critical care anesthesiologist, as the procedure is not without risks. Ovarian hyperstimulation syndrome occurs when the ovaries are hyperstimulated by exogenously administered gonadotropins before egg retrieval. It is a serious and potentially fatal complication of assisted reproductive technology. Complications seen in the setting of ovarian hyperstimulation syndrome include volume overload with ascites, pericardial effusion, pleural and effusions, and thromboembolic complications.[50,51] These complications can be life-threatening in PAH patients with an already compromised cardiopulmonary status.

ROLE OF ADVANCED MECHANICAL CIRCULATORY SUPPORT

The use of mechanical circulatory support in the form of extracorporeal membrane oxygenation (ECMO) as a bridge to transplantation or recovery in PAH has been reported and is further discussed in the Critical Care Management of the Pulmonary Hypertension Patient article in this issue.[52] The data available on the of ECMO support in PH during pregnancy or the past partum period are limited,[53,54] and at present, while there are no guidelines established for the use of ECMO in the pregnant or postpartum, the authors would utilize support if needed. Use of ECMO tends to be reserved for patients with severe PAH and hemodynamic collapse. In 1 study of 49 patients with PAH and pregnancy at tertiary sites in North America, all 6 patients who received ECMO ultimately died.[55] The elevated maternal mortality in these patients is likely secondary to severe PH and right heart failure rather than the ECMO itself. One case series on use of ECMO in pregnancy and postpartum includes an Eisenmenger patient cannulated at 34 weeks' gestation who ultimately survived to decannulation postpartum and was discharged home.[54] A more recent series looking at 98 patients with PAH requiring ECMO as either bridge to transplant or nonbridge to transplant demonstrated an overall survival to hospital discharge of 54.1%.[56] Although these were not pregnant patients with PAH, it is important to note that as expertise in this area grows, successful outcomes using ECMO is more possible.

DISCLOSURE

The authors have nothing to disclose.

REFERENCES

1. Humbert M, Sitbon O, Chaouat A, et al. Pulmonary arterial hypertension in France: results from a national registry. Am J Respir Crit Care Med 2006; 173(9):1023–30.
2. Badesch DB, Raskob GE, Elliott CG, et al. Pulmonary arterial hypertension: baseline characteristics from the REVEAL Registry. Chest 2010;137(2):376–87.
3. Weiss BM, Zemp L, Seifert B, et al. Outcome of pulmonary vascular disease in pregnancy: a systematic overview from 1978 through 1996. J Am Coll Cardiol 1998;31(7):1650–7.
4. Soma-Pillay P, Nelson-Piercy C, Tolppanen H, et al. Physiological changes in pregnancy. Cardiovasc J Afr 2016;27(2):89–94.
5. Miller MA, Chalhoub M, Bourjeily G. Peripartum pulmonary embolism. Clin Chest Med 2011;32(1): 147–64.
6. Hemnes AR, Kiely DG, Cockrill BA, et al. Statement on pregnancy in pulmonary hypertension from the Pulmonary Vascular Research Institute. Pulm Circ 2015;5(3):435–65.
7. Schrier RW. Pathogenesis of sodium and water retention in high-output and low-output cardiac failure, nephrotic syndrome, cirrhosis, and pregnancy (2). N Engl J Med 1988;319(17):1127–34.
8. Nadel AS, Ballermann BJ, Anderson S, et al. Interrelationships among atrial peptides, renin, and blood volume in pregnant rats. Am J Physiol 1988;254(5 Pt 2):R793–800.
9. Lindheimer MD, Katz AI. Sodium and diuretics in pregnancy. N Engl J Med 1973;288(17):891–4.
10. Comp PC, Thurnau GR, Welsh J, et al. Functional and immunologic protein S levels are decreased during pregnancy. Blood 1986;68(4):881–5.
11. Clark P, Brennand J, Conkie JA, et al. Activated protein C sensitivity, protein C, protein S and coagulation in normal pregnancy. Thromb Haemost 1998; 79(6):1166–70.
12. Mesa A, Jessurun C, Hernandez A, et al. Left ventricular diastolic function in normal human pregnancy. Circulation 1999;99(4):511–7.
13. Katz R, Karliner JS, Resnik R. Effects of a natural volume overload state (pregnancy) on left ventricular performance in normal human subjects. Circulation 1978;58(3 Pt 1):434–41.
14. Poppas A, Shroff SG, Korcarz CE, et al. Serial assessment of the cardiovascular system in normal pregnancy. Role of arterial compliance and pulsatile arterial load. Circulation 1997;95(10):2407–15.
15. Simmons LA, Gillin AG, Jeremy RW. Structural and functional changes in left ventricle during normotensive and preeclamptic pregnancy. Am J Physiol Heart Circ Physiol 2002;283(4):H1627–33.
16. Crystal GJ, Salem MR. The Bainbridge and the "reverse" Bainbridge reflexes: history, physiology,

and clinical relevance. Anesth Analg 2012;114(3): 520–32.
17. Moran AM, Colan SD, Mauer MB, et al. Adaptive mechanisms of left ventricular diastolic function to the physiologic load of pregnancy. Clin Cardiol 2002;25(3):124–31.
18. Schannwell CM, Zimmermann T, Schneppenheim M, et al. Left ventricular hypertrophy and diastolic dysfunction in healthy pregnant women. Cardiology 2002;97(2):73–8.
19. Mahendru AA, Everett TR, Wilkinson IB, et al. A longitudinal study of maternal cardiovascular function from preconception to the postpartum period. J Hypertens 2014;32(4):849–56.
20. Clapham KR, Singh I, Capuano IS, et al. MEF2 and the right ventricle: from development to disease. Front Cardiovasc Med 2019;6:29.
21. Lahm T, Douglas IS, Archer SL, et al. Assessment of right ventricular function in the research setting: knowledge gaps and pathways forward. An official American Thoracic Society Research Statement. Am J Respir Crit Care Med 2018; 198(4):e15–43.
22. Singh I, Oliveira RKF, Naeije R, et al. Pulmonary vascular distensibility and early pulmonary vascular remodeling in pulmonary hypertension. Chest 2019; 156(4):724–32.
23. Sharma R, Kumar A, Aneja GK. Serial changes in pulmonary hemodynamics during pregnancy: a non-invasive study using Doppler echocardiography. Cardiol Res 2016;7(1):25–31.
24. Berlin D, Singh I, Barjaktarevic I, et al. A technique for bronchoscopic intubation during high-flow nasal cannula oxygen therapy. J Intensive Care Med 2016; 31(3):213–5.
25. Prowse CM, Gaensler EA. Respiratory and acid-base changes during pregnancy. Anesthesiology 1965;26:381–92.
26. Piao L, Fang YH, Parikh KS, et al. GRK2-mediated inhibition of adrenergic and dopaminergic signaling in right ventricular hypertrophy: therapeutic implications in pulmonary hypertension. Circulation 2012; 126(24):2859–69.
27. Morgan JM, Griffiths M, du Bois RM, et al. Hypoxic pulmonary vasoconstriction in systemic sclerosis and primary pulmonary hypertension. Chest 1991; 99(3):551–6.
28. Melot C, Naeije R, Hallemans R, et al. Hypoxic pulmonary vasoconstriction and pulmonary gas exchange in normal man. Respir Physiol 1987;68(1):11–27.
29. Presbitero P, Somerville J, Stone S, et al. Pregnancy in cyanotic congenital heart disease. Outcome of mother and fetus. Circulation 1994;89(6):2673–6.
30. Madden BP. Pulmonary hypertension and pregnancy. Int J Obstet Anesth 2009;18(2):156–64.
31. Manikandan K, Raghavan S. Amniotic fluid volume changes in response to frusemide induced maternal

fluid shifts. J Pharmacol Pharmacother 2014;5(2): 153–4.

32. Jain JK, Mishell DR Jr. A comparison of intravaginal misoprostol with prostaglandin E2 for termination of second-trimester pregnancy. N Engl J Med 1994; 331(5):290–3.

33. European Society of G, Association for European Paediatric C, German Society for Gender M, et al. ESC guidelines on the management of cardiovascular diseases during pregnancy: the Task Force on the Management of Cardiovascular Diseases During Pregnancy of the European Society of Cardiology (ESC). Eur Heart J 2011;32(24): 3147–97.

34. Bedard E, Dimopoulos K, Gatzoulis MA. Has there been any progress made on pregnancy outcomes among women with pulmonary arterial hypertension? Eur Heart J 2009;30(3):256–65.

35. George RB, Olufolabi AJ, Muir HA. Critical arrhythmia associated with pulmonary artery catheterization in a parturient with severe pulmonary hypertension. Can J Anaesth 2007;54(6):486–7.

36. Richter JA, Barankay A. Pulmonary hypertension and right ventricular dysfunction after operations for congenital heart disease. Acta Anaesthesiol Scand Suppl 1997;111:31–3.

37. Power KJ, Avery AF. Extradural analgesia in the intrapartum management of a patient with pulmonary hypertension. Br J Anaesth 1989;63(1):116–20.

38. Munnur U, de Boisblanc B, Suresh MS. Airway problems in pregnancy. Crit Care Med 2005;33(10 Suppl):S259–68.

39. Ciofolo MJ, Reiz S. Circulatory effects of volatile anesthetic agents. Minerva Anestesiol 1999;65(5): 232–8.

40. Ewalenko P, Brimioulle S, Delcroix M, et al. Comparison of the effects of isoflurane with those of propofol on pulmonary vascular impedance in experimental embolic pulmonary hypertension. Br J Anaesth 1997;79(5):625–30.

41. Duggan AB, Katz SG. Combined spinal and epidural anaesthesia for caesarean section in a parturient with severe primary pulmonary hypertension. Anaesth Intensive Care 2003;31(5):565–9.

42. Uebing A, Steer PJ, Yentis SM, et al. Pregnancy and congenital heart disease. BMJ 2006;332(7538): 401–6.

43. Metkus TS, Mullin CJ, Grandin EW, et al. Heart rate dependence of the pulmonary resistance x compliance (RC) time and impact on right ventricular load. PLoS One 2016;11(11):e0166463.

44. Roberts NV, Keast PJ, Brodeky V, et al. The effects of oxytocin on the pulmonary and systemic circulation in pregnant ewes. Anaesth Intensive Care 1992; 20(2):199–202.

45. Ratwatte S, Anderson J, Strange G, et al. Pulmonary arterial hypertension with below threshold pulmonary vascular resistance. Eur Respir J 2020;56(1): 1901654.

46. Jais X, Olsson KM, Barbera JA, et al. Pregnancy outcomes in pulmonary arterial hypertension in the modern management era. Eur Respir J 2012;40(4): 881–5.

47. Easterling TR, Ralph DD, Schmucker BC. Pulmonary hypertension in pregnancy: treatment with pulmonary vasodilators. Obstet Gynecol 1999;93(4): 494–8.

48. Huang S, DeSantis ER. Treatment of pulmonary arterial hypertension in pregnancy. Am J Health Syst Pharm 2007;64(18):1922–6.

49. Metzler E, Ginsburg E, Tsen LC. Use of assisted reproductive technologies and anesthesia in a patient with primary pulmonary hypertension. Fertil Steril 2004;81(6):1684–7.

50. Stewart JA, Hamilton PJ, Murdoch AP. Thromboembolic disease associated with ovarian stimulation and assisted conception techniques. Hum Reprod 1997;12(10):2167–73.

51. Abramov Y, Elchalal U, Schenker JG. Pulmonary manifestations of severe ovarian hyperstimulation syndrome: a multicenter study. Fertil Steril 1999; 71(4):645–51.

52. Rosenzweig EB, Brodie D, Abrams DC, et al. Extracorporeal membrane oxygenation as a novel bridging strategy for acute right heart failure in group 1 pulmonary arterial hypertension. ASAIO J 2014;60(1):129–33.

53. Abid Memon H, Safdar Z, Goodarzi A. Use of extracorporeal membrane oxygenation in postpartum management of a patient with pulmonary arterial hypertension. Case Rep Pulmonol 2018;2018: 7031731.

54. Agerstrand C, Abrams D, Biscotti M, et al. Extracorporeal membrane oxygenation for cardiopulmonary failure during pregnancy and postpartum. Ann Thorac Surg 2016;102(3):774–9.

55. Meng ML, Landau R, Viktorsdottir O, et al. Pulmonary hypertension in pregnancy: a report of 49 cases at four tertiary North American sites. Obstet Gynecol 2017;129(3):511–20.

56. Rosenzweig EB, Gannon WD, Madahar P, et al. Extracorporeal life support bridge for pulmonary hypertension: a high-volume single-center experience. J Heart Lung Transplant 2019;38(12):1275–85.

Section III: Advanced Diagnostics

Advanced Imaging in Pulmonary Vascular Disease

Eileen M. Harder, MD[a],*, Rebecca Vanderpool, PhD[b],
Farbod N. Rahaghi, MD, PhD[a]

KEYWORDS

- Advanced imaging • Pulmonary hypertension • MRI • Computed tomography

KEY POINTS

- Imaging is critical in the noninvasive screening, classification, and monitoring of pulmonary vascular disease (PVD).
- Beyond the standard computed tomography (CT) chest, there are multiple options to assess pulmonary perfusion, including dual-energy CT and single-photon emission CT.
- MRI provides the most detailed cardiopulmonary assessment, including pulmonary arterial stiffness, blood flow patterns, and right ventricular coupling.
- Multiple parameters on advanced imaging correlate with hemodynamics and outcomes, and these modalities will likely play an increasingly important role in PVD treatment.

INTRODUCTION

Imaging plays a central role in the screening, classification, and monitoring of pulmonary vascular disease (PVD). In patients with diagnosed PVD, it allows noninvasive quantification of structural changes to the heart and lungs and measurement of functional parameters of the pulmonary circulation. Improvements in acquisition and processing have dramatically increased imaging capabilities, and a host of emerging modalities offer the potential to significantly improve the ability to phenotype PVD and monitor subtle treatment effects. Furthermore, the development of symptoms in PVD indicates that disease is already advanced and so imaging that can assist in early and noninvasive diagnosis is also of interest.

This article reviews the current role of advanced imaging in the clinical assessment of PVD, as well as the emerging techniques that may ultimately be used in diagnosis and evaluation. This article starts in the lung parenchyma, where various modalities can be used to quantify parenchymal changes, examine perfusion, and assess vascular properties. It then moves toward the central pulmonary arteries, examining flow and their relationship with the right heart, and concludes by discussing developments in cardiac imaging.

IMAGING THE LUNG PARENCHYMA AND VASCULATURE
Computed Tomography

Given that dyspnea, particularly during exertion, is a common presenting symptom of pulmonary hypertension (PH), a computed tomography (CT) scan of the chest is often an early diagnostic test. Parenchymal abnormalities may occur, including fibrotic or emphysematous changes in World Health Organization (WHO) group 3 PH.[1] A mosaic attenuation pattern may develop in pulmonary arterial hypertension (PAH) or chronic

[a] Division of Pulmonary and Critical Care Medicine, Department of Medicine, Brigham and Women's Hospital, 15 Francis Street, Boston, MA 02115, USA; [b] Division of Translational and Regenerative Medicine, Department of Medicine, University of Arizona, 1656 East Mabel Street, Tucson, AZ 85721, USA
* Corresponding author.
E-mail address: eharder1@bwh.harvard.edu
Twitter: @rrvdpool (R.V.)

Clin Chest Med 42 (2021) 101–112
https://doi.org/10.1016/j.ccm.2020.11.004

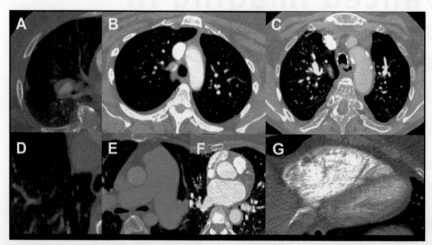

Fig. 1. (*A*) Filling defect in a dilated proximal pulmonary artery (PA) with contrast visible in CTEPH. (*B, C*) Mosaicism in CTEPH (*B*) and PAH (*C*). (*D*) Thickened septal lines are characteristic findings in pulmonary veno-occlusive disease. (*E, F*) Dilated main pulmonary arteries indicate increased PA pressures (*E*), with enlarged left atrium suggesting contribution from left-sided heart disease (*F*). (*G*) An enlarged right ventricle may develop in advanced PH, particularly compared with the left ventricle.

thromboembolic pulmonary hypertension (CTEPH)[2] (**Fig. 1**). In pulmonary veno-occlusive disease, a rare subgroup of WHO group 1 PAH, CT may show the characteristic findings of interlobular septal thickening, mediastinal lymphadenopathy, and centrilobular ground-glass opacities.[3]

Certain nonparenchymal features on CT chest may also suggest the presence of PVD. Pulmonary artery (PA) enlargement greater than or equal to 29 mm is concerning for PH (see **Fig. 1**).[4] Although this feature alone is considered to be only moderately sensitive and specific for disease, its specificity increases when segmental artery-to-bronchus ratio is also greater than 1:1 in 3 or 4 lobes.[4,5] A ratio of the PA diameter normalized by the ascending aorta diameter greater than 1 also suggests PH.[5]

CT angiography (CTA) allows more detailed evaluation of the pulmonary vasculature. Apart from its role in identifying acute pulmonary emboli (PEs), it is an essential diagnostic tool in CTEPH, where organizing thrombi may appear as eccentric wall-adherent clots, intraluminal webs or bands, or intimal thickening.[6] Clot burden and location on CTA are also important in determining candidacy for pulmonary endarterectomy in CTEPH. CTA can also quantify the degree and distribution of the distal pulmonary arterial vascular pruning in PH (**Fig. 2**). On CT, decreased total two-dimensional (2D) cross-sectional area of small vessels correlated with the severity of PH in smokers with chronic obstructive pulmonary disease (COPD).[7] On three-dimensional (3D) CTA

reconstructions, patients with CTEPH had significantly greater pruning of the distal arterial vasculature compared with normal controls, with corresponding proximal artery dilatation and depressed cardiac index.[8] Increased vessel tortuosity on CT also correlates with higher mean PA pressure (mPAP), pulmonary vascular resistance (PVR), and WHO functional class.[9]

The utility of cardiac CT in PH is growing, although it is often limited by the need for electrocardiogram gating and contrast. Right ventricle (RV) volume on CT correlated inversely with right ventricular systolic pressure (RVSP) on echocardiogram, such that it may predict RV dysfunction and failure.[10] Left atrial and ventricular volumes on CT may also predict the presence of WHO group 2 PH.[11]

Dual Energy Computed Tomography

Dual energy CT (DECT) has a growing role in the evaluation of pulmonary structure and perfusion. DECT uses iodinated contrast and photons of 2 different energies to estimate iodine density as a surrogate for blood density, which can be superimposed onto standard weighted-average CT images to evaluate relative perfusion.[12] DECT requires additional software technology but no additional scanning time, contrast, or radiation exposure. It agrees well with V/Q scans in detecting CTEPH and offers the added advantage of anatomic visualization.[3] Perfusion patterns on DECT may be useful in PH classification, with patchy defects in PAH compared with mixed patchy and PE-like abnormalities in CTEPH.[13]

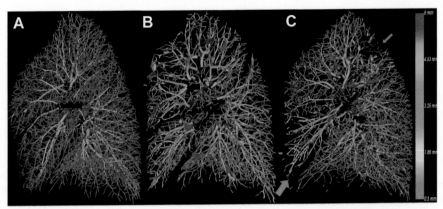

Fig. 2. Vascular reconstructions from CT angiograms (CT PE protocol). Color indicates the vessel radius. (*A*) A patient with no evident pulmonary or cardiac disease. (*B*) A patient with resting PAH with proximal vessel dilatation and loss of small vasculature. (*C*) A patient with CTEPH with regional loss of small vessels (*arrows*).

DECT can also monitor therapy response, with restoration of perfusion noted after treatment[14] (**Fig. 3**).

Nuclear Imaging

Single-photon emission computed tomography

Single-photon emission CT (SPECT) can evaluate regional pulmonary perfusion, particularly when merged with CT.[3] The presence of PH is associated with a significant decrease in gravity-dependent perfusion distribution on SPECT/CT, which correlates with 6-minute walk distance (6MWD) and may be used to quantify response of mPAP to balloon angioplasty in CTEPH.[15,16]

PET

In PAH, there is increased uptake of ^{18}F-labeled fluorodeoxyglucose (FDG) in the RV and pulmonary vasculature, consistent with a transition from oxidative to glycolytic metabolism.[17] Increased FDG uptake occurs early in the course of disease and correlates with hemodynamics and time to clinical worsening, such that it may be a potential marker of severity.[18,19] In patients who respond to treatment, decreases in FDG uptake correlate with improvements in invasive parameters such as PVR and noninvasive metrics such as RV ejection fraction (RVEF) and 6MWD.[18,20] Additional radioligands may also be useful: after the administration of [13]NN-saline, patients with exercise PAH had increased spatial heterogeneity of perfusion compared with normal and resting controls with PAH, suggesting that this group may have a distinct imaging pattern[21] (**Fig. 4**).

Contrast-Enhanced Magnetic Resonance Angiography

Contrast-enhanced magnetic resonance angiography (MRA) provides a detailed structural assessment of pulmonary vessels, although parenchymal resolution is limited. Like CT, PH classes may have distinct patterns on MRA: PAH is often associated with vascular pruning, whereas lung hyperinflation causes splayed vessels in COPD-associated PH.[22] In CTEPH, contrasted MRA can identify more stenoses, poststenotic dilatations, and occlusions than CTA.[23]

MRA can also provide functional information on pulmonary perfusion. Mean transit time (MTT) is the time required for blood to pass from the RV

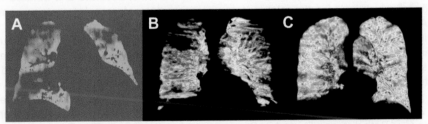

Fig. 3. (*A*) Two-dimensional iodine density map normalized by the contrast density in the main PA and with the large vessels removed in CTEPH. There are patchy areas of decreased perfusion. (*B, C*) Three-dimensional iodine map reconstructions in a patient with clots before (*B*) and after (*C*) treatment.

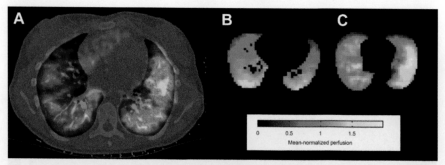

Fig. 4. (A) PET-CT imaging can be used to assess perfusion and its spatial heterogeneity. (B) An example of spatial heterogeneity shows a gradient associated with gravity in a control patient. (C) Loss of this gravity dependence in a patient with exercise PAH. (Images courtesy of Dr. Tilo Winkler, Massachusetts General Hospital.)

to left ventricle (LV), which is calculated as the ratio of pulmonary blood volume to pulmonary blood flow. Flow decreases with increased PVR, although blood volume remains relatively unchanged.[24] MTT is therefore prolonged in PH and correlates with mPAP and PVR, such that it may be useful in noninvasive assessment of disease severity and treatment monitoring.[24]

IMAGING OF PROXIMAL ARTERIES AND RIGHT VENTRICLE–PULMONARY ARTERY COUPLING
Two-Dimensional Phase Contrast MRI

Abnormalities in blood flow can be evaluated with phase contrast MRI (PC-MRI). The phase contrast technique relies on magnetic field gradients that produce phase shifts in nonstationary protons, and not intravenous contrast, to show moving fluid. Two-dimensional PC-MRI quantifies blood flow and velocity through 1 plane, and it can provide detailed information on PA stiffness, pressures, and velocity, as well as RV-PA coupling.[25] Because signal data can be reconstructed into magnitude sequences, PC-MRI also allows anatomic evaluation.[25]

An early hallmark of PH is abnormal pulmonary vasculature stiffness. Increased PA stiffness correlates with functional capacity and mortality in PH and can be assessed by multiple indices on 2D PC-MRI,[25,26] which includes the relative area change (RAC; also termed pulsatility) in the PA lumen during the cardiac cycle. RAC declines with increasing PH severity, with a value of less than 40% sensitive for disease.[26,27] Similarly, PA distensibility (the change in PA area relative to change in pulse pressure) decreases in PH and correlates well with mPAP, RV hypertrophy, and RV dilatation.[27–29] Both distensibility and RAC predict mortality.[29,30] Compliance and capacitance are additional stiffness parameters that correlate

with invasive hemodynamics and carry prognostic significance in PH.[27,28]

Increased PA stiffness promotes pressure increases in PH, and studies have attempted to noninvasively quantify these abnormalities on PC-MRI. Recent analyses defined equations to estimate mPAP based largely on the ventricular mass index (VMI) and the interventricular septal angle.[31,32] Similarly, multiple models for pulmonary capillary wedge pressure (PCWP) have been derived based on either MRI-measured E/e' (peak early mitral inflow velocity divided by peak early diastolic mitral annular velocity) or indexed left atrial volume.[32,33] Furthermore, PVR can also be calculated using MRI-estimated cardiac output and PCWP; an additional model based on RVEF and average PA blood velocity has also been proposed.[32–34] Although these models for mPAP, PCWP, and PVR have moderate to good correlation with hemodynamics on right heart catheterization (RHC), they require validation in large prospective cohorts before widespread use.[32]

Four-Dimensional Phase Contrast MRI

Four-dimensional (4D) PC-MRI is one of the most novel imaging modalities in PH. This sequence uses phase contrast with 3D velocity encoding to evaluate flow in 3 dimensions and time. It can provide the most accurate and detailed noninvasive assessment of vascular anatomy, complex flow patterns, and hemodynamics.[25,35] Four-dimensional PC-MRI can precisely visualize structural abnormalities, including endovascular obstructions such as clots and webs.[36] Furthermore, this imaging modality can reveal the main PA vortices that may develop in PH; these correlate with disease severity and diastolic dysfunction[35,37,38] (**Fig. 5**). Helicity, a measure of laminar flow stability, decreases in PH and correlates with ventricular-vascular coupling.[39] In

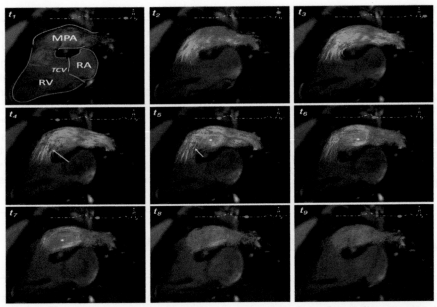

Fig. 5. Two-axis long chamber view of the right heart with superimposed 4D-flow MRI-generated path lines depicting flow through the PA. In midsystole (t4), the generation of physiologic vortices becomes noticeable near the pulmonary valve leaflet (*white arrows*). Further in late systole (T5–T6), a large vortex forms along the inferior aspect of the main PA (*white asterisks*), representing a key finding in PH. This vortex typically prevails for the remainder of the cardiac cycle. The strength and duration of the vortex have been investigated in multiple studies as a potential marker of clinical and hemodynamic outcomes. (Images courtesy of Drs. Michal Schafer and Alex J Barker, University of Colorado, Anschutz Medical Campus.)

addition, 4D PC-MRI shows that wall shear stress (WSS; the force that blood flow exerts on vascular endothelium) is decreased in the proximal vasculature in PH.[40–42] Because low WSS promotes cellular proliferation, this finding is associated with increased arterial stiffness and worsened hemodynamics in PH.[41]

Right Ventricle/Pulmonary Artery Coupling

Abnormal PA stiffness has an early impact on the RV.[26] RV-PA coupling describes the relationship between RV contractility and afterload: when PVR and therefore afterload increases, RV contractility adapts to maintain function and cardiac output until it can no longer compensate.[43] RV-PA coupling is traditionally derived from measurements of pressure, volume, and flow on RHC, but it can be estimated on cardiac MRI (cMRI) by the noninvasive surrogate of RV stroke volume (SV) divided by end-systolic volume (ESV; SV/ESV).[30,43,44]

RV/PA uncoupling occurs early in PH and worsens with increasing disease severity.[43,45] In a small PH cohort, progressive RV-PA uncoupling, reflected by reduced RV SV/ESV, correlated strongly with RVEF less than 35% and was potentially superior to the invasive coupling measurement.[43] Decreased RV SV/ESV is associated with worse survival.[30,46] Because RV-PA uncoupling may precede overt RV failure, it may be useful in early diagnosis, treatment monitoring, and prognostication.

IMAGING OF THE HEART
Transthoracic Echocardiography

Two-dimensional echocardiography

Transthoracic echocardiography (TTE) is the recommended initial screening test for PH.[3,47] RVSP and PA systolic pressure (PASP) are the most commonly assessed parameters in PH and are derived using the peak tricuspid regurgitant jet velocity and the modified Bernoulli equation. Assuming a normal right atrial (RA) pressure, a maximal PASP of 36 mm Hg or 40 mm Hg is generally accepted, although values may be higher in older or obese patients.[48] Correlation between TTE PASP and invasive hemodynamics is variable and is unreliable in some situations.[3,49,50]

Sustained pressure overload in PH results in cardiac remodeling. Increased RA area is associated with worse survival in PAH.[47] RV hypertrophy with subsequent dilatation are common and suggest long-standing disease. Interventricular septal flattening may occur in systole and diastole from RV pressure and volume overload, respectively, and can be measured by the left ventricular eccentricity index. This index correlates with mortality, as does the presence of a pericardial effusion.[48,51]

RV function predicts survival in PH and can also be assessed by multiple parameters on TTE. Although the estimation of RVEF is difficult on 2D echocardiography, the surrogate metric of RV fractional area change (FAC) correlates with treatment response and prognosis.[48] RV longitudinal function is measured by the tricuspid annular plane systolic excursion (TAPSE), the systolic

Strain Imaging

Strain imaging techniques can be used in both 2D and 3D echocardiography. Measured by color tissue Doppler imaging or speckle tracking, strain is the change in myocardial length that reflects myocardial deformation. Decreases in longitudinal RV strain and strain rate correlate with RV dysfunction and mortality.[56,57] Moreover, in a series of 37 patients with PAH, 2D RV strain and strain rate improved with vasodilator treatment (as did symptoms and hemodynamics) such that these markers may reflect therapeutic response.[56]

$$Tei\ index = \frac{RV\ isovolumetric\ contraction\ time + RV\ isovolumetric\ relaxation\ time}{ejection\ time}$$

displacement of the tricuspid annulus toward the RV apex. A value less than 1.6 cm is abnormal; however, even a TAPSE less than 1.8 cm is associated with RV systolic dysfunction, higher PVR, and shorter survival in PH.[52] In addition, the RV myocardial performance index (Tei index) measures both systolic and diastolic RV function:

A higher Tei index indicates RV dysfunction and correlates with worse hemodynamics and survival in PAH, as well as treatment response.[48]

Three-dimensional echocardiography

Three-dimensional echocardiography is an emerging advanced technique to evaluate right-sided geometry and function. With sustained pressure overload, RA dilatation occurs predominantly along the short axis, toward the free wall.[53] Although dilatation can be assessed by length, diameter, or area on 2D echocardiography, the RA sphericity index has been proposed as a 3D surrogate. It incorporates both length and diameter and is measured as the RA short axis parallel to the tricuspid annulus at the midcavity, divided by the RA long axis perpendicular to the tricuspid annulus at end systole. In 62 patients with PAH, an increase in RA sphericity index greater than 0.24 correlated with clinical deterioration.[53] Other parameters of remodeling can also be assessed. Three-dimensional echocardiography is more accurate than the 2D modality in estimating RV volumes and RVEF, using cardiac MRI as the reference.[48,54] Moreover, 3D TTE suggests that patterns of remodeling vary between PH subgroups: among 141 patients with PH, RV diastolic dilatation and RVEF reductions were greater in PAH than in CTEPH and mitral regurgitation–related PH.[55]

Different types of PH have distinct RV strain patterns on 3D speckle tracking[58] (**Fig. 6**). Although strain imaging is less load and geometry dependent than other echocardiographic techniques, there is variation between systems, and accurate assessment depends on resolution.[58] Two-dimensional strain imaging is also limited by cardiac movement that restricts the plane of view.[58]

Cardiac MRI

cMRI is the gold standard for the assessment of cardiac structure and function. Because it is highly accurate and reproducible, it also has a growing role in determining prognosis and treatment response.[59] Although the exact sequences vary between institutions and imaging indications, standard cMRI protocols usually incorporate both anatomic and functional assessments.[60]

Structural Parameters

As PH worsens, structural abnormalities that relate to risk and prognosis become common. RV hypertrophy is an early change that is reflected by an increased VMI[36,61]:

$$VMI = \frac{RV\ mass}{LV\ mass}$$

In 233 patients with suspected PH, VMI was the cMRI parameter that correlated most strongly with mPAP and that had the highest diagnostic accuracy for PH.[62]

After initial adaptation, including hypertrophy, the RV dilates in response to a continued afterload.[63] This dilatation leads to larger RV end-diastolic and end-systolic volumes on cMRI.[64] In 64 patients with idiopathic PAH (IPAH), an RV

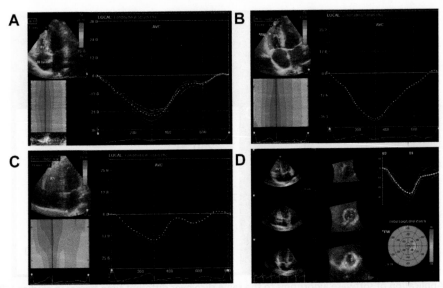

Fig. 6. Representative images using speckle tracking to estimate local strain by tracking the relative motion of features (speckles) in the cardiac cycle. (*A*) Global longitudinal right ventricular strain in a normal patient with maximum strain estimated as 28%. (*B*) Regional free wall (FW) strain in a normal patient, estimated as 36%. (*C*) There is a reduction in the global FW strain in PH, with estimated strain of 13%. (*D*) These data can be summarized in a multiview format (shown for a normal patient). FW is labeled by asterisks. AVC, aortic valve closure; ED, end diastolic; ES, end systolic. (Adapted with permission from Vitarelli et al. (Vitarelli A, Mangieri E, Terzano C, et al. 'Three-Dimensional Echocardiography and 2D-3D Speckle-Tracking Imaging in Chronic Pulmonary Hypertension: Diagnostic Accuracy in Detecting Hemodynamic Signs of Right Ventricular Failure; Journal of American Heart Association; Wiley. ©2015 The Authors. Published on behalf of the American Heart Association, Inc., by Wiley Blackwell).)

end-diastolic volume index greater than or equal to 84 mL/m² on cMRI correlated with worse survival, and progressive RV dilatation was one of the strongest predictors of 1-year mortality.[65] RV end-systolic volume is also an independent predictor of death in PH, which likely reflects depressed systolic function.[30]

Right heart failure drives septal and LV dysfunction. Septal curvature correlates with systolic PA pressure (sPAP) on RHC, with the presence of any leftward bowing indicating an sPAP greater than 67 mm Hg.[66] Leftward septal displacement promotes LV underfilling, which results in decreased LV SV, peak filling rate, and end-diastolic volume, the last of which is associated with mortality.[64,65,67] Valvular structures can also be evaluated on cMRI.

Functional Parameters

Multiple RV functional parameters can be examined on cMRI. Reduced RVEF is a predictor of mortality, potentially even stronger than PVR, and has prognostic implications during follow-up.[59,68,69] Additional functional surrogates on cMRI include TAPSE and RV FAC, the latter of which predicts survival.[69,70] Similarly, RV SV may

be reduced in PH. Diminished SV correlates with mortality in IPAH, and a progressive decrease despite treatment predicts therapeutic failure.[65] A change in SV as small as 10 cm³ has been identified as clinically significant.[71] Because cardiac chamber volumes can be assessed throughout the cardiac cycle, complex functional parameters, including RV-PA coupling, can also be evaluated (**Fig. 7**).

Advanced Techniques

Advanced MRI techniques can be applied to evaluate cardiac parameters. Similar to its use in evaluating the pulmonary vasculature, 4D PC-MRI can measure multiple cardiac parameters, including shunt fraction, RV kinetic work, and tricuspid regurgitation flow and volume.[25,72] Peak velocity of the regurgitant tricuspid jet can be used to calculate sPAP, which correlates well with invasive hemodynamics.[25]

Myocardial abnormalities can be evaluated with late gadolinium enhancement (LGE). LGE generally appears on T1-weighted pulse sequences as enhancement at the anterior and posterior insertion points of the RV into the interventricular septum shortly after contrast administration. The

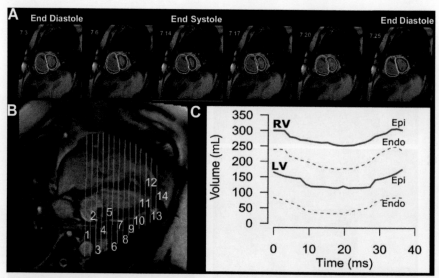

Fig. 7. (*A*) Application of software algorithms to the same slice over different time frames in cardiac MRI. Can be used (*B*) to measure the endocardial and epicardial boundaries of the ventricles and (*C*) to estimate ventricular volumes over the cardiac cycle. In addition to deriving measures such as right ventricular ejection fraction and end-diastolic volumes, this can be used to construct pressure-volume loops and assess complex metrics, including RV-arterial coupling. Endo, endocardial; Epi, epicardial.

mass of late-enhancing myocardium correlates with mPAP, cardiac index, and clinical worsening, suggesting LGE may be a noninvasive tool to assess the degree of RV remodeling and dysfunction.[73,74]

T1 mapping is an emerging technique to measure myocardial relaxation time. Higher T1 times reflect fibrosis; in PH, this may be diffuse or focal at ventricular insertion points.[35] Higher relaxation T1 mapping correlates with worse hemodynamics and coupling in animals; its utility in humans, including predicting prognosis, is unclear.[75,76]

Strain may also be evaluated with feature tracking on cMRI. Depressed RV longitudinal strain and rate correlate with worse outcomes, including clinical decompensation, transplant, and death in PH.[77]

Advantages and Limitations

cMRI is highly reproducible and sensitive to small changes, such that it is ideal for monitoring treatment response in PH. Patients are not exposed to ionizing radiation, and the contrast agents are nontoxic unless an allergy or concurrent renal disease is present.[64] Limitations include duration of breath hold and potential for MRI-incompatible implants. Patients with arrhythmias and chronic kidney disease require special consideration, including use of prospective gating and avoidance of contrast, respectively.[22] Other factors that have limited its use include lack of widespread availability, significant protocol variability between centers,

and potential for prohibitive cost. However, these limitations are evolving and represent progressively less of a barrier.

SUMMARY AND FUTURE DIRECTIONS

Imaging plays an important role in the diagnosis and monitoring of PH. Reliance on patient symptoms alone often leads to the diagnosis of advanced PVD, and noninvasive imaging is a key tool for earlier detection. A growing awareness of the importance of timely diagnosis has also led to the recognition of exercise PH (EPH), an inappropriate pulmonary vascular response to exertion that is potentially a precursor to manifest disease. On cMRI, patients with EPH have PA stiffening with reduced compliance and capacitance and infrequent main PA vortices, both of which are absent in healthy controls.[26,37] Although the current diagnosis of both EPH and borderline PH requires invasive exercise testing, imaging may ultimately provide a noninvasive bridge to screening and early recognition. Furthermore, cMRI will likely also be important in monitoring treatment response, given its correlations with hemodynamics and prognosis.

There is also growing interest in the noninvasive classification of PH. Although cMRI is useful for heart and central pulmonary vessel evaluation, CT imaging, particularly DECT, is likely to be useful in phenotyping PH in the distal vasculature. Nuclear studies such as PET scans may play a role in understanding the molecular basis of disease.

In conjunction with genetic and environmental data, imaging will likely be an important part of personalized medicine in PH.

Imaging is essential in the noninvasive assessment, treatment monitoring, and risk stratification of patients with PVD. Advanced imaging techniques have led to an improved understanding of disease pathophysiology, the ability to perform highly accurate and detailed cardiopulmonary evaluations, and the advent of early noninvasive biomarkers for predicting prognosis. As the treatment of PVD continues toward personalized medicine, imaging will likely play a critical role in early disease recognition, therapeutic monitoring, risk stratification, and prognostication.

CLINICS CARE POINTS

- The advent of advanced imaging modalities has allowed for detailed anatomical visualization and functional assessment of the cardiopulmonary circuit in pulmonary vascular disease.
- Cardiac magnetic resonance imaging (MRI) in particular is highly accurate, sensitive, and reproducible and correlates well with clinical outcomes. As such, it likely will serve a particularly important role in evaluating RV function and may ultimately be a useful noninvasive clinical metric.
- The use of advanced imaging techniques to noninvasively assess hemodynamics is also under investigation.
- The use of cardiac MRI and other techniques is currently limited by the lack of widespread availability and variation between protocols; however, these barriers continue to evolve.

DISCLOSURE

The authors have nothing to disclose.

REFERENCES

1. Nathan SD, Barbera JA, Gaine SP, et al. Pulmonary hypertension in chronic lung disease and hypoxia. Eur Respir J 2019;53(1):1801914.
2. Kligerman SJ, Henry T, Lin CT, et al. Mosaic attenuation: etiology, methods of differentiation, and pitfalls. Radiographics 2015;35(5):1360–80.
3. Kiely DG, Levin D, Hassoun P, et al. EXPRESS: statement on imaging and pulmonary hypertension from the pulmonary vascular research institute (PVRI). Pulm Circ 2019;9(3). 2045894019841990.
4. Tan RT, Kuzo R, Goodman LR, et al. Utility of CT scan evaluation for predicting pulmonary hypertension in patients with parenchymal lung disease. Medical college of Wisconsin lung transplant group. Chest 1998;113(5):1250–6.
5. Shen Y, Wan C, Tian P, et al. CT-base pulmonary artery measurement in the detection of pulmonary hypertension: a meta-analysis and systematic review. Medicine 2014;93(27):e256.
6. Grosse A, Grosse C, Lang IM. Distinguishing chronic thromboembolic pulmonary hypertension from other causes of pulmonary hypertension using CT. Am J Roentgenol 2017;209(6):1228–38.
7. Matsuoka S, Washko GR, Yamashiro T, et al. Pulmonary hypertension and computed tomography measurement of small pulmonary vessels in severe emphysema. Am J Respir Crit Care Med 2010;181(3):218–25.
8. Rahaghi FN, Ross JC, Agarwal M, et al. Pulmonary vascular morphology as an imaging biomarker in chronic thromboembolic pulmonary hypertension. Pulm Circ 2016;6(1):70–81.
9. Helmberger M, Pienn M, Urschler M, et al. Quantification of tortuosity and fractal dimension of the lung vessels in pulmonary hypertension patients. PloS one 2014;9(1):e87515.
10. Rahaghi FN, Vegas-Sanchez-Ferrero G, Minhas JK, et al. Ventricular geometry from non-contrast Non-ECG-gated CT Scans: an imaging marker of cardiopulmonary disease in smokers. Acad Radiol 2017; 24(5):594–602.
11. Aviram G, Rozenbaum Z, Ziv-Baran T, et al. Identification of pulmonary hypertension caused by left-sided heart disease (world health organization group 2) based on cardiac chamber volumes derived from chest CT imaging. Chest 2017;152(4):792–9.
12. Ameli-Renani S, Rahman F, Nair A, et al. Dual-energy CT for imaging of pulmonary hypertension: challenges and opportunities. RadioGraphics 2014;34(7):1769–90.
13. Giordano J, Khung S, Duhamel A, et al. Lung perfusion characteristics in pulmonary arterial hypertension (PAH) and peripheral forms of chronic thromboembolic pulmonary hypertension (pCTEPH): dual-energy CT experience in 31 patients. Eur Radiol 2017;27(4):1631–9.
14. Koike H, Sueyoshi E, Sakamoto I, et al. Comparative clinical and predictive value of lung perfusion blood volume CT, lung perfusion SPECT and catheter pulmonary angiography images in patients with chronic thromboembolic pulmonary hypertension before and after balloon pulmonary angioplasty. Eur Radiol 2018;28(12):5091–9.
15. Lau EM, Bailey DL, Bailey EA, et al. Pulmonary hypertension leads to a loss of gravity dependent redistribution of regional lung perfusion: a SPECT/CT study. Heart 2014;100(1):47–53.
16. Maruoka Y, Nagao M, Baba S, et al. Three-dimensional fractal analysis of 99mTc-MAA SPECT images in chronic thromboembolic pulmonary hypertension for evaluation of response to balloon

pulmonary angioplasty: association with pulmonary arterial pressure. Nucl Med Commun 2017;38(6): 480–6.

17. Boucherat O, Vitry G, Trinh I, et al. The cancer theory of pulmonary arterial hypertension. Pulm Circ 2017; 7(2):285–99.

18. Oikawa M, Kagaya Y, Otani H, et al. Increased [18F] fluorodeoxyglucose accumulation in right ventricular free wall in patients with pulmonary hypertension and the effect of epoprostenol. J Am Coll Cardiol 2005;45(11):1849–55.

19. Tatebe S, Fukumoto Y, Oikawa-Wakayama M, et al. Enhanced [18F]fluorodeoxyglucose accumulation in the right ventricular free wall predicts long-term prognosis of patients with pulmonary hypertension: a preliminary observational study. Eur Heart J Cardiovasc Imaging 2014;15(6):666–72.

20. Saygin D, Highland KB, Farha S, et al. Metabolic and functional evaluation of the heart and lungs in pulmonary hypertension by gated 2-[18F]-Fluoro-2-deoxy-D-glucose positron emission tomography. Pulm Circ 2017;7(2):428–38.

21. Kohli P, Kelly VJ, Kehl EG, et al. Perfusion imaging distinguishes exercise pulmonary arterial hypertension at rest. Am J Respir Crit Care Med 2019; 199(11):1438–41.

22. Swift AJ, Wild JM, Nagle SK, et al. Quantitative magnetic resonance imaging of pulmonary hypertension: a practical approach to the current state of the art. J Thorac Imaging 2014;29(2):68–79.

23. Rajaram S, Swift AJ, Capener D, et al. Diagnostic accuracy of contrast-enhanced MR angiography and unenhanced proton MR imaging compared with CT pulmonary angiography in chronic thromboembolic pulmonary hypertension. Eur Radiol 2012; 22(2):310–7.

24. Ohno Y, Hatabu H, Murase K, et al. Primary pulmonary hypertension: 3D dynamic perfusion MRI for quantitative analysis of regional pulmonary perfusion. AJR Am J Roentgenol 2007;188(1): 48–56.

25. Reiter U, Reiter G, Fuchsjäger M. MR phase-contrast imaging in pulmonary hypertension. Br J Radiol 2016;89(1063):20150995.

26. Sanz J, Kariisa M, Dellegrottaglie S, et al. Evaluation of pulmonary artery stiffness in pulmonary hypertension with cardiac magnetic resonance. JACC Cardiovasc Imaging 2009;2(3):286–95.

27. Ray JC, Burger C, Mergo P, et al. Pulmonary arterial stiffness assessed by cardiovascular magnetic resonance imaging is a predictor of mild pulmonary arterial hypertension. Int J Cardiovasc Imaging 2019;35(10):1881–92.

28. Stevens GR, Garcia-Alvarez A, Sahni S, et al. RV dysfunction in pulmonary hypertension is independently related to pulmonary artery stiffness. JACC Cardiovasc Imaging 2012;5(4):378–87.

29. Gan CT, Lankhaar JW, Westerhof N, et al. Noninvasively assessed pulmonary artery stiffness predicts mortality in pulmonary arterial hypertension. Chest 2007;132(6):1906–12.

30. Swift AJ, Capener D, Johns C, et al. Magnetic resonance imaging in the prognostic evaluation of patients with pulmonary arterial hypertension. Am J Respir Crit Care Med 2017;196(2):228–39.

31. Johns CS, Kiely DG, Rajaram S, et al. Diagnosis of pulmonary hypertension with cardiac MRI: derivation and validation of regression models. Radiology 2019;290(1):61–8.

32. Swift AJ, Rajaram S, Hurdman J, et al. Noninvasive estimation of PA pressure, flow, and resistance with CMR imaging: derivation and prospective validation study from the ASPIRE registry. JACC Cardiovasc Imaging 2013;6(10):1036–47.

33. Bane O, Shah SJ, Cuttica MJ, et al. A non-invasive assessment of cardiopulmonary hemodynamics with sMRI in pulmonary hypertension. Magn Reson Imaging 2015;33(10):1224–35.

34. García-Alvarez A, Fernández-Friera L, Mirelis JG, et al. Non-invasive estimation of pulmonary vascular resistance with cardiac magnetic resonance. Eur Heart J 2011;32(19):2438–45.

35. Freed BH, Collins JD, François CJ, et al. MR and CT imaging for the evaluation of pulmonary hypertension. JACC Cardiovasc Imaging 2016;9(6): 715–32.

36. Peacock AJ, Vonk Noordegraaf A. Cardiac magnetic resonance imaging in pulmonary arterial hypertension. Eur Respir Rev 2013;22(130):526.

37. Reiter G, Reiter U, Kovacs G, et al. Magnetic resonance-derived 3-dimensional blood flow patterns in the main pulmonary artery as a marker of pulmonary hypertension and a measure of elevated mean pulmonary arterial pressure. Circ Cardiovasc Imaging 2008;1(1):23–30.

38. Reiter G, Reiter U, Kovacs G, et al. Blood flow vortices along the main pulmonary artery measured with MR imaging for diagnosis of pulmonary hypertension. Radiology 2015;275(1):71–9.

39. Schafer M, Barker AJ, Kheyfets V, et al. Helicity and vorticity of pulmonary arterial flow in patients with pulmonary hypertension: quantitative analysis of flow formations. J Am Heart Assoc 2017;6(12): e007010.

40. Paszkowiak JJ, Dardik A. Arterial wall shear stress: observations from the bench to the bedside. Vasc Endovascular Surg 2003;37(1):47–57.

41. Schäfer M, Kheyfets VO, Schroeder JD, et al. Main pulmonary arterial wall shear stress correlates with invasive hemodynamics and stiffness in pulmonary hypertension. Pulm Circ 2016;6(1):37–45.

42. Tang BT, Pickard SS, Chan FP, et al. Wall shear stress is decreased in the pulmonary arteries of patients with pulmonary arterial hypertension: an

image-based, computational fluid dynamics study. Pulm Circ 2012;2(4):470–6.

43. Tello K, Dalmer A, Axmann J, et al. Reserve of right ventricular-arterial coupling in the setting of chronic overload. Circ Heart Fail 2019;12(1):e005512.

44. Sanz J, Garcia-Alvarez A, Fernandez-Friera L, et al. Right ventriculo-arterial coupling in pulmonary hypertension: a magnetic resonance study. Heart 2012;98(3):238–43.

45. Singh I, Rahaghi FN, Naeije R, et al. Dynamic right ventricular-pulmonary arterial uncoupling during maximum incremental exercise in exercise pulmonary hypertension and pulmonary arterial hypertension. Pulm Circ 2019;9(3). 2045894019862435-2045894019862435.

46. Vanderpool RR, Pinsky MR, Naeije R, et al. RV-pulmonary arterial coupling predicts outcome in patients referred for pulmonary hypertension. Heart 2015;101(1):37–43.

47. Galiè N, Humbert M, Vachiery J-L, et al. 2015 ESC/ERS Guidelines for the diagnosis and treatment of pulmonary hypertension. Eur Respir J 2015;46(4):903.

48. Bossone E, D'Andrea A, D'Alto M, et al. Echocardiography in pulmonary arterial hypertension: from diagnosis to prognosis. J Am Soc Echocardiogr 2013;26(1):1–14.

49. Taleb M, Khuder S, Tinkel J, et al. The diagnostic accuracy of Doppler echocardiography in assessment of pulmonary artery systolic pressure: a meta-analysis. Echocardiography 2013;30(3):258–65.

50. Parasuraman S, Walker S, Loudon BL, et al. Assessment of pulmonary artery pressure by echocardiography-A comprehensive review. Int J Cardiol Heart Vasc 2016;12:45–51.

51. Ghio S, Klersy C, Magrini G, et al. Prognostic relevance of the echocardiographic assessment of right ventricular function in patients with idiopathic pulmonary arterial hypertension. Int J Cardiol 2010;140(3):272–8.

52. Forfia PR, Fisher MR, Mathai SC, et al. Tricuspid annular displacement predicts survival in pulmonary hypertension. Am J Respir Crit Care Med 2006;174(9):1034–41.

53. Grapsa J, Gibbs JS, Cabrita IZ, et al. The association of clinical outcome with right atrial and ventricular remodelling in patients with pulmonary arterial hypertension: study with real-time three-dimensional echocardiography. Eur Heart J Cardiovasc Imaging 2012;13(8):666–72.

54. Grapsa J, O'Regan DP, Pavlopoulos H, et al. Right ventricular remodelling in pulmonary arterial hypertension with three-dimensional echocardiography: comparison with cardiac magnetic resonance imaging. Eur J Echocardiogr 2010;11(1):64–73.

55. Grapsa J, Gibbs JS, Dawson D, et al. Morphologic and functional remodeling of the right ventricle in pulmonary hypertension by real time three dimensional echocardiography. Am J Cardiol 2012;109(6):906–13.

56. Borges AC, Knebel F, Eddicks S, et al. Right ventricular function assessed by two-dimensional strain and tissue Doppler echocardiography in patients with pulmonary arterial hypertension and effect of vasodilator therapy. Am J Cardiol 2006;98(4):530–4.

57. Sachdev A, Villarraga HR, Frantz RP, et al. Right ventricular strain for prediction of survival in patients with pulmonary arterial hypertension. Chest 2011;139(6):1299–309.

58. Vitarelli A, Mangieri E, Terzano C, et al. Three-dimensional echocardiography and 2D-3D speckle-tracking imaging in chronic pulmonary hypertension: diagnostic accuracy in detecting hemodynamic signs of right ventricular (RV) failure. J Am Heart Assoc 2015;4(3):e001584.

59. Peacock AJ, Crawley S, McLure L, et al. Changes in right ventricular function measured by cardiac magnetic resonance imaging in patients receiving pulmonary arterial hypertension-targeted therapy: the EURO-MR study. Circ Cardiovasc Imaging 2014;7(1):107–14.

60. Kramer CM, Barkhausen J, Flamm SD, et al. Standardized cardiovascular magnetic resonance (CMR) protocols 2013 update. J Cardiovasc Magn Reson 2013;15:91.

61. Wang N, Hu X, Liu C, et al. A systematic review of the diagnostic accuracy of cardiovascular magnetic resonance for pulmonary hypertension. Can J Cardiol 2014;30(4):455–63.

62. Swift AJ, Rajaram S, Condliffe R, et al. Diagnostic accuracy of cardiovascular magnetic resonance imaging of right ventricular morphology and function in the assessment of suspected pulmonary hypertension results from the ASPIRE registry. J Cardiovasc Magn Reson 2012;14(1):40.

63. Voelkel NF, Quaife RA, Leinwand LA, et al. Right ventricular function and failure. Circulation 2006;114(17):1883–91.

64. McLure LER, Peacock AJ. Cardiac magnetic resonance imaging for the assessment of the heart and pulmonary circulation in pulmonary hypertension. Eur Respir J 2009;33(6):1454.

65. van Wolferen SA, Marcus JT, Boonstra A, et al. Prognostic value of right ventricular mass, volume, and function in idiopathic pulmonary arterial hypertension. Eur Heart J 2007;28(10):1250–7.

66. Roeleveld RJ, Marcus JT, Faes TJ, et al. Interventricular septal configuration at mr imaging and pulmonary arterial pressure in pulmonary hypertension. Radiology 2005;234(3):710–7.

67. Gan C, Lankhaar JW, Marcus JT, et al. Impaired left ventricular filling due to right-to-left ventricular interaction in patients with pulmonary arterial

hypertension. Am J Physiol Heart Circ Physiol 2006; 290(4):H1528–33.

68. van de Veerdonk MC, Kind T, Marcus JT, et al. Progressive right ventricular dysfunction in patients with pulmonary arterial hypertension responding to therapy. J Am Coll Cardiol 2011;58(24):2511–9.

69. Mauritz GJ, Kind T, Marcus JT, et al. Progressive changes in right ventricular geometric shortening and long-term survival in pulmonary arterial hypertension. Chest 2012;141(4):935–43.

70. Nijveldt R, Germans T, McCann GP, et al. Semiquantitative assessment of right ventricular function in comparison to a 3D volumetric approach: a cardiovascular magnetic resonance study. Eur Radiol 2008;18(11):2399–405.

71. van Wolferen SA, van de Veerdonk MC, Mauritz GJ, et al. Clinically significant change in stroke volume in pulmonary hypertension. Chest 2011;139(5): 1003–9.

72. Westenberg JJ, Roes SD, Ajmone Marsan N, et al. Mitral valve and tricuspid valve blood flow: accurate quantification with 3D velocity-encoded MR imaging with retrospective valve tracking. Radiology 2008; 249(3):792–800.

73. Shehata ML, Lossnitzer D, Skrok J, et al. Myocardial delayed enhancement in pulmonary hypertension:

pulmonary hemodynamics, right ventricular function, and remodeling. AJR Am J Roentgenol 2011; 196(1):87–94.

74. Freed BH, Gomberg-Maitland M, Chandra S, et al. Late gadolinium enhancement cardiovascular magnetic resonance predicts clinical worsening in patients with pulmonary hypertension. J Cardiovasc Magn Reson 2012;14:11.

75. Garcia-Alvarez A, Garcia-Lunar I, Pereda D, et al. Association of myocardial T1-mapping CMR with hemodynamics and RV performance in pulmonary hypertension. JACC Cardiovasc Imaging 2015;8(1): 76–82.

76. Saunders LC, Johns CS, Stewart NJ, et al. Diagnostic and prognostic significance of cardiovascular magnetic resonance native myocardial T1 mapping in patients with pulmonary hypertension. J Cardiovasc Magn Reson 2018;20(1):78.

77. de Siqueira MEM, Pozo E, Fernandes VR, et al. Characterization and clinical significance of right ventricular mechanics in pulmonary hypertension evaluated with cardiovascular magnetic resonance feature tracking. J Cardiovasc Magn Reson 2016; 18(1):39.

The Role of Exercise Testing in Pulmonary Vascular Disease
Diagnosis and Management

David Systrom, MD[a,1], Arabella Warren[a,1], Robert Naeije, MD, PhD[b,*]

KEYWORDS

- Exercise intolerance • Pulmonary hypertension • Exercise capacity • Cardiopulmonary exercise test
- Unexplained dyspnea • Pulmonary vascular disease

KEY POINTS

- Because of the quasilinear correlations between oxygen uptake, speed, and workload, 12-minute run or 6-minute walk distances can be used as simple surrogates of VO2max.
- Pulmonary hypertension is associated with a decreased aerobic exercise capacity. Exercise testing in pulmonary hypertension allows for the assessment of functional impairment and prognostication.
- Combining hemodynamic measurements and CPET allows for the diagnosis of early or latent pulmonary hypertension and exercise-induced right heart failure.

INTRODUCTION

Pulmonary vascular disease is a common complication of cardiac and pulmonary disease, but may occur independently as pulmonary arterial hypertension (PAH) or chronic thromboembolic pulmonary hypertension (CTEPH). PAH is a disease of the resistive vessels of the pulmonary circulation. CTEPH is caused by organized clots, which predominate in the proximal part of the pulmonary arterial tree, but often extend to the periphery and combine with pulmonary vascular remodeling in nonobstructed areas. Symptoms of dyspnea and fatigue are common to pulmonary vascular disease and causal cardiac or pulmonary conditions.[1] This article focuses on PAH and analyzes the special influence of pulmonary vascular disease on exercise capacity. The derived notions are often transposable to CTEPH and left heart failure.

Although the principles of exercise testing were established several decades ago,[2] this article summarizes their modern applications in supporting evidence that pulmonary vascular disease is a cause of pulmonary hypertension (PH) and exercise intolerance.

BASIC NOTIONS
Aerobic Exercise Capacity

The body's ability to deliver oxygen to exercising muscles via the integration of connective and diffusive transport systems involving the heart, lungs, and circulation is critical for performing daily activities. Muscle work may be transiently performed in lactic or alactic anaerobic resistive

Solve ME/CFS initiative Open Medicine Foundation (Dr. David Systrom and Arabella Warren).
[a] Brigham and Women's Hospital, Harvard Medical School, Boston, MA, USA; [b] Free University of Brussels, Brussels, Belgium
[1] Present address: 75 Francis Street, PBB CA-3, Boston 02115.
* Corresponding author. Department of Pathophysiology, Faculty of Medicine, Free University of Brussels, Lennik Road 808, Brussels B-1070, Belgium,
E-mail address: rnaeije@gmail.com

conditions. However, this is accompanied by an eventual increase in metabolic rate, increased oxygen uptake (Vo_2), output of carbon dioxide (Vco_2), and proportional increases in cardiac output (Q) and ventilation (V_E), all characteristic of aerobic exercise.

If the typical plateau for Vo_2 versus work rate cannot be demonstrated at maximal exercise, an individual's capacity for aerobic work is defined by a symptom-limited maximum O_2 uptake (Vo_{2max}), or peak O_2 uptake (Vo_{2peak}). Vo_{2max} and Vo_{2peak} are usually in agreement, provided care is taken to accept the measurement at a respiratory exchange ratio (RER) of at least 1.1.

According to the Fick principle, a Vo_{2max} is equal to the product of the maximal values of Q and the arteriovenous oxygen content difference, $C(a - v)$ O_2.

$$Vo_{2max} = Q_{max} \times C(a - v)O_{2max}$$

Although Vo_2 is measured in liters per minute, it is also expressed as per kilogram of body weight to allow for intersubject comparisons. Resting energy expenditure corresponds to a Vo_2 of approximately 3.5 mL/kg/min. Maximal Vo_2 is affected by age, sex, conditioning status, and the presence of disease. World-class male endurance athletes may achieve a Vo_{2max} of 80 to 90 mL/kg/min. Healthy young adults present with a Vo_{2max} of 35 to 45 mL/kg/min. Aerobic exercise capacity decreases by 8% to 10% per decade. With the exception of very old subjects, a Vo_{2max} should normally exceed 20 to 25 mL/kg/min. Vo_{2max} is in the range of 10 to 15 mL/kg/min in advanced PAH. The Vo_{2max} may also be expressed as a percent of predicted, derived from normative population studies and adjusted for age, gender, and an estimate of lean muscle mass drive from height.

Vo_{2max} is achieved by exercise involving approximately half of the body's total musculature. Therefore, it is reasonable to assume that maximal aerobic exercise capacity is determined by maximal cardiac output, rather than by peripheral factors. Furthermore, the oxyhemoglobin dissociation curve has a sigmoidal shape, whereby the flattening of the curve at low- and high-partial pressures of O_2 (Po_2) correspond to increased affinity of hemoglobin for O_2. There are upper and lower limits for O_2 content, with extremes for low Cvo_2 that are similar in healthy athletes and cardiac patients. At maximal exercise, Cvo_2 becomes a constant in the Fick equation, and Vo_{2max} is exclusively dependent on the product of Q and CaO_2, or DO_2, which expresses convectional O_2 transport to exercising muscles.

$$DO_{2max} = Q_{max} \times Cao_2$$

Flow dependency of skeletal muscle Vo_2 in healthy subjects and heart failure patients has been repeatedly demonstrated.[3] Jondeau and colleagues[4] reasoned that a skeletal muscle limitation to aerobic exercise capacity in heart failure permitted the adding of more muscle during a standard incremental cardiopulmonary exercise test (CPET) to increase Vo_{2max}. The investigators showed that combining arm ergometry with a standard bicycle ergometer incremental CPET did not increase Vo_{2max}, with the exception of the most severely ill patients. The Vo_{2max} measurement can be explained by either an alteration in O_2 extraction by skeletal muscle or by insufficient remaining leg muscle mass in cachectic cardiac patients. A maximal challenge of the cardiovascular O_2 transport system requires at least 10 to 12 kg of working muscle. A very low femoral Cvo_2 was observed in heart failure patients with either preserved or reduced ejection fraction (HFpEF and HFrEF) at peak exercise[5] in the range reported in endurance-trained athletes.[6] A low Cvo_2 provides some evidence against a skeletal muscle limitation to Vo_{2max} in heart failure.

The Ventilatory Limitation to Exercise Capacity

Although exercise capacity is primarily limited by cardiac output (or O_2 delivery) in normal subjects and in patients with cardiac conditions, lung diseases may be associated with a mechanical limitation to increased ventilation. In normal conditions, maximum exercise V_E (V_{Emax}) averages at 50% to 80% of a 12- to 15-second maximum voluntary ventilation (MVV). MMV can be estimated from the forced expiratory volume in 1 second (FEV1) in the equation:

$$MVV = 40 \times FEV1$$

The average difference between MVV and V_{Emax} is normally around 40 L/min. Whether MVV is directly measured or estimated from the FEV1 produces no significant difference. A patient is described as ventilatory limited when the ventilatory reserve is less than 11 L/min or V_E/MVV is greater than 70%. Patients with chronic obstructive pulmonary disease (COPD) typically present with a V_{Emax} that is equal or close to MVV, with a maximal RER lower than 1.1.[7,8] In the absence of coexistent parenchymal lung disease, patients with congestive heart failure or PAH have a preserved ventilatory reserve.[9]

Measurements at the Ventilatory Threshold

Most daily activities do not require a maximal effort. Therefore, a widely used submaximal index of exercise capacity is the lactate, anaerobic, or ventilatory threshold (VT), defined by the exercise level at which ventilation begins to increase exponentially for a given increment in Vo_2. This increase in ventilation is necessary for the elimination of excess CO_2 produced during the buffering of lactate and the muscle metabolic reflex, which contributes to increased chemosensitivity. The VT usually occurs at 50% to 65% of the Vo_{2max} in healthy untrained subjects but increases with endurance training. Interestingly, the VT expressed in % of VO_{2peak} is increased in PAH and severe congestive heart failure.[9] The measurement of VT relies on the V-slope method, based on the departure of Vco_2 from a line of identity drawn through a plot of Vco_2 versus Vo_2. Measuring Vo_2 at the VT instead of Vo_{2max} requires a less strenuous test and improves safety. However, identifying VT can be difficult, particularly in patients with severe heart failure or those experiencing early lactic acidosis. It should be noted that VT is less reproducible than VO_{2peak} or Vo_{2max}.

During a CPET, V_E/Vco_2 is measured as a slope, or preferably as a fraction at the VT. V_E/Vco_2 is expressed as a function of arterial Pco_2 and provides a measure of chemosensitivity. The expression of V_E/Vco_2 as a function of end-tidal Pco_2 integrates the effects of physiologic dead space and chemosensitivity during the ventilatory response to exercise.[10] The ventilatory equivalent for CO_2 is preferably measured at the VT because the anatomic dead space decreases with respect to tidal volume along with exercise-induced increase in V_E, which allows for improved estimation of physiologic dead space. However, above the VT, an increase in V_E is no longer proportional to metabolic demand owing to muscle metaboreflex and the chemoreflex effects of acidosis. Therefore, V_E/Vco_2 expressed as a function of workload or Vo_2 produces a U shape in normal subjects. This U shape is less apparent in patients with cardiopulmonary conditions.

The 6-Minute Walk Test

The linear relationship between Vo_2, Q, and workload permits the substitution of VO_{2peak} with running or walking speed, measured as a 12-minute run distance in normal subjects[11] or as a 6-minute walk distance (6MWD) by patients in hospital corridors.[12] However, Vo_{2peak} and the 6MWD are not consistently tightly related, with coefficient correlations of 0.5 to 0.7 depending on studies and population sizes. A lack of consistency is due to the individual variability in the mechanical efficiency of running or walking.[12] The measurement of a 6MWD is simple, safe, and relatively inexpensive. 6MWD has been shown to correlate to functional state, is sensitive to therapeutic interventions, and is useful for predicting survival.

For the 6MWD to be reproducible, intrasubject coefficients of variation should average less than 10%. Modest improvement up to 10% on repeated initial testing requires at least 2 (preferably 3) tests to produce reliable results. However, the 6MWD presents a problem referred to as the "ceiling effect" in cardiac and pulmonary patients. This effect is caused by maximal speed of walk between the distances of 450 and 500 m.[13] It is likely that the 6MWD would retain its predictive capability of Vo_{2max} if running in hospital corridors were possible.[12]

Development of portable ergospirometric equipment in recent years has allowed for the measurement of ventilation and gas exchange during walk tests. One would expect 12-minute runners or 6-minute walkers, whose maximum speed is compatible with minimal dyspnea and prolonged preservation of glycogen stores, to stabilize at a level of gas exchange at, or just below, VT. COPD and PAH patients with an RER slightly less than 1 and a Vo_2 value close to or equal to Vo_{2max},[14,15] walk at a constant speed, but only stabilize their VE, Vo_2, and Vco_2 after 2 to 3 minutes.

A higher Vo_2 is achieved at a lower RER during the 6-minute walk test compared with CPET; this is likely explained by altered Vo_2 kinetics with respect to rapid increases in workload during traditional "ramp" protocols. Most of these protocols rely on increments in workload every minute, whereas Vo_2 requires approximately 2 to 3 minutes to stabilize in patients with severe chronic cardiorespiratory conditions. Joseph and colleagues[19] have recently related a short 6MWD in patients with suspected pulmonary vascular disease to directly measured impaired systemic oxygen delivery, With O_2 delivery most heavily by indices of right heart afterload.[16]

PULMONARY ARTERIAL HYPERTENSION
Cardiopulmonary Exercise Test Profile in Pulmonary Arterial Hypertension

PH is a (right) heart failure syndrome.[17] It is therefore not surprising that the CPET profiles in heart failure and PAH are strikingly similar, with decreased maximal values of Vo_2, workload, O_2 pulse, and Vo_2 at the VT, decreased rate of change of Vo_2 per rate of change in work rate, early lactic acidosis, increased V_E/Vco_2, decreased maximal heart rate, and slow heart rate recovery.[9,18] Typical measurements are presented in **Fig. 1** and in **Table 1**.

It should be noted that Vo_{2peak} and maximal O_2 pulse tend to be lower in PAH compared with congestive heart failure with similar functional impairment. This finding is explained by a greater limitation of maximal cardiac output caused by predominant right ventricle (RV) dysfunction. On the other hand, PAH patients present with a higher level of ventilation and decreased arterial Pco_2, suggesting increased chemosensitivity.

Impaired Ventilation and Pulmonary Gas Exchange as a Limiting Factor

Do impaired lung mechanics limit exercise capacity in PAH? In the absence of significant pulmonary parenchymal disease, the answer is usually no. There is little or no perturbation in spirometry or lung volumes in patients with idiopathic PAH. Increased physiologic dead space additionally accounted for exercise hyperpnea, but did not limit exercise capacity, as ventilatory reserve is preserved in PAH.[9,18]

Dynamic hypoxemia can contribute to a reduced Vo_{2max} through the Fick principle. A diffusion defect associated with rapid red cell transit time through the pulmonary capillary may be further exacerbated by a low mixed venous Po_2, a consequence of low cardiac output.[19–23] In some patients, hypoxemia is caused by right-to-left shunting through a patent foramen ovale.[22,24] Interestingly, a recent randomized placebo-controlled study of supplemental O_2 in PAH demonstrated improved exercise capacity.[25]

Thus, it is likely that although PAH patients do not generally reach a ventilatory limit, exertional hypoxemia can limit Vo_{2max} and contribute to symptoms.

Hyperventilation

Patients with severe PH hyperventilate during exercise, rest, and even sleep. Hyperventilation is explained in some by exertional hypoxemia but in others by an increased chemosensitivity in proportion to disease severity, as seen in congestive heart failure.[10] However, a major difference with heart failure is that ventilatory oscillations characteristic of advanced left heart failure do not occur in PAH.[25] Hypocapnia, V_EVco_2 at exercise, and sympathetic nervous system hyperactivity are predictors of decreased survival in PAH.[26,27] Increased chemosensitivity contributes to dyspnea. The reason for increased chemosensitivity and related sympathetic nervous system activation in PAH is not exactly known. Increased filling pressures of the right heart and altered baroreflex control are thought to be involved.[10] Sympathetic nervous system activation has deleterious effects in the long term on the heart and the pulmonary circulation.

Peripheral Factors

Skeletal muscle dysfunction is a possible cause for the symptoms of PAH, which are typically triggered by physical activity. Studies demonstrate a

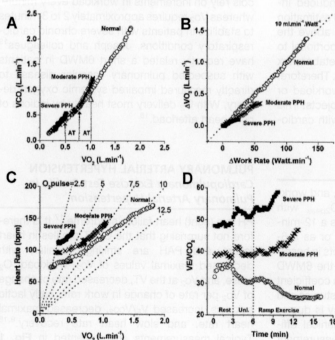

Fig. 1. Panels show carbon dioxide (Co_2) production (A) (Vco_2) and heart rate as a function of oxygen uptake (Vo_2) left (C), changes in Vo_2 as a function of change in work rate (B), and ventilatory equivalent for Co_2 (V_E/Vco_2) as a function of time left (D). Empty circles represent a normal control subject; crosses represent a patient with moderately severe idiopathic pulmonary arterial hypertension (PPH); filled-in squares represent a patient with very severe PPH. Patients with PPH show decreased Vco_2 and Vo_2, increased resting heart rate but decreased maximal heart rate, decreased rate of increase in Vo_2 as a function of rate of increase in work rate, and increased ventilatory equivalents for Co_2 in proportion to disease severity. Unl, unloaded cycling. (with permission from ref.[19])

Table 1
Cardiopulmonary exercise test variables in 19 patients with pulmonary arterial hypertension and 19 patients with congestive heart failure

Variables	PAH	CHF	P	Limits of Normal
NYHA	2.7 ± 0.1	2.8 ± 0.2	NS	
6MWD, m	395 ± 30	419 ± 20	NS	
Peak workload, W	53 ± 5	73 ± 6	<.05	129–241
Vo_{2peak}, mL/kg/min	10.1 ± 0.6	12.8 ± 0.8	<.01	23–32
VT, % Vo_{2peak}	74 ± 3	71 ± 3	NS	45–65
Peak O_2 pulse, mL/beat	5.9 ± 0.4	8.7 ± 0.5	<.001	9.1–16.5
Peak RER	1.15 ± 0.02	1.19 ± 0.02	NS	1.15–1.25
Resting V_E, L/min	14.3 ± 1.0	11.4 ± 0.8	<.03	4.8–7.2
Peak V_E, L/min	55 ± 5	55 ± 3	NS	70–108
Peak HR, beats/min	131 ± 5	115 ± 5	.06	150–178
Resting V_E/Vco_2	59 ± 2	49 ± 3	<.01	33–35
VT V_E/Vco_2	58 ± 3	44 ± 3	<.01	26–30
$\Delta Vo_2/\Delta WR$ above AT	5.3 ± 2.3	8.4 ± 3.8	<.02	9–11
HR recovery, beats	11 ± 2	10 ± 2	NS	>12

Values are mean $\pm$ SE. The CPET profile of PAH and CHF is of similar functional state, 6MWD is similar; with lower peak Vo_{2peak}, workload; O_2 pulse, and rate of Vo_2 per rate of workload and increased ventilatory equivalents. Chronotropic responses and recoveries appear similarly altered.

Abbreviations: CHF, congestive heart failure; HR, heart rate; NS, nonsignificant; NYHA, New York Heart Association; SE, standard error; WR, work rate.

From Deboeck G, Niset G, Lamotte M, Vachiery JL, Naeije R. Exercise testing in pulmonary arterial hypertension and in chronic heart failure. Eur Respir J. 2004;23(5):747-751. with permission.

decreased skeletal muscle strength in PAH,[28,29] but this is more likely related to brief alactic or lactic anaerobic efforts than it is to endurance aerobic exercise. Muscle phosphorus spectroscopy and biopsy studies have suggested abnormalities of microcirculatory O_2 delivery to the skeletal muscle mitochondrion in PAH.[30] Others have uncovered abnormalities of capillary density and intrinsic mitochondrial biogenesis and bioenergetics.[31]

An invasive hemodynamic study compared maximal aerobic exercise capacity in PAH patients with heart failure patients. PAH patients presented with a decreased maximal O_2 extraction, resulting in cardiac output limitations and a lower maximal aerobic exercise capacity.[32] A similar argument has been made for HFpEF when compared with normal.[33]

Peripheral limitation to exercise capacity is commonly evaluated by the extent of decrease in $C(a-v)O_2$, based on the principle that O_2 content difference is directly affected by O_2 extraction at any given value of CaO_2.

$$O_2 \text{ extraction} = Vo_2/DO_2 = C(a-v)O_2/CaO_2$$

However, this reasoning overlooks the fact that Q and $C(a-v)O_2$ are not truly independent variables. Muscle Vo_2 depends on convectional and

diffusional O_2 transport systems, described respectively by the Fick principle and Fick law of diffusion, which determines the flow of O_2 from muscle capillaries (c) to mitochondria (mit).

$$Vo_2 = D \times P(c - mit)Po_2$$

Muscle capillary Po_2 can be assumed near equal to venous Po_2 (Pvo_2), and Pmit neglected as being in the order of 1 mm Hg. Therefore:

$$Vo_2 = K \times Pvo_2$$

These relationships can be combined on a diagram relating Vo_2 to Pvo_2 (or Cvo_2), which are common to Fick principle and Fick law equations, illustrated in **Fig. 2**.

According to the Fick principle, an increase in Pvo_2 decreases Vo_2, whereas the Fick law of diffusion states an increase in Pvo_2 increases Vo_2. The 2 relationships couple at unique values for Vo_2 and Pvo_2.[35]

The convectional/diffusional O_2 transport diagram was applied to exercise studies with catheterization of the leg in 8 healthy volunteers and 12 HFrEF patients.[36] After an 8-week period of quadricep muscle training, 6 of the HFrEF patients restored muscle O_2 diffusing capacity. However, Vo_{2peak} remained decreased as a result of decreased maximum cardiac output.[37] These results demonstrate that in heart failure, a decrease in Vo_{2peak} is decreased not only by a decline in cardiac output but also by an alteration in O_2 muscle diffusion. This analysis was transposed to the entire body, assuming an exercise-induced increase in Vo_2 and decrease in Pvo_2 or Cvo_2 would predominantly be determined by changes in muscle metabolic rate. Forty-eight HFpEF and 56 HFrEF patients confirmed a major skeletal muscle contribution to the limitation of aerobic exercise capacity when compared with a control group of 24 subjects (see **Fig. 2**).[34] In another study comprising 79 HFpEF patients and 55 controls, HFpEF patients showed decreased VO_{2peak} as a result of a decreased maximum O_2 transport and an O_2 extraction of 26% and 36% of that of the control group.[38] Correction of maximum cardiac output restored only 7% of predicted Vo_{2max}, but the investigators insisted on the limitations of such modeling owing to the physiologic interdependence of all successive steps of O_2 transport from the lungs to the muscle mitochondria.

This analysis has not yet been transposed to patients with PAH. In a randomized controlled trial in 87 patients with either PAH or CTEPH, a 12-week exercise training program increased peak Vo_2 by an average of only 3.1 mL/kg/min. Maximum cardiac output increased on average by 1.1 L/min along with a decreased pulmonary vascular resistance (PVR), suggesting predominant central effects.[39]

Interestingly, systemic O_2 extraction during exercise may worsen with successful pulmonary vasodilator treatment of pulmonary hemodynamics,[1] raising the question: can improved cardiac output unmask a preexisting peripheral limit to exercise? The latter could include abnormal systemic vascular structure and function as well as intrinsic mitochondrial dysfunction in limb skeletal muscle[31]

Cardiopulmonary Exercise Tests Combined with Hemodynamic Measurements

There is a growing interest in combining CPET invasive and noninvasive assessments of cardiac function with pulmonary circulation. Invasive CPET combined with right heart catheterization is mainly used for the assessment of unexplained dyspnea.[40,41] It allows for the identification of 3 main causes of unexplained dyspnea: early pulmonary vascular disease, latent heart failure, and preload insufficiency.

Identification of pulmonary vascular disease versus latent left heart failure by exercise hemodynamic measurements requires robust definitions of normal limits based on data collected over the last decade. Experts have agreed on, and established, a set of mean values for CPET data for the diagnosis of cardiac and pulmonary abnormalities. Mean pulmonary artery pressure (mPAP) should not exceed 30 mm Hg at a cardiac output of less than 10 L/min. The upper limit for PVR is 3 Woods units,[42–44] and PAWP (Pulmonary Artery Wedge Pressure) should not go beyond 25 mm Hg or 2 mm Hg/L of increase in cardiac output.[44,45] Age-related upper limits of normal for pulmonary artery pressure, pulmonary capillary wedge pressure, and PVR have been published.[46]

Measurements of pulmonary vascular pressures at increasing levels of workload and cardiac output allow for the derivation of a distensibility factor α.

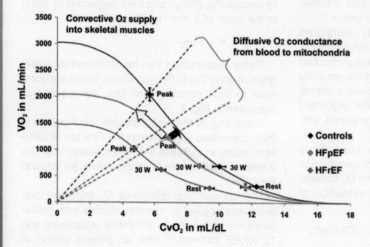

Fig. 2. The convective and diffusive components that interact to determine exercise capacity (Vo_2) in heart failure and controls. Mean values for Cvo_2 and Vo_2 at rest, 30 W, and peak exercise are used to construct Fick principle lines, which indicate convective O_2 delivery and are curvilinear because they directly reflect the hemoglobin dissociation curve. The vertical lines extending from the origin to the Vo_2-Cvo_2 plot at peak exercise indicate maximum diffusive oxygen delivery as determined by the Fick law, with a steeper relationship indicating better O_2 diffusion. The black arrow indicates the increment in peak Vo_2 in HFpEF if convective O_2 delivery was corrected to that of normal controls. White arrow indicates the increment in peak Vo_2 if O_2 diffusion was normalized in HFpEF. CvO2, oxygen content in venous blood; Vo_2, oxygen consumption. (with permission from ref[34].)

Distensibility factor α quantifies the distensibility of resistive vessels and is measured in % change in diameter per mm Hg.[42] The distensibility factor α has been shown to decrease in early and latent pulmonary vascular disease.[47] In the same study, α was on average of 0.25%/mm Hg in patients with overt PH and pulmonary vascular disease, 0.45%/mm Hg in patients with abnormal lung scintigraphy but no PH, and 1.40%/mm Hg in healthy controls. Interestingly, distensibility factor α was able to discriminate pulmonary vascular disease with no PH from normal hemodynamic conditions, at a sensitivity of 88% and a specificity of 100%. MPAP-flow relationships in healthy subjects with a normal distensibility factor α of 2%/mm Hg and a decreased distensibility factor α of 0.5%/mm Hg in pulmonary vascular disease are shown in **Fig. 3**. The graph indicates that stiffening of pulmonary resistive vessels considerably increases mPAP during exercise.[42]

In another study, α was shown to decrease to an average of 0.4%/mm Hg in PAH and 0.8% to 0.9%/mm Hg in heart failure, compared with 1.4%/mm Hg in age-matched controls.[48] These results have been independently confirmed. A low α is associated with a decreased exercise capacity, altered coupling of RV function to the pulmonary circulation, and a shorter survival.[48–50] Decreased resistive vessel distensibility limits exercise-induced decrease in PVR, which may be another indicator of pulmonary vascular disease.[42]

Exercise hemodynamics has multiple methodological constraints.[43] Exercise has to be dynamic, as static or resistive exercise does not sufficiently increase cardiac output.[50] Measurements must be done during, not after, exercise, as pulmonary vascular pressures and cardiac output return to normal in only a few minutes.[51] Care must be taken to zero the leveling of pressure transducers, and reading pulmonary vascular pressures in hyperventilating patients is challenging.[52] Averaging pulmonary vascular pressures during the cardiac cycle avoids overestimation of end-expiratory reading and provides values close to those corrected for intrathoracic pressure swings.[53] Hemodynamic assessments can be done using echocardiography with reasonable accuracy, but these lack precision, and results are difficult to use for individual decision making. An advantage of exercise stress echocardiography is that it allows for assessment of the right heart in addition to pulmonary circulation.[44,54] Cardiac output can be indirectly assessed by either workload[55,56] or Vo_2 measurements.[57] The measurements are quasilinearly correlated, so that the following equations can be used[58]:

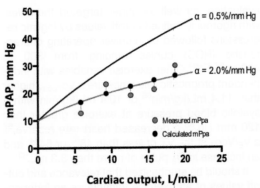

Fig. 3. Distensible model of pulmonary circulation. mPAP-flow relationships are depicted at 2 different levels of pulmonary vascular distensibility α (0.5%/ mm Hg, *black line*; and 2.0%/mm Hg, *gray line*) according to the distensible model of the pulmonary circulation. Higher values of α are associated with maintaining lower pulmonary artery pressures at increasing cardiac output (CO), despite the same values for pulmonary artery wedge pressure and PVR at rest. The distensible model provides an explanation for the slight curvilinear shape of normal pressure-flow relationships. The method of successive iterations with minimization of the differences between measured (*in gray*) and calculated (*in black*) pulmonary artery pressures was used to find a single value of α from a set of pressure-flow data obtained during exercise. mPpa, resting mean pulmonary artery pressure levels. (with permission from ref[43].)

$$Q \text{ (L/min)} = 0.34 \times Vo_2 \text{ (mL/kg/min)} + 5.4.$$

$$Q \text{ (L/min)} = 0.06 \text{ Workload (W)} + 6.5.$$

However, these correlations are not tight so that cardiac output may vary considerably at any level of workload or Vo_2. For example, cardiac output may vary between 15 and 25 L/min at a workload of 200 W or a Vo_2 of 40 mL/kg/min.[51,58] Pulmonary vascular pressures are flow dependent, rather than workload or Vo_2 dependent, so directly measuring cardiac output is preferable during exercise.

Decreased aerobic exercise capacity by limitation of maximum cardiac output is caused by exercise-induced PH.[59] Exercise hemodynamics, combined with CPET, allows for the identification of early-stage pulmonary vascular disease,[60] latent HFrEF or HFpEF treatment adjustments, and prediction of outcome.[43]

PREDICTIVE VALUE OF EXERCISE TESTING IN PULMONARY ARTERIAL HYPERTENSION

The 6MWD has been shown to be a powerful and independent predictor of survival in PAH at initial evaluation, as well as under targeted therapies, with rigorously defined cutoff values by logistic regressions followed by receiver operating characteristic (ROC) curves ranging from 300 to 400 m.[27,61–64] Other exercise variables with independent prognostic relevance are a Vo_{2peak} higher than 11.4 mL/kg/min[65] or 10.4 mL/kg/min with a systolic blood pressure at exercise greater than 120 mm Hg,[66] a decreased heart rate reserve,[67] a V_E/Vco_2 at the VT of less than 48[63] or 54[64], and an increase in O_2 pulse of more than 3.3 mL.[63]

It should be emphasized that relevance and cutoff values of an exercise variable as an independent predictor of outcome depends on the study population, which is sometimes either exclusively composed of idiopathic PAH,[28,60,61,66] PAH with associated conditions,[64] or IPAH (Idiopathic Pulmonary Arterial Hypertension) mixed with CTEPH.[62] None of these studies was prospective. The predictive capability of exercise measurements was higher for idiopathic PAH than PAH with associated conditions.[63] Rigorous calculation of threshold values from univariate and multivariate analysis and ROC analysis produced different results depending on sample size and number of variables taken into consideration. It is however interesting that rigorously determined cutoff values to discriminate good versus bad prognosis are very low for the 6MWD and Vo_{2peak} (around 300–330 m and 10–11 mL/kg/min, respectively), yet very high for V_E/Vco_2.[56–63]

Cutoff values to define low-, intermediate-, and high-risk exercise variables in European Respiratory and Cardiology Societies guidelines were 440, 400 to 165, and 165 m, respectively, for the 6MWD, 11, 11 to 15, and 15 mL/kg/min for VO_{2peak}, and 36, 36 to 45, and 45 for V_E/Vco_2.[68] These guidelines were based on expert consensus rather than rigorous univariable/multivariable analysis, and ROC curves were only used for independent predictors. Only the 6MWD is incorporated in contemporary risk assessment scores in PAH.[69–72]

The 6MWD was used in PAH drug trials as a primary endpoint in 3- to 6-months' duration studies, or incorporated in a composite clinical deterioration endpoint in event-driven studies.[73] Peak Vo_2 was used as a primary endpoint in 2 PAH drug trials. The peak Vo_2 values produced were negative, whereas an improvement in the 6MWD as a secondary endpoint was significant.[74,75] These negative values could be the result of an effect size (difference in means divided by pooled standard deviations) too small for the tested drugs.

It has been argued that changes in variables over time matter more than absolute values for predicting outcome in PAH.[76] However, when changes in variables over time are small with respect to standard deviation, the statistics performed on time change are blurred by excessive noise. Therefore, comparisons of absolute values before and after treatment versus placebo may be more relevant.

For this reason, metaanalysis of drug studies showed that absolute values of right atrial pressure, cardiac index, and PVR, but not changes of 6MWD, were sensitive to targeted therapies.[77,78]

Invasive CPET has been used to follow up the treatment of exercise PAH.[40,79] Only 1 study reported on the added value of CPET variables to hemodynamics in the follow-up of resting PAH.[80]

PERSPECTIVE

In summary, PH is typically associated with a decreased aerobic exercise capacity, which is largely explained by a limited oxygen delivery in response to peripheral oxygen demand, with a possible contribution of decreased muscle oxygen extraction. Exercise capacity in PAH is simply measured by a 6MWD. Like for any test, the 6MWD has intrinsic limitations: individual variability of the mechanical efficiency of the walk and a ceiling effect. The CPET is useful for refining the measurement of decreased exercise capacity and its differential diagnosis. When combined with hemodynamic assessment, CPET allows for the diagnosis of exercise-induced PH caused by either pulmonary vascular disease, heart failure, or both. The 6MWD is rightly integrated in clinical decision making, goal-oriented treatment strategies, and newly designed event-driven trials for the diagnosis of clinical deterioration.

However, more research is needed. Questions remain unanswered regarding directly measured maximal cardiac output as a major determinant of aerobic exercise capacity, skeletal muscle oxygen extraction and coupling of convectional and diffusional O_2 delivery, the role of physiologic dead space versus chemosensitivity in determining dyspnea symptoms, the effects of resistive exercise testing with measurements of anaerobic lactic and alactic power output, and whether the prognostic relevance of exercise variables is similar in idiopathic PAH, PAH with associated conditions, and CTEPH. Although exercise testing is for functional, not disease-specific diagnosis, a large-scale multicenter study would be needed to assess the relevance of CPET variables when added to clinical evaluation, right heart catheterization, and imaging in pulmonary vascular disease risk assessment.

CLINICS CARE POINTS

- Pulmonary hypertension is associated with a decreased aerobic exercise capacity. Exercise testing in pulmonary hypertension allows for the assessment of functional impairment and prognostication.
- Combining hemodynamic measurements and CPET allows for the diagnosis of early or latent pulmonary hypertension and exercise-induced right heart failure.

REFERENCES

1. Oliveira RKF, Waxman AB, Hoover PJ, et al. Pulmonary vascular and right ventricular burden during exercise in interstitial lung disease. Chest 2020; 158(1):350–8.
2. Wasserman K, Whipp BJ. Excercise physiology in health and disease. Am Rev Respir Dis 1975; 112(2):219–49.
3. LeJemtel TH, Testa M, Jondeau G. Direct and indirect assessment of skeletal muscle blood flow in patients with congestive heart failure. J Mol Cell Cardiol 1996;28(11):2249–54.
4. Jondeau G, Katz SD, Zohman L, et al. Active skeletal muscle mass and cardiopulmonary reserve. Failure to attain peak aerobic capacity during maximal bicycle exercise in patients with severe congestive heart failure. Circulation 1992;86(5):1351–6.
5. Katz SD, Maskin C, Jondeau G, et al. Near-maximal fractional oxygen extraction by active skeletal muscle in patients with chronic heart failure. J Appl Physiol (1985) 2000;88(6):2138–42.
6. Richardson RS, Knight DR, Poole DC, et al. Determinants of maximal exercise VO2 during single leg knee-extensor exercise in humans. Am J Physiol 1995;268(4 Pt 2):H1453–61.
7. Pynnaert C, Lamotte M, Naeije R. Aerobic exercise capacity in COPD patients with and without pulmonary hypertension. Respir Med 2010; 104(1):121–6.
8. Cote CG, Pinto-Plata V, Kasprzyk K, et al. The 6-min walk distance, peak oxygen uptake, and mortality in COPD. Chest 2007;132(6):1778–85.
9. Deboeck G, Niset G, Lamotte M, et al. Exercise testing in pulmonary arterial hypertension and in chronic heart failure. Eur Respir J 2004;23(5): 747–51.
10. Naeije R, Faoro V. The great breathlessness of cardiopulmonary diseases. Eur Respir J 2018;51(2): 1702517.
11. Cooper KH. A means of assessing maximal oxygen intake. Correlation between field and treadmill testing. JAMA 1968;203(3):201–4.
12. Naeije R. The 6-min walk distance in pulmonary arterial hypertension: "Je t'aime, moi non plus. Chest 2010;137(6):1258–60.
13. Lipkin DP, Scriven AJ, Crake T, et al. Six minute walking test for assessing exercise capacity in chronic heart failure. Br Med J (Clin Res Ed) 1986; 292(6521):653–5.
14. Deboeck G, Niset G, Vachiery JL, et al. Physiological response to the six-minute walk test in pulmonary arterial hypertension. Eur Respir J 2005;26(4): 667–72.
15. Troosters T, Vilaro J, Rabinovich R, et al. Physiological responses to the 6-min walk test in patients with chronic obstructive pulmonary disease. Eur Respir J 2002;20(3):564–9.
16. Joseph P, Oliveira RKF, Eslam RB, et al. Fick principle and exercise pulmonary hemodynamic determinants of the six-minute walk distance in pulmonary hypertension. Pulm Circ 2020;10(3). 2045894020957576.
17. Sanz J, Sanchez-Quintana D, Bossone E, et al. Anatomy, function, and dysfunction of the right ventricle: JACC s tate-of-the-art review. J Am Coll Cardiol 2019;73(12):1463–82.
18. Sun XG, Hansen JE, Oudiz RJ, et al. Exercise pathophysiology in patients with primary pulmonary hypertension. Circulation 2001;104(4):429–35.
19. Jujo T, Tanabe N, Sakao S, et al. Severe pulmonary arteriopathy is associated with persistent hypoxemia after pulmonary endarterectomy in chronic thromboembolic pulmonary hypertension. PLoS One 2016; 11(8):e0161827.
20. Farber HW, Badesch DB, Benza RL, et al. Use of supplemental oxygen in patients with pulmonary arterial hypertension in REVEAL. J Heart Lung Transplant 2018;37(8):948–55.
21. Dantzker DR, Bower JS. Mechanisms of gas exchange abnormality in patients with chronic obliterative pulmonary vascular disease. J Clin Invest 1979; 64(4):1050–5.
22. Melot C, Naeije R, Mols P, et al. Effects of nifedipine on ventilation/perfusion matching in primary pulmonary hypertension. Chest 1983;83(2):203–7.
23. Dantzker DR, D'Alonzo GE, Bower JS, et al. Pulmonary gas exchange during exercise in patients with chronic obliterative pulmonary hypertension. Am Rev Respir Dis 1984;130(3):412–6.
24. Ulrich S, Saxer S, Hasler ED, et al. Effect of domiciliary oxygen therapy on exercise capacity and quality of life in patients with pulmonary arterial or chronic thromboembolic pulmonary hypertension: a randomised, placebo-controlled trial. Eur Respir J 2019;54(2):1900276.
25. Vicenzi M, Deboeck G, Faoro V, et al. Exercise oscillatory ventilation in heart failure and in pulmonary arterial hypertension. Int J Cardiol 2016;202:736–40.
26. Hoeper MM, Pletz MW, Golpon H, et al. Prognostic value of blood gas analyses in patients with

idiopathic pulmonary arterial hypertension. Eur Respir J 2007;29(5):944–50.

27. Ciarka A, Doan V, Velez-Roa S, et al. Prognostic significance of sympathetic nervous system activation in pulmonary arterial hypertension. Am J Respir Crit Care Med 2010;181(11):1269–75.

28. Meyer FJ, Lossnitzer D, Kristen AV, et al. Respiratory muscle dysfunction in idiopathic pulmonary arterial hypertension. Eur Respir J 2005;25(1):125–30.

29. Bauer R, Dehnert C, Schoene P, et al. Skeletal muscle dysfunction in patients with idiopathic pulmonary arterial hypertension. Respir Med 2007;101(11): 2366–9.

30. Sithamparanathan S, Rocha MC, Parikh JD, et al. Skeletal muscle mitochondrial oxidative phosphorylation function in idiopathic pulmonary arterial hypertension: in vivo and in vitro study. Pulm Circ 2018; 8(2). 2045894018768290.

31. Batt J, Ahmed SS, Correa J, et al. Skeletal muscle dysfunction in idiopathic pulmonary arterial hypertension. Am J Respir Cell Mol Biol 2014;50(1):74–86.

32. Tolle J, Waxman A, Systrom D. Impaired systemic oxygen extraction at maximum exercise in pulmonary hypertension. Med Sci Sports Exerc 2008; 40(1):3–8.

33. Wong YY, van der Laarse WJ, Vonk-Noordegraaf A. Reduced systemic oxygen extraction does not prove muscle dysfunction in PAH. Med Sci Sports Exerc 2008;40(8):1554. author reply 1555.

34. Dhakal BP, Malhotra R, Murphy RM, et al. Mechanisms of exercise intolerance in heart failure with preserved ejection fraction: the role of abnormal peripheral oxygen extraction. Circ Heart Fail 2015;8(2):286–94.

35. Wagner PD. New ideas on limitations to VO2max. Exerc Sport Sci Rev 2000;28(1):10–4.

36. Esposito F, Mathieu-Costello O, Shabetai R, et al. Limited maximal exercise capacity in patients with chronic heart failure: partitioning the contributors. J Am Coll Cardiol 2010;55(18):1945–54.

37. Esposito F, Reese V, Shabetai R, et al. Isolated quadriceps training increases maximal exercise capacity in chronic heart failure: the role of skeletal muscle convective and diffusive oxygen transport. J Am Coll Cardiol 2011;58(13):1353–62.

38. Faria-Urbina M, Oliveira RKF, Segrera SA, et al. Impaired systemic oxygen extraction in treated exercise pulmonary hypertension: a new engine in an old car? Pulm Circ 2018;8(1). 2045893218755325.

39. Houstis NE, Eisman AS, Pappagianopoulos PP, et al. Exercise intolerance in heart failure with preserved ejection fraction: diagnosing and ranking its causes using personalized O_2 pathway analysis. Circulation 2018;137(2):148–61.

40. Ehlken N, Lichtblau M, Klose H, et al. Exercise training improves peak oxygen consumption and haemodynamics in patients with severe pulmonary arterial hypertension and inoperable chronic

thrombo-embolic pulmonary hypertension: a prospective, randomized, controlled trial. Eur Heart J 2016;37(1):35–44.

41. Maron BA, Cockrill BA, Waxman AB, et al. The invasive cardiopulmonary exercise test. Circulation 2013;127(10):1157–64.

42. Naeije R, Vanderpool R, Dhakal BP, et al. Exercise-induced pulmonary hypertension: physiological basis and methodological concerns. Am J Respir Crit Care Med 2013;187(6):576–83.

43. Kovacs G, Herve P, Barbera JA, et al. An official European Respiratory Society statement: pulmonary haemodynamics during exercise. Eur Respir J 2017;50(5):1700578.

44. Naeije R, Saggar R, Badesch D, et al. Exercise-induced pulmonary hypertension: translating pathophysiological concepts into clinical practice. Chest 2018;154(1):10–5.

45. Eisman AS, Shah RV, Dhakal BP, et al. Pulmonary capillary wedge pressure patterns during exercise predict exercise capacity and incident heart failure. Circ Heart Fail 2018;11(5):e004750.

46. Oliveira RK, Agarwal M, Tracy JA, et al. Age-related upper limits of normal for maximum upright exercise pulmonary haemodynamics. Eur Respir J 2016; 47(4):1179–88.

47. Lau EMT, Chemla D, Godinas L, et al. Loss of vascular distensibility during exercise is an early hemodynamic marker of pulmonary vascular disease. Chest 2016;149(2):353–61.

48. Malhotra R, Dhakal BP, Eisman AS, et al. Pulmonary vascular distensibility predicts pulmonary hypertension severity, exercise capacity, and survival in heart failure. Circ Heart Fail 2016;9(6). https://doi.org/10.1161/CIRCHEARTFAILURE.115.003011.

49. Singh I, Oliveira RKF, Naeije R, et al. Pulmonary vascular distensibility and early pulmonary vascular remodeling in pulmonary hypertension. Chest 2019; 156(4):724–32.

50. Motoji Y, Forton K, Pezzuto B, et al. Resistive or dynamic exercise stress testing of the pulmonary circulation and the right heart. Eur Respir J 2017; 50(1):1700151.

51. Oliveira RK, Waxman AB, Agarwal M, et al. Pulmonary haemodynamics during recovery from maximum incremental cycling exercise. Eur Respir J 2016;48(1):158–67.

52. Argiento P, Vanderpool RR, Mule M, et al. Exercise stress echocardiography of the pulmonary circulation: limits of normal and sex differences. Chest 2012;142(5):1158–65.

53. Kovacs G, Avian A, Pienn M, et al. Reading pulmonary vascular pressure tracings. How to handle the problems of zero leveling and respiratory swings. Am J Respir Crit Care Med 2014;190(3): 252–7.

54. Guazzi M, Bandera F, Ozemek C, et al. Cardiopulmonary exercise testing: what is its value? J Am Coll Cardiol 2017;70(13):1618–36.

55. Claessen G, La Gerche A, Voigt JU, et al. Accuracy of echocardiography to evaluate pulmonary vascular and RV function during exercise. JACC Cardiovasc Imaging 2016;9(5):532–43.

56. van Riel AC, Opotowsky AR, Santos M, et al. Accuracy of echocardiography to estimate pulmonary artery pressures with exercise: a simultaneous invasive- noninvasive comparison. Circ Cardiovasc Imaging 2017;10(4):e005711.

57. Tolle JJ, Waxman AB, Van Horn TL, et al. Exercise-induced pulmonary arterial hypertension. Circulation 2008;118(21):2183–9.

58. Forton K, Motoji Y, Deboeck G, et al. Effects of body position on exercise capacity and pulmonary vascular pressure-flow relationships. J Appl Physiol (1985) 2016;121(5):1145–50.

59. Santos M, Opotowsky AR, Shah AM, et al. Central cardiac limit to aerobic capacity in patients with exertional pulmonary venous hypertension: implications for heart failure with preserved ejection fraction. Circ Heart Fail 2015;8(2):278–85.

60. Singh I, Rahaghi F, Naeije R, et al. EXPRESS: dynamic right ventricular-pulmonary arterial uncoupling during maximum incremental exercise in exercise pulmonary hypertension and pulmonary arterial hypertension. Pulm Circ 2019;9(3). 2045894019862435.

61. Miyamoto S, Nagaya N, Satoh T, et al. Clinical correlates and prognostic significance of six-minute walk test in patients with primary pulmonary hypertension. Comparison with cardiopulmonary exercise testing. Am J Respir Crit Care Med 2000;161(2 Pt 1):487–92.

62. Sitbon O, Humbert M, Nunes H, et al. Long-term intravenous epoprostenol infusion in primary pulmonary hypertension: prognostic factors and survival. J Am Coll Cardiol 2002;40(4):780–8.

63. Groepenhoff H, Vonk-Noordegraaf A, Boonstra A, et al. Exercise testing to estimate survival in pulmonary hypertension. Med Sci Sports Exerc 2008; 40(10):1725–32.

64. Deboeck G, Scoditti C, Huez S, et al. Exercise testing to predict outcome in idiopathic versus associated pulmonary arterial hypertension. Eur Respir J 2012;40(6):1410–9.

65. Huez S, Brimioulle S, Naeije R, et al. Feasibility of routine pulmonary arterial impedance measurements in pulmonary hypertension. Chest 2004;125(6): 2121–8.

66. Wensel R, Opitz CF, Anker SD, et al. Assessment of survival in patients with primary pulmonary hypertension: importance of cardiopulmonary exercise testing. Circulation 2002;106(3):319–24.

67. Wensel R, Francis DP, Meyer FJ, et al. Incremental prognostic value of cardiopulmonary exercise testing and resting haemodynamics in pulmonary arterial hypertension. Int J Cardiol 2013;167(4):1193–8.

68. Galie N, Humbert M, Vachiery JL, et al. [2015 ESC/ERS Guidelines for the diagnosis and treatment of pulmonary hypertension]. Kardiol Pol 2015;73(12):1127–206.

69. Hoeper MM, Kramer T, Pan Z, et al. Mortality in pulmonary arterial hypertension: prediction by the 2015 European Pulmonary Hypertension Guidelines Risk Stratification Model. Eur Respir J 2017;50(2):1700740.

70. Kylhammar D, Kjellstrom B, Hjalmarsson C, et al. A comprehensive risk stratification at early follow-up determines prognosis in pulmonary arterial hypertension. Eur Heart J 2018;39(47):4175–81.

71. Boucly A, Weatherald J, Savale L, et al. Risk assessment, prognosis and guideline implementation in pulmonary arterial hypertension. Eur Respir J 2017;50(2):1700889.

72. Benza RL, Gomberg-Maitland M, Elliott CG, et al. Predicting survival in patients with pulmonary arterial hypertension: the REVEAL risk score calculator 2.0 and comparison with ESC/ERS-based risk assessment strategies. Chest 2019;156(2):323–37.

73. Galie N, Channick RN, Frantz RP, et al. Risk stratification and medical therapy of pulmonary arterial hypertension. Eur Respir J 2019;53(1):1801889.

74. Barst RJ, McGoon M, McLaughlin V, et al. Beraprost therapy for pulmonary arterial hypertension. J Am Coll Cardiol 2003;41(12):2119–25.

75. Barst RJ, Langleben D, Frost A, et al. Sitaxsentan therapy for pulmonary arterial hypertension. Am J Respir Crit Care Med 2004;169(4):441–7.

76. Nickel N, Golpon H, Greer M, et al. The prognostic impact of follow-up assessments in patients with idiopathic pulmonary arterial hypertension. Eur Respir J 2012;39(3):589–96.

77. Savarese G, Musella F, D'Amore C, et al. Haemodynamics, exercise capacity and clinical events in pulmonary arterial hypertension. Eur Respir J 2013; 42(2):414–24.

78. Savarese G, Paolillo S, Costanzo P, et al. Do changes of 6-minute walk distance predict clinical events in patients with pulmonary arterial hypertension? A meta-analysis of 22 randomized trials. J Am Coll Cardiol 2012;60(13):1192–201.

79. Segrera SA, Lawler L, Opotowsky AR, et al. Open label study of ambrisentan in patients with exercise pulmonary hypertension. Pulm Circ 2017;7(2):531–8.

80. Badagliacca R, Papa S, Poscia R, et al. The added value of cardiopulmonary exercise testing in the follow-up of pulmonary arterial hypertension. J Heart Lung Transplant 2019;38(3):306–14.

Section IV: Management of the Pulmonary Hypertension Patient

Contemporary Pharmacotherapeutic Approach in Pulmonary Arterial Hypertension

Jalil Ahari, MD, Akshay Bhatnagar, MD, Anna Johnson, BS,
Mardi Gomberg-Maitland, MD, MSc*

KEYWORDS

- Prostacyclin • Prostanoid • Endothelial antagonist • Phosphodiesterase inhibitor
- Guanylate cyclase stimulator • Clinical trials • Pharmacologic treatment approach

KEY POINTS

- Pulmonary arterial hypertension management has advanced with multiple oral, inhaled, and parenteral therapeutic options.
- Pulmonary arterial hypertension trial design is more sophisticated, as placebo-controlled trials with no background therapy are unethical.
- Research will need to address other pathologic mechanisms that drive vascular remodeling and the right ventricle.

INTRODUCTION

In 1973, experts convened in Geneva, Switzerland, at the First World Symposium on Pulmonary Hypertension (PH). Classification schema, pathophysiology, and clinical features were discussed, among other aspects of PH.[1] Importantly, however, their published report in 1975 did not mention pharmacotherapy; it would only be 20 years later in 1995 that epoprostenol[2] would become the first medication to gain approval by the Food and Drug Administration (FDA) as a specific treatment for what was then known as primary PH,[3] now referred to as idiopathic pulmonary arterial hypertension (PAH).

Following this breakthrough, a multitude of pharmaceutical company–sponsored randomized, placebo-controlled trials (RCTs) over the next 2 decades led to the availability of drugs targeting different pathophysiologic pathways. The main 3 pathways are the endothelin pathway, the nitric oxide pathway, and the prostacyclin pathway. With this pharmacologic advancement and medication options, a consensus approach to treatment was required. Physicians worldwide needed a guide to understand how to best use these agents for individual patients, understanding that not all patients would have a similar response.[4]

To appreciate where we are now in terms of contemporary management strategy, we must understand the history of our journey in drug development (**Fig. 1**). The evolution of this overall clinical approach with continued refinement is the focus of this review.

EARLY TREATMENT OPTIONS

Before 1995, management of PAH consisted only of a combination of nonspecific therapies now referred to as "standard" or "general" therapies.[5] These included supplemental oxygen, diuretics, anticoagulation, vasodilators such as hydralazine, and digoxin.[6] One of our first successful

George Washington University School of Medicine and Health Sciences, 2150 Pennsylvania Avenue 4th Floor, Washington, DC 20037, USA
* Corresponding author.
E-mail address: mgomberg@mfa.gwu.edu

Clin Chest Med 42 (2021) 125–131
https://doi.org/10.1016/j.ccm.2020.10.002

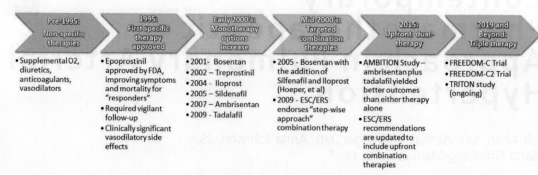

Fig. 1. Progression of pharmacotherapeutic options for PAH.

discoveries was the calcium channel blocker (CCB) cohort. In 1992, Rich and colleagues[7] demonstrated a subclass of patients who, when treated with high doses of CCBs, had marked improvement in acute hemodynamics. With the continuation of these medications, they noted a survival benefit in those with a continued response to therapy. Unfortunately, over time we learned that this "dramatic" response is not often long term. In the original reports from the French group, 12.5% of patients with idiopathic PAH had a reduction of mean pulmonary arterial pressure (mPAP) $\geq$ 10 mm Hg to reach a value $\leq$ 40 mm Hg with an increased or unchanged cardiac output. At 1 year, only 6.8% had a sustained response,[8] defined as clinical improvement to New York Heart Association Functional Class I/II, with sustained hemodynamic improvement (same or better than achieved in the acute test usually with mPAP<30 mm Hg).[9] Patients with this phenotype continue to have a better prognosis compared with nonresponders even in present day.[9]

FDA approval of epoprostenol in 1995 transformed care by improving patient outcomes. Compared with standard therapy, epoprostenol improved symptoms of heart failure and low perfusion, exercise capacity, and hemodynamics. It is the only therapy that prospectively improved mortality in a clinical trial.[10] Nevertheless, treatment options for PAH remained limited during the 1990s. Clinicians caring for these patients faced a simple choice. Those with mild to moderate PAH who had a positive vasodilator response test[11] were considered "responders," and CCBs could be prescribed with mandatory vigilant follow-up. For those who did not meet the definition of a "responder," epoprostenol was the alternative option but required sophisticated coordination among the patient, family, and physician/nurse team to administer via a continuous intravenous infusion. Epoprostenol had to be

prepared using sterile mixing procedures and therapy needed to be kept cold with ice packs for it to be effective. Administration required a permanent central venous catheter and associated catheter care, which could be quite cumbersome. In addition, managing vasodilatory side effects associated with prostacyclin derivatives again required a coordinated team approach.[12]

MONOTHERAPY APPROACH

At the Second World Symposium on PH in 1998 in Evian, France, experts constructed a detailed classification scheme[4] reflecting the advanced comprehension of disease pathogenesis. Viewed originally as predominant pulmonary vasoconstrictive disease, further histologic and molecular studies illustrated that PH also had a vasoproliferative process with abnormal vascular remodeling and cellular proliferation at the center of its pathophysiology.[8,13]

The early 2000s gave rise to the first RCTs in PAH. Enrollment consisted of newly diagnosed and untreated subjects. In 2001, bosentan,[14] a nonspecific endothelin receptor antagonist (ERA), became the first oral therapy, and second overall therapeutic, to be approved by the FDA for use in PAH. Bosentan also benefited patients with Eisenmenger syndrome secondary to congenital heart disease.[15] Subsequently, a myriad of seminal trials were completed within a relatively short period and resulted in regulatory approvals of additional agents for this orphan disease. These included 2 other prostacyclin analogues: intravenous and subcutaneous formulations of treprostinil[16] in 2002 and iloprost,[17] delivered via an aerosolized route of administration, in 2004. Next approved, sildenafil,[18] a phosphodiesterase-5 inhibitor (PDE-5I), in 2005 and ambrisentan,[19] a selective ERA, in 2007, followed by tadalafil,[20] a long-acting PDE-5I, in 2009, and riociguat, a soluble guanylate cyclase stimulator in 2013.[21] Based on these trials, an upfront initial monotherapy approach with the sequential addition of medications targeting different pathways became standard of care. Contemporary guidelines focused on World Health Organization functional class (WHO FC) III, with emphasis on intravenous prostaglandins for patients with WHO FC IV.[22,23] With difficulty in performing monotherapy trials with multiple classes of therapies and novel routes of delivery of approved therapies, the previously mentioned guidelines briefly commented on the possibility/need of combination therapy.[24] However, data regarding the use of combination therapy were too limited at the time to make official recommendations.

COMBINATION THERAPY: GOAL-ORIENTED APPROACH

In 2005, Hoeper and colleagues[25] published a pivotal study examining the use of combination therapy in a goal-oriented approach at a single center. Criteria for initiating combination therapy were predefined by the group. They included specific treatment goals regarding the 6-minute walk test (<380 m), peak oxygen uptake on cardiopulmonary exercise testing (>10.4 mL/min per kg), and peak systolic blood pressure (>120 mm Hg) during exercise. Combination therapy was instituted per a predefined algorithm: first-line treatment consisted of bosentan, and, if treatment goals were not met with bosentan monotherapy, sildenafil was added, followed by inhaled iloprost. The latter was switched to intravenous iloprost in patients with progressive disease (ie, WHO IV and/or right heart failure signs/symptoms). The goal-oriented approach benefited patients over a historical control group of patients with PAH treated at the same center. Nearly half of the patients advanced to requiring combination therapy, reflecting the lack of sustained efficacy of monotherapy at 3 years.[25]

COMBINATION THERAPY: SEQUENTIAL APPROACH

Over the past decade, data emerged from subsequent RCTs supporting the use of combination therapy, either as initial or upfront combination therapy versus sequential combination therapy.[26–28] The pivotal sequential study was a double-blind placebo-controlled trial of sildenafil added to patients on stable epoprostenol.[26] This study proved benefit in combination therapy in a prevalent patient cohort. Physician practice varied worldwide without data on the management of combination therapy. Some physicians started a second agent if patients were not at treatment

goal at 3 months or if there was evidence of disease progression (ie, worsening objective measures of WHO FC, 6-minute walk distance, echocardiographic right ventricular function, and/or hemodynamics). Others switched to an alternative agent and stopped the original therapy altogether. Sequential combination therapy, nonetheless, became the standard of care during this time,[29,30] with supporting evidence from a number of RCTs.[31] The 2009 European Society of Cardiology/European Respiratory Society (ESC/ERS) guidelines[32] endorsed this approach, recommending goal-oriented combination therapy in a "stepwise approach" in patients who were not responding to monotherapy.

Despite advancements in treatment, patients presented late during their clinical course (FC III/IV) to centers in Europe and the United States and mortality rates for PAH remained high.[33] This could, in part, be explained by physicians outside of large centers not escalating therapies appropriately and improper diagnostic evaluations.[34–37] Analysis of the US Registry to Evaluate Early and Long-term PAH Disease Management (REVEAL) registry in 2013[38] indicated that a substantial percentage of patients with WHO FC IV PAH were still receiving only monotherapy at time of death. Even in the sickest patients, physicians throughout North America failed to escalate to combination therapy including intravenous medication.

COMBINATION THERAPY: UPFRONT DUAL THERAPY

The first study that examined upfront combination PAH therapy was the BREATHE-2 study.[39] Patients initiated on intravenous epoprostenol were randomized to either placebo or bosentan. There was no statistically significant difference between the 2 groups in the primary endpoint of change in total pulmonary resistance. This nonsignificant result halted further studies looking at combination therapy as a potential therapeutic approach in PAH.

The concept reemerged a decade later with the reports of the 2015 AMBITION study comparing the use of upfront combination therapy with ambrisentan (selective ERA) plus tadalafil (PDE5-I) to either monotherapy alone.[40] The study demonstrated a significant benefit of initial combination therapy with respect to all evaluated outcome measures: risk of clinical-failure events, N-terminal pro-brain natriuretic peptide (BNP), and improved exercise capacity as measured by 6-minute walk distance. A subsequent retrospective analysis assessing real-world data regarding upfront dual combination therapy with an ERA and a PDE-5 I from the French registry on patients with newly diagnosed PAH also demonstrated improved WHO FC, exercise capacity, and hemodynamics.[41] As a result of these pivotal trials, the 2015 ESC/ERS guidelines modified recommendations from a sequential approach based on predefined clinical goals to initial combination therapy, recommending either a sequential or upfront approach.[42] The only absolute contraindication for use of this approach is the specific combination of riociguat and PDE-5 I. The combination of these 2 drugs on the nitric oxide pathway can result in severe hypotension.[43]

CLINICAL TRIALS: SHORT-TERM VERSUS LONG-TERM OUTCOME MEASURES

Early RCTs involving PAH focused primarily on short-term outcomes (eg, improvement in 12/16 weeks, 6-minute walk test, BNP). Whether PAH targeted therapy achieved disease modification with long-term hemodynamic and clinical benefits remained uncertain.[44,45] This led to development of endpoint-driven RCTs with particular focus on long-term morbidity and mortality. SERAPHIN[46] (Macitentan and Morbidity and Mortality in Pulmonary Arterial Hypertension) and GRIPHON[47] (Selexipag for the Treatment of Pulmonary Arterial Hypertension) studies evaluated double and triple sequential combination therapy in the context of event-driven RCTs. These trials, however, did not provide enough data to determine formal recommendations for combination therapy.

COMBINATION THERAPY: TRIPLE THERAPY

The Freedom C (Oral Treprostinil in Combination With an Endothelin Receptor Antagonist [ERA] and/or a Phosphodiesterase-5 [PDE-5] Inhibitor for the Treatment of Pulmonary Arterial Hypertension [PAH])[48] and Freedom C2 (Oral Treprostinil for the Treatment of Pulmonary Arterial Hypertension in Patients Receiving Background Endothelin Receptor Antagonist and Phosphodiesterase Type 5 Inhibitor Therapy)[49] trials began the investigation into triple combination therapy.

Class IV patients require aggressive management, especially if the patient is presenting as a new diagnosis of PAH. Patients need a fast, efficient evaluation and ultimately may need an emergent lung transplantation. A retrospective pilot study[50] within French national centers reported the outcomes of 19 newly diagnosed patients presenting with WHO FC III or IV PAH who were started on upfront triple combination therapy while in the hospital. WHO FC, exercise capacity, and

hemodynamics improved. Patients did experience worsening liver function, likely due to combination therapy that consisted of the use of bosentan. Based on this preliminary evidence, the TRITON study (The Efficacy and Safety of Initial Triple vs Initial Dual Oral Combination Therapy in Patients with Newly Diagnosed Pulmonary Arterial Hypertension) was initiated to compare upfront triple combination therapy (macitentan, tadalafil, selexipag) versus dual combination therapy (macitentan, tadalafil, placebo) in patients with newly diagnosed PAH. The trial is completed and reported in abstract form and did not meet its primary outcome of pulmonary vascular resistance.[51] Current consensus and guidelines recommend triple therapy added sequentially in high-risk patients for whom combination dual therapy has proved to be clinically inadequate and should remain despite this study.[52] But, understanding which combinations work best together needs to be further investigated.

NOVEL APPROACHES TO DELIVERY OF THERAPY

Medications are only effective in clinical practice if patients can easily comply with the therapy's dosing and administration. Some of our therapeutic advances can be attributed to dosing adjustments and/or switching the mode of delivery (intravenous, subcutaneous, inhaled, oral) with same class agents, limiting the side effects and potential toxicity. Innovative systems for approved therapies continue to evolve. The internal catheter-pump (implantable) system developed by Medtronic for intravenous treprostinil had fewer catheter-related infections, improved quality of life, and long-term safety. It is FDA approved but not yet marketed in the United States.[53–55]

SUMMARY

The management of PAH has advanced from the use of standard therapies alone, to intravenous prostacyclin therapy, followed by monotherapy with a choice between a variety of oral agents, to use of dual and triple combination therapy in sequential and upfront approaches, and more recently with novel methods of medication delivery. Trial designs are now more sophisticated, as PAH drug development can no longer perform trials in newly diagnosed patients with a placebo, nor an open-label study like the pivotal epoprostenol study. Our endpoints have evolved from short-term improvement in exercise capacity and functional class to longer-term event-driven outcomes.

The field needs new endpoints and better phenotyping of patients to assist in future drug development. As the medical arsenal from which therapeutic agents for PAH can be selected has expanded over the past 3 decades, the treatment approach in terms of which parameters to target as a measurement of success continues to evolve.

There is no cure for PAH and thus despite our advances, there is still a need for new drugs to address other pathologic mechanisms that drive vascular remodeling and ultimately right ventricular failure. As laboratory scientists uncover more mechanistic pathways, there is no shortage of novel drug targets of potential therapeutic interest[56] (**Table 1**). Understanding which target/drug has a higher likelihood of success and which patients will respond to particular therapies is unclear and is an important next step in the pharmacotherapeutic approach.

DISCLOSURE

Dr M. Gomberg-Maitland is a consultant on steering committees/data safety monitoring for Acceleron, Actelion/Janssen, Altavant, Complexa,

Reata, and United Therapeutics. George Washington University Medical Faculty Practice receives money for research grants from United Therapeutics and Altavant. Drs J. Ahari and A. Bhatnagar, and Ms A. Johnson have nothing to disclose.

REFERENCES

1. Hatano S, Strasser T. Primary pulmonary hypertension. Geneva, Switzerland: Report on a WHO Meeting, World Health Organization; 1975. p. 7–45.
2. Barst RJ, Rubin LJ, Long WA, et al. A comparison of continuous intravenous epoprostenol (prostacyclin) with conventional therapy for primary pulmonary hypertension. N Engl J Med 1996;334(5):296–301.
3. Dresdale DT, Schultz M, Michtom RJ. Primary pulmonary hypertension. I. Clinical and hemodynamic study. Am J Med 1951;11(6):686–705.
4. Oudiz RJ. Evolution in PH care: 3 decades of milestones. Adv Pulm Hypertens 2018;16(4):169. https://doi.org/10.21693/1933-088X-16.4.165. Available at:.
5. Alam S, Palevsky HI. Standard therapies for pulmonary arterial hypertension. Clin Chest Med 2007; 28(1):91–115, viii.
6. Sitbon O, Vonk Noordegraaf A. Epoprostenol and pulmonary arterial hypertension: 20 years of clinical experience. Eur Respir Rev 2017;26(143):160055.
7. Rich S, Kaufmann E, Levy PS. The effect of high doses of calcium-channel blockers on survival in primary pulmonary hypertension. N Engl J Med 1992; 327(2):76–81.
8. Sitbon O, Humbert M, Jais X, et al. Long-term response to calcium channel blockers in idiopathic pulmonary arterial hypertension. Circulation 2005; 111(23):3105–11.
9. Simonneau G, Montani D, Celermajer DS, et al. Haemodynamic definitions and updated clinical classification of pulmonary hypertension. Eur Respir J 2019;53.
10. McLaughlin VV, Shillington A, Rich S. Survival in primary pulmonary hypertension: the impact of epoprostenol therapy. Circulation 2002;106(12): 1477–82.
11. Hoeper MM, Ghofrani HA, Grunig E, et al. Pulmonary hypertension. Dtsch Arztebl Int 2017;114(5):73–84.
12. Kingman M, Archer-Chicko C, Bartlett M, et al. Management of prostacyclin side effects in adult patients with pulmonary arterial hypertension. Pulm Circ 2017;7(3):598–608.
13. Hoeper MM, Galie N, Simonneau G, et al. New treatments for pulmonary arterial hypertension. Am J Respir Crit Care Med 2002;165(9):1209–16.
14. Rubin LJ, Badesch DB, Barst RJ, et al. Bosentan therapy for pulmonary arterial hypertension. N Engl J Med 2002;346(12):896–903.

Table 1
Potential targets for the drug development in pulmonary arterial hypertension

Mechanism	Target	Drug
Genetic	BMPR2	Tacrolimus
	TGFb (ligand trap)	Sotatercept
Inflammation	CD20	Rituximab
	IL6 receptors	Tocilizumab
	IL1	Anakira
Metabolic	AMPK	Metformin
	Nf2 and NFκB	Bardoxolone
Estrogen signaling	Aromatase	Anastrozole
Humoral	ACE2	Recombinant ACE2
	Mineralocorticoid receptor	Spironolactone
DNA repair	PARP1	Olaparib
Tyrosine kinase inhibitor	VEGFR1,2,3, RAF, PDGR-β	Sorafenib
	c-kit, PDGRF	Imatinib
	mTOR	Rapamycin (intravenous)

15. Galie N, Beghetti M, Gatzoulis MA, et al. Bosentan therapy in patients with Eisenmenger syndrome: a multicenter, double-blind, randomized, placebo-controlled study. Circulation 2006;114(1):48–54.

16. Simonneau G, Barst RJ, Galie N, et al. Continuous subcutaneous infusion of treprostinil, a prostacyclin analogue, in patients with pulmonary arterial hypertension: a double-blind, randomized, placebo-controlled trial. Am J Respir Crit Care Med 2002; 165(6):800–4.

17. Olschewski H, Simonneau G, Galie N, et al. Inhaled iloprost for severe pulmonary hypertension. N Engl J Med 2002;347(5):322–9.

18. Galie N, Ghofrani HA, Torbicki A, et al. Sildenafil citrate therapy for pulmonary arterial hypertension. N Engl J Med 2005;353(20):2148–57.

19. Galie N, Olschewski H, Oudiz RJ, et al. Ambrisentan for the treatment of pulmonary arterial hypertension: results of the ambrisentan in pulmonary arterial hypertension, randomized, double-blind, placebo-controlled, multicenter, efficacy (ARIES) study 1 and 2. Circulation 2008;117(23):3010–9.

20. Galie N, Brundage BH, Ghofrani HA, et al. Tadalafil therapy for pulmonary arterial hypertension. Circulation 2009;119(22):2894–903.

21. Ghofrani HA, Galie N, Grimminger F, et al. Riociguat for the treatment of pulmonary arterial hypertension. N Engl J Med 2013;369:330–40.

22. Galie N, Seeger W, Naeije R, et al. Comparative analysis of clinical trials and evidence-based treatment algorithm in pulmonary arterial hypertension. J Am Coll Cardiol 2004;43(12 Suppl S): 81S–8S.

23. Galie N, Torbicki A, Barst R, et al. Guidelines on diagnosis and treatment of pulmonary arterial hypertension. The task force on diagnosis and treatment of pulmonary arterial hypertension of the European Society of Cardiology. Eur Heart J 2004;25(24): 2243–78.

24. Badesch DB, Abman SH, Ahearn GS, et al. Medical therapy for pulmonary arterial hypertension: ACCP evidence-based clinical practice guidelines. Chest 2004;126(1 Suppl):35S–62S.

25. Hoeper MM, Markevych I, Spiekerkoetter E, et al. Goal-oriented treatment and combination therapy for pulmonary arterial hypertension. Eur Respir J 2005;26(5):858–63.

26. Simonneau G, Rubin LJ, Galie N, et al. Addition of sildenafil to long-term intravenous epoprostenol therapy in patients with pulmonary arterial hypertension: a randomized trial. Ann Intern Med 2008; 149(8):521–30.

27. McLaughlin VV, Benza RL, Rubin LJ, et al. Addition of inhaled treprostinil to oral therapy for pulmonary arterial hypertension: a randomized controlled clinical trial. J Am Coll Cardiol 2010;55(18):1915–22.

28. Galie N, Corris PA, Frost A, et al. Updated treatment algorithm of pulmonary arterial hypertension. J Am Coll Cardiol 2013;62(25 Suppl):D60–72.

29. McLaughlin VV, Shah SJ, Souza R, et al. Management of pulmonary arterial hypertension. J Am Coll Cardiol 2015;65(18):1976–97.

30. Fallah F. Recent strategies in treatment of pulmonary arterial hypertension, a review. Glob J Health Sci 2015;7(4):307–22.

31. Ghofrani HA, Humbert M. The role of combination therapy in managing pulmonary arterial hypertension. Eur Respir Rev 2014;23(134):469–75.

32. Galie N, Hoeper MM, Humbert M, et al. Guidelines for the diagnosis and treatment of pulmonary hypertension: the task force for the diagnosis and treatment of pulmonary hypertension of the European Society of Cardiology (ESC) and the European Respiratory Society (ERS), endorsed by the International Society of Heart and Lung Transplantation (ISHLT). Eur Heart J 2009;30(20):2493–537.

33. Oudiz RJ. Death in pulmonary arterial hypertension. Am J Respir Crit Care Med 2013;188(3):269–70.

34. Badesch DB, Raskob GE, Elliott CG, et al. Pulmonary arterial hypertension: baseline characteristics from the REVEAL Registry. Chest 2010;137(2): 376–87.

35. Humbert M, Sitbon O, Chaouat A, et al. Pulmonary arterial hypertension in France: results from a national registry. Am J Respir Crit Care Med 2006; 173(9):1023–30.

36. McLaughlin VV, Langer A, Tan M, et al. Contemporary trends in the diagnosis and management of pulmonary arterial hypertension: an initiative to close the care gap. Chest 2013;143(2):324–32.

37. Thenappan T, Shah SJ, Rich S, et al. A USA-based registry for pulmonary arterial hypertension: 1982–2006. Eur Respir J 2007;30(6):1103–10.

38. Farber HW, Miller DP, Meltzer LA, et al. Treatment of patients with pulmonary arterial hypertension at the time of death or deterioration to functional class IV: insights from the REVEAL registry. J Heart Lung Transplant 2013;32(11):1114–22.

39. Humbert M, Barst RJ, Robbins IM, et al. Combination of bosentan with epoprostenol in pulmonary arterial hypertension: BREATHE-2. Eur Respir J 2004;24(3):353–9.

40. Galie N, Barbera JA, Frost AE, et al. Initial use of ambrisentan plus tadalafil in pulmonary arterial hypertension. N Engl J Med 2015;373(9):834–44.

41. Sitbon O, Sattler C, Bertoletti L, et al. Initial dual oral combination therapy in pulmonary arterial hypertension. Eur Respir J 2016;47(6):1727–36.

42. Galie N, Humbert M, Vachiery JL, et al. 2015 ESC/ ERS guidelines for the diagnosis and treatment of pulmonary hypertension: the joint task force for the diagnosis and treatment of pulmonary hypertension of the European Society of Cardiology (ESC) and the

European Respiratory Society (ERS): endorsed by: Association for European Paediatric and Congenital Cardiology (AEPC), International Society for Heart and Lung Transplantation (ISHLT). Eur Heart J 2016;37(1):67–119.

43. Galie N, Muller K, Scalise AV, et al. PATENT PLUS: a blinded, randomised and extension study of riociguat plus sildenafil in pulmonary arterial hypertension. Eur Respir J 2015;45(5):1314–22.

44. Rich S. The current treatment of pulmonary arterial hypertension: time to redefine success. Chest 2006;130(4):1198–202.

45. Galie N, Simonneau G, Barst RJ, et al. Clinical worsening in trials of pulmonary arterial hypertension: results and implications. Curr Opin Pulm Med 2010; 16(Suppl 1):S11–9.

46. Pulido T, Adzerikho I, Channick RN, et al. Macitentan and morbidity and mortality in pulmonary arterial hypertension. N Engl J Med 2013;369(9):809–18.

47. Sitbon O, Channick R, Chin KM, et al. Selexipag for the treatment of pulmonary arterial hypertension. N Engl J Med 2015;373(26):2522–33.

48. Tapson VF, Torres F, Kermeen F, et al. Oral treprostinil for the treatment of pulmonary arterial hypertension in patients on background endothelin receptor antagonist and/or phosphodiesterase type 5 inhibitor therapy (the FREEDOM-C study): a randomized controlled trial. Chest 2012;142(6):1383–90.

49. Tapson VF, Jing ZC, Xu KF, et al. Oral treprostinil for the treatment of pulmonary arterial hypertension in patients receiving background endothelin receptor antagonist and phosphodiesterase type 5 inhibitor therapy (the FREEDOM-C2 study): a randomized controlled trial. Chest 2013;144(3):952–8.

50. Sitbon O, Jais X, Savale L, et al. Upfront triple combination therapy in pulmonary arterial hypertension: a pilot study. Eur Respir J 2014;43(6):1691–7.

51. Actelion. The efficacy and safety of initial triple versus initial dual oral combination therapy in patients with newly diagnosed pulmonary arterial hypertension: a multi-center, double-blind, placebo-controlled, phase 3b study. NLM identifier NCT02558231. Available at: https://clinicaltrials.gov/ct2/show/NCT02558231. Accessed August 1, 2020.

52. Klinger JR, Elliott CG, Levine DJ, et al. Therapy for pulmonary arterial hypertension in adults: update of the CHEST guideline and expert panel report. Chest 2019;155(3):565–86.

53. Waxman AB, McElderry HT, Gomberg-Maitland M, et al. Totally implantable IV treprostinil therapy in pulmonary hypertension assessment of the implantation procedure. Chest 2017;152(6):1128–34.

54. Gomberg-Maitland M, Bourge RC, Shapiro SM, et al. Long-term results of the delivery for pulmonary arterial hypertension trial. Pulm Circ 2019;9(4). 2045894019878615.

55. Shapiro SM, Bourge RC, Pozella P, et al. Implantable system for treprostinil: a real-world patient experience study. Pulm Circ 2020;10(2):1–10.

56. Sitbon O, Gomberg-Maitland M, Granton J, et al. Clinical trial design and new therapies for pulmonary arterial hypertension. Eur Respir J 2019;53(1): 1801908.

Preoperative Assessment and Perioperative Management of the Patient with Pulmonary Vascular Disease

Jochen Steppan, MD, DESA[a],*, Paul M. Heerdt, MD, PhD[b]

KEYWORDS

• Pulmonary hypertension • Anesthesia • Surgery

KEY POINTS

• Pulmonary Hypertension is a significant contributor to peri-operative morbidity and mortality.
• The exact incidence and impact of occult disease is unknown.
• Perioperative management of high risk patients should be conducted by a dedicated perioperative team who has the skills and experience to take care of those patients.
• Preoperative optimization and intra-operative management that focuses on lowering pulmonary vascular resistance and supporting right ventricular function are key in caring for those patients.

BACKGROUND

Pulmonary hypertension (PH) is a disease of the lung vasculature, whose definition currently is in flux. It has been defined as a mean pulmonary artery pressure (mPAP) greater than or equal to 25 mm Hg during resting right heart catheterization (RHC).[1] At the recent sixth World Symposium on Pulmonary Hypertension, however, it was proposed that this definition should be expanded to include patients with a mPAP of greater than 20 mm Hg and a pulmonary vascular resistance (PVR) of greater than or equal to 3 Wood units for all forms of precapillary PH.[1] Elevated mPAP can be due to increased PVR, high cardiac output, or increased pulmonary venous pressure secondary to left heart disease. Consequently, PH can be classified into 5 distinct groups incorporating both precapillary and postcapillary pathology: pulmonary arterial (PA) hypertension (group I); left heart disease (group II); chronic lung disease and/or hypoxia (group III); chronic thromboembolic disease (group IV); and unclear or multifactorial mechanisms (group V).[1,2] Currently, therapy for patients with known PA hypertension remains focused on pulmonary vasodilators targeting 3 mechanistic pathways and their modulators: endothelin, nitric oxide, and prostacyclin.[3]

PERIOPERATIVE IMPACT

Estimating the true incidence of PH in surgical populations is complicated due to variant etiology, method of diagnosis, occult disease, and influence of anesthesia and surgery on mPAP. The perioperative incidence of PH in patients undergoing major noncardiac surgery was estimated to be less than 1% (0.81%) in the Healthcare Cost and Utilization Project's National Inpatient Sample data set that included more than 17 million hospitalizations in the United States.[4] This incidence was not static,

[a] Johns Hopkins University, School of Medicine, Department of Anesthesiology and Critical Care Medicine, Baltimore, MD, USA; [b] Department of Anesthesiology Yale School of Medicine, Division of Applied Hemodynamics, New Haven, CT, USA

* Corresponding author. Johns Hopkins University, 1800 Orleans Street, Zayed 6208C, Baltimore, MD 21287.
E-mail address: J.Steppan@jhmi.edu

Clin Chest Med 42 (2021) 133–141
https://doi.org/10.1016/j.ccm.2020.11.013

however, and it increased steadily over the study period, with the latest incidence in 2014 being estimated as 1.2%.[4,5]

Perioperative Risk and Pulmonary Hypertension

It is well established that PH is a deadly disease; patients with PH have a significantly lower survival and a higher rate of major adverse cardiovascular events than patients without PH.[5,6] A diagnosis of PH increases 1-year standardized mortality by more than 7-fold.[5] Not surprisingly, superimposing the stresses of anesthesia and surgery on top of preexisting PH is not trivial. Studies evaluating PH as a specific risk factor for adverse outcomes after surgery still are evolving, but available data clearly demonstrate that patients with PH are at significantly higher risk for perioperative morbidity and mortality.[4,7–13] Quantitative interpretation of available data is complicated by factors such as differences in study methodology, how PH was defined and/or diagnosed (echocardiography vs *Internal Classification of Diseases, Ninth Revision,* coding vs right heart catheterization), disease classification, and therapeutic options. Nevertheless, mortality and morbidity among patients with PH are consistently high, with reported mortality for noncardiac surgery as high as 10%.[7] Although a recent noncardiac surgery database analysis indicated a lower mortality rate (4.4% in PH patients compared with 1.1% in the non-PH population), this study demonstrated that major adverse cardiovascular events (death, acute myocardial infarction, and stroke) occurred in more than 8% of hospitalizations with PH compared with 2.0% of those without PH.[4] Other cardiovascular complications, such as pulmonary embolism, cardiogenic shock, and cardiac arrest, also were much more likely in the PH group compared with those without PH (6.1% vs 0.7%, respectively).[4] Although large database analysis does not lend itself to pinpointing the specific cause of death, in smaller studies postoperative mortality was frequently due to right ventricular (RV) failure and occurred within 48 hours of the operation.[13] Other morbidities frequently include respiratory failure (21%–28%), cardiac dysrhythmias (3%–21%), hypotension (7%–14%), and congestive heart failure (6%–11%).[8–10,12–14] The types of surgery associated with higher mortality generally ranged from minimally invasive procedures (eg, laparoscopic cholecystectomy), to major surgery (eg, major bowel resection), and to obstetric procedures. Lastly, emergency surgeries were consistently associated with a higher rate of perioperative mortality.[10,12,13]

Occult Disease

Although the increased risk of perioperative complications in patients with known PH is well established, these data may underestimate the actual impact because the true incidence of PH in the noncardiac surgical population is unknown. This uncertainty is influenced by the variability imposed by both underdiagnosis and overdiagnosis. For example, patients with PH presenting for surgery are more likely to be older and male and have a history of smoking, obstructive sleep apnea, obesity, systemic hypertension, chronic pulmonary disease, and/or valvular heart disease.[4,15] These demographics and comorbidities are common in the surgical population. This raises the prospect of occult PH that, although subclinical preoperatively, can have significant perioperative implications. The incidence of PH overall has been reported to be relatively low in patients with left heart disease (<4%) or pulmonary disease (<1%), suggesting that PH is a surprisingly rare complication overall.[5] Alternatively, patients increasingly are labeled as having PH not based on the gold standard RHC but by echocardiographic criteria alone (RV systolic pressure estimation using Doppler).[16] The incidence of PH by echocardiographic evaluation alone, however, has been reported to be as high as 20%.[17] It must be born in mind, however, that the correlation between echocardiography-derived pressure estimates for PA pressures is far from perfect, with Doppler echocardiography being inaccurate (defined as deviating more than 10 mm Hg from the invasive measurement) in approximately 48% of cases.[18] A more recent study reported the sensitivity and specificity of echo-derived estimates detecting RV systolic pressures greater than 52 mm Hg, at 81% and 69%, respectively.[19]

PREOPERATIVE ASSESSMENT

Multiple risk-assessment tools of varying complexity are available and long have been used to predict outcomes in patients undergoing noncardiac surgery.[20–24] Despite the clearly elevated perioperative risk associated with PH, however, none specifically accounts for the presence or severity of PH.[25] It, therefore, is critical for the preoperative evaluation to consider these risks and plan perioperative management accordingly, ideally using a multidisciplinary and systemic approach that includes all team members.[7]

Although absolute PA pressure values (either systolic or mean PA pressure) are used to make a diagnosis of PH, they are of limited value in defining severity in a functional sense.[26] For example, functional capacity independent of absolute mPAP has been linked to long-term outcomes and correlates well with survival.[27] Ultimately, a patient's symptoms and mortality are dictated by how effectively the RV adapts to a chronically elevated afterload.[28] This balance, or coupling, between contractility and afterload initially may be preserved despite markedly elevated mPAP with subsequent uncoupling predictive of cardiovascular decompensation.[29] In this context, indices of functional capacity (eg, 6-minute walk test or New York Heart Association functional class), and cardiac reserve (eg, cardiac index) are more reliable predictors of perioperative outcomes than mPAP in isolation.

In general, perioperative risk factors can be separated as procedure-related (emergency surgery, intermediate-risk to high-risk surgery, or surgery longer than 3 hours) and patient related (American Society of Anesthesiologists class III or IV, functional capacity, additional cardiovascular disease, or abnormal hemodynamics).[9,10,12,13,30,31] Broadly, PH patients with RV to pulmonary vascular uncoupling, which manifests as reduced exercise capacity, rapid progression of symptoms, and elevated right heart filling pressure, have the highest risk for perioperative complications (**Box 1**). In addition,

other echocardiographic measures of RV function have been described, but the predictive value in PH remains unclear.[32]

PERIOPERATIVE MANAGEMENT
A Team Approach

The perioperative period in general presents technical challenges and multiple insults that potentially are detrimental in the setting of PH (**Box 2**).[33] Accordingly, optimal patient care starts with the formulation of a management plan, ideally by a multidisciplinary team that incorporates preoperative evaluation, intraoperative management, and postoperative care. Recommendations for constructing such a team have been described and suggest the designation of an anesthesiologist specializing in PH as the focal point for integrating input from referring physicians, PH specialists, surgeons, anesthesiologists, and critical care staff, with the logistical considerations of the operating room.[7] This approach facilitates a preoperative multidisciplinary discussion of key factors by all stakeholders to ensure the patient is optimized and the approach is ideal. For example, contingency plans may be required for procedures

---

Box 1
Perioperative predictors of mortality and morbidity

Exercise capacity

Rapid progression of symptoms

Elevated right heart filling pressure

Presence of RV failure

Syncope

Functional class IV

Six-minute walk test distance of less than 399 m

Tricuspid annular plane systolic excursion of less than 1.5 cm

Presence of a pericardial effusion,

Right atrial pressure of more than 15 mm Hg

Cardiac index of less than 2.0 L/min/m^2

Peak Vo_2 <1 mL/min/kg

VE/Vco_2 ≥45

Adopted from Leuchte HH, Ten Freyhaus H, Gall H, et al. Risk stratification strategy and assessment of disease progression in patients with pulmonary arterial hypertension: Updated Recommendations from the Cologne Consensus Conference 2018. Int J Cardiol. 2018;272S:20-29.

Box 2
Perioperative changes that increase pulmonary vascular resistance

Hypoxemia and hypercapnia

- Due to sedation, analgesia, inadequate mask ventilation, delayed intubation

Acidosis

- Secondary to hypovolemia, infection, decreased cardiac output, hypoventilation

Hypothermia

- Caused by cold intravenous fluids or ambient temperature

Atelectasis and hyperinflation

- Tidal volume, positive end-expiratory pressure

Catecholamine release

- Pain, inadequate anesthesia, anxiety

Medications

- Pure α-agonists

From Steppan J, Diaz-Rodriguez N, Barodka VM, et al. Focused Review of Perioperative Care of Patients with Pulmonary Hypertension and Proposal of a Perioperative Pathway. Cureus. 2018;10(1):e2072; with permission.

known to acutely impact RV to pulmonary vascular coupling, such as laparoscopy, joint replacement, and intrathoracic surgery requiring single-lung ventilation. In addition, for high-risk procedures, the availability of extracorporeal membrane oxygenation (ECMO) can be discussed (**Box 3**).

Preoperative Evaluation and Optimization

Priory to surgery, patient evaluation should encompass consideration of 3 broad questions: (1) Is the etiology of PH sufficiently defined? (2) What is the patient's functional status relative to the planned procedure? and (3) Are there modifiable risk factors within the surgical time frame?[34,35] Preoperative echocardiography represents an important screening tool for elevated RV systolic pressure, valve pathology, and biventricular function but may not be sufficient to define whether the etiology of PH is precapillary/postcapillary or combined. In that this distinction has value in formulating plans for perioperative management in patients undergoing elective major surgery, RHC with vasoreactivity testing has been advocated.[34] In addition to physical examination, echocardiography, and routine assessments, such as

electrocardiogram, pulmonary function testing, and serum brain natriuretic peptide measurement, a 6-minute walk test readily can be performed. Although specific interpretation across the wide spectrum of PH etiology and surgical procedures can be difficult, a distance of less than 399 m has been shown to be associated with perioperative complications in patients undergoing major noncardiac and nonobstetric surgery.[13] The potential role of preoperative cardiopulmonary exercise testing remains unclear. Although cardiopulmonary exercise testing may characterize functional capacity more fully, there currently are no established parameter levels specifically linked to perioperative risk or postoperative outcome in patients with PH.[35] Preoperative optimization should focus on maximizing functional capacity by targeting modifiable factors, such as PH therapy, including nonpharmacologic interventions such as oxygen therapy and continuous positive airway pressure at night, and optimizing volume status. Importantly, surgical urgency needs to be considered when formulating an optimization strategy. Many therapies can take weeks or even months for optimal effect; thus, the risk of delaying surgery (eg, an oncological procedure) needs to be carefully weighed against the benefit of postponement for further optimization. Management of pulmonary vasodilators can be challenging particularly because functional improvement after preoperative dose adjustment is not instantaneous. Perioperatively, every effort should be made to maintain vasodilator therapy without interruption.[36,37] That said, administration may have to be adjusted to account for considerations, such as platelet dysfunction. Lastly, there should be a plan for how to handle parenteral application devices, because providers might not be familiar with their management.

Intraoperative Management

Several reviews have been written on anesthetic management for patients with PH undergoing both cardiac and noncardiac surgery, and, although there is no firm consensus regarding specific drugs and techniques, the basic principle of preventing RV to pulmonary vascular uncoupling is universal.[7,38] Fundamentally, this entails maintaining RV contractility while minimizing increases in afterload imposed by mechanical, physiologic, and pharmacologic factors (**Box 4**). The operating room represents a unique environment in that transient episodes of hypotension are relatively common, and, although well tolerated in most patients, for

---

Box 3
Standardized preoperative planning questions to be addressed

Do the benefits of the surgery outweigh the PH-associated risks of the procedure?

Is the patient medically optimized?

How will PH medications be managed in the perioperative period?

Are procedural modifications necessary to mitigate PH-associated risk?

Should the procedure be moved from its usual location?

How should anesthesia staffing be allocated?

What is the optimal postoperative disposition?

Is the patient a candidate for ECMO?

Are there special circumstances requiring additional expert input?

Is the plan communicated to every member of the team/stakeholders?

Modified from Steppan J, Diaz-Rodriguez N, Barodka VM, et al. Focused Review of Perioperative Care of Patients with Pulmonary Hypertension and Proposal of a Perioperative Pathway. Cureus. 2018;10(1):e2072; with permission.

Box 4
Optimizing right ventricular function

Preload

- Euvolemia
- Avoid volume loading (especially large fluid boluses)

Contractility

- Maintain coronary blood flow (normal or elevated systemic afterload)
- Support with drugs as needed (eg, β-agonists)
- Optimize metabolic factors (avoid acidosis, hypothermia, hypocalcemia, etc.)

Afterload

- High inspired oxygen concentration
- Mild hypocarbia
- Treat acidosis early
- Normothermia
- Low mean airway pressures (decrease tidal volumes, extend expiratory time; ideally, spontaneous ventilation, although be aware of hypercarbia)
- Avoid catecholamine release (eg, due to pain or anxiety)
- Use medications that either decrease PVR (eg, milrinone or inhaled nitric oxide) directly, or use medications that do not affect PVR (eg, vasopressin)

Rate and rhythm

- Maintain normal sinus rhythm

---

those with PH the consequences can be profound. High RV pressures increase myocardial oxygen demand while at the same time shifting coronary perfusion from the normal pattern of flow in both systole and diastole to predominantly diastole alone. Ultimately, if coronary perfusion pressure in the aortic root falls below a critical threshold whereas RV pressure and oxygen demand remain high, myocardial contractility rapidly declines due to ischemia and RV failure ensues. Accordingly, maintaining systemic blood pressure with norepinephrine or vasopressin is a key component of intraoperative management along with inotropic augmentation and avoidance of metabolic or pharmacologic myocardial depressants.

The operating room also represents an environment where events commonly occur that can precipitate acute changes in RV afterload that, although usually well tolerated in most patients, can elicit exaggerated responses with significant consequences in patients with PH (see **Box 2**). For example, during positive pressure ventilation, there is a U-shaped relationship between PVR and lung volume. At low volumes, PVR rises due to atelectasis and hypoxic pulmonary vasoconstriction (HPV), whereas hyperinflation increases PVR by compression of the intra-alveolar vessels. Additionally, hypercapnic acidosis resulting from even modest hypoventilation, as may occur with common lung protective ventilation strategies, may increase PVR. In this context, careful attention to optimal titration of tidal volume and positive end-expiratory pressure in patients with PH is important. Similarly, air bubbles or other small venous emboli that would be relatively innocuous in normal patients may elicit a significant response in those with PH.[39] Superimposed is the potential for marked fluid shifts, lateral or prone positioning, and components of the surgical procedure, such as steep head-down tilt and pneumoperitoneum for laparoscopy.[38] Until relatively recently, intrathoracic noncardiac surgery in patients with PH was limited largely to lung biopsy or transplantation.[40,41] With improved minimally invasive surgical techniques, however, anatomic resections (segmentectomy and lobectomy) are becoming more common. These procedures often require single-lung ventilation to optimize exposure, thereby producing atelectasis among other undesired consequences. Implications in terms of RV to pulmonary vascular coupling are largely related to elevated afterload secondary to increased airway pressure in the ventilated lung, modest hypoxemia and hypercapnia, and extensive HPV in the nonventilated lung. Pulmonary vasodilators used therapeutically diminish HPV to varying degrees as do volatile anesthetics.[42] There currently are no data, however, specifically defining any interaction with single-lung ventilation in terms of hypoxic risk, and anecdotal evidence to suggest altering therapy preoperatively is lacking. Nonetheless, in patients receiving pulmonary vasodilator therapy either chronically or initiated preoperatively, intraoperative addition of inhaled nitric oxide or prostacyclins has been recommended as a means of maximizing dilation of the ventilated lung and optimize the matching of ventilation and perfusion.[38,41]

Technique

The choice of anesthetic technique is based on disease severity, surgical requirements, and planned interventions/medications to maximize

RV function (see **Box 4**). For example, regional anesthesia with an awake, comfortable, and sufficiently breathing patient can be the ideal anesthetic if appropriate for the planned surgery. That said, avoiding tracheal intubation and mechanical ventilation at all cost not always is beneficial; interventions, such as spinal anesthesia, can produce significant hypotension, and sedation may compromise ventilation, resulting in hypercapnia. Ultimately, many patients require general anesthesia, and a variety of approaches for induction and maintenance have been described.[7,43,44] There is no fixed recipe, with experience of the anesthesiologist more important than specific drugs. Clinical experience has prompted re-examination of firmly held beliefs, such as the concept that ketamine is contraindicated in patients with PH. The combination of ketamine with a benzodiazepine and sufficient ventilation now has been described as beneficial for maintaining RV contractility without increasing PVR.[45–47] Other well-tolerated drugs are opioids, dexmedetomidine, and lidocaine to facilitate a balanced anesthetic technique, incorporating a combination of low-dose intravenous and inhaled anesthetics with muscle relaxants.[48,49] Systemic blood pressure ideally should be maintained with drugs that are devoid of direct effects on PVR (eg, vasopressin) or that have both α-adrenergic and β-adrenergic agonist effects (eg, norepinephrine or ephedrine), to augment both inotropy and systemic vascular tone.[50–52] Using norepinephrine alone often is sufficient, and there is evidence supporting its use in models of RV failure.[53,54] Inotropic support also can be provided with low-dose dobutamine or milrinone. Both drugs can increase cardiac output and reduce PVR but also produce simultaneous systemic vasodilation and hypotension.[53] Targeted afterload reduction can be achieved with inhaled nitric oxide or prostacyclins in both intubated and spontaneously breathing patients, although there are insufficient data regarding how their intraoperative use affects long-term outcomes.[54,55]

Monitoring

The decision regarding intraoperative monitoring largely is dictated by preoperative assessment of disease severity, comorbidities, exercise capacity, and the planned surgical procedure. In general, placement of an intra-arterial catheter under local anesthesia is recommended for continuous blood pressure monitoring and intermittent blood gas analysis given the

benefit relative to the low risk of complications.[56] Similarly, although placing a central venous catheter is not without risk, the benefit for reliably administering vasoactive drugs centrally is clear, and many clinicians find monitoring of central venous pressure useful. In contrast, PA catheters generally are not indicated because the risks probably outweigh the benefits. As discussed previously, even seemingly simple minimally invasive procedures can impose acute intraoperative challenges that mandate consideration. In cases of significant blood loss or marked changes in RV afterload anticipated, PA catheter insertion prior to beginning the procedure may be helpful in selected patients, guiding pulmonary vasodilator therapy and fluid administration. Increasingly, adjunctive intraoperative monitoring with transesophageal echocardiography provides direct visualization of biventricular filling and qualitative assessment. When considered in the context of simultaneous measurements of systemic arterial and central venous pressures, transesophageal echocardiography can facilitate differentiation of hypovolemia and right heart failure.

Postoperative Management

Given the high rate of postoperative RV failure and respiratory complications in patients with PH, postoperative management in a monitored setting or intensive care unit is recommended. For some patients, the experience of the medical team in managing PH may outweigh any inexperience in managing postoperative needs (eg, patients with severe PH undergoing minor surgery). Thus, patients on parenteral therapy may benefit from postoperative care in a location staffed by providers experienced in the management of pulmonary vasodilators.[7]

SUMMARY

Current outcome prediction models fail to adequately capture PH as a specific factor. It is well established, however, that patients with PH are at increased perioperative risk. It, therefore, is important to apply a systematic approach for identifying these patients early and optimizing both their physical status and perioperative care plan prior to surgery. In general, patients with symptomatic PH, reduced exercise tolerance, and elevated right heart filling pressures are at the greatest perioperative risk. Therefore, perioperative management should prioritize factors that maintain or improve RV to pulmonary vascular coupling.

CLINICS CARE POINTS

- Interpret a preoperative diagnosis of PH based exclusively on echocardiography carefully – elevated RV systolic pressure by Doppler is not a definitive diagnosis.

- Preoperative optimization of volume status and an adequate medical regimen are key to maximize exercise tolerance before the procedure.

- Intraoperatively, anticipation and early intervention are key factors – relatively common events such as transient hypotension or hypo/hyperventilation can have serious consequences.

- Minimally invasive can be maximally challenging – interventions such as pneumoperitoneum for laparoscopy can rapidly alter the balance between RV contractility and afterload.

DISCLOSURE

P.M. Heerdt: Consultant, Baxter International and Baudax Bio; Jochen steppan is funded by the NHLBI grant K08HL145132.

REFERENCES

1. Simonneau G, Montani D, Celermajer DS, et al. Haemodynamic definitions and updated clinical classification of pulmonary hypertension. Eur Respir J 2019;53(1):1801913.

2. Simonneau G, Gatzoulis MA, Adatia I, et al. Updated clinical classification of pulmonary hypertension. J Am Coll Cardiol 2013;62(25 Suppl):D34–41.

3. Lau EMT, Giannoulatou E, Celermajer DS, et al. Epidemiology and treatment of pulmonary arterial hypertension. Nat Rev Cardiol 2017;14(10):603–14.

4. Smilowitz NR, Armanious A, Bangalore S, et al. Cardiovascular outcomes of patients with pulmonary hypertension undergoing noncardiac surgery. Am J Cardiol 2019;123(9):1532–7.

5. Wijeratne DT, Lajkosz K, Brogly SB, et al. Increasing incidence and prevalence of World Health Organization groups 1 to 4 pulmonary hypertension: a population-based cohort study in Ontario, Canada. Circ Cardiovasc Qual Outcomes 2018;11(2): e003973.

6. Strange G, Lau EM, Giannoulatou E, et al. Survival of idiopathic pulmonary arterial hypertension patients in the modern era in Australia and New Zealand. Heart Lung Circ 2018;27(11):1368–75.

7. Steppan J, Diaz-Rodriguez N, Barodka VM, et al. Focused review of perioperative care of patients with pulmonary hypertension and proposal of a perioperative pathway. Cureus 2018;10(1):e2072.

8. Ramakrishna G, Sprung J, Ravi BS, et al. Impact of pulmonary hypertension on the outcomes of noncardiac surgery: predictors of perioperative morbidity and mortality. J Am Coll Cardiol 2005;45(10):1691–9.

9. Lai HC, Lai HC, Wang KY, et al. Severe pulmonary hypertension complicates postoperative outcome of non-cardiac surgery. Br J Anaesth 2007;99(2): 184–90.

10. Price LC, Montani D, Jais X, et al. Noncardiothoracic nonobstetric surgery in mild-to-moderate pulmonary hypertension. Eur Respir J 2010;35(6):1294–302.

11. Memtsoudis SG, Ma Y, Chiu YL, et al. Perioperative mortality in patients with pulmonary hypertension undergoing major joint replacement. Anesth Analg 2010;111(5):1110–6.

12. Kaw R, Pasupuleti V, Deshpande A, et al. Pulmonary hypertension: an important predictor of outcomes in patients undergoing non-cardiac surgery. Respir Med 2011;105(4):619–24.

13. Meyer S, McLaughlin VV, Seyfarth HJ, et al. Outcomes of noncardiac, nonobstetric surgery in patients with PAH: an international prospective survey. Eur Respir J 2013;41(6):1302–7.

14. Deljou A, Sabov M, Kane GC, et al. Outcomes after noncardiac surgery for patients with pulmonary hypertension: a historical cohort study. J Cardiothorac Vasc Anesth 2020;34(6):1506–13.

15. Whelton PK, Carey RM, Aronow WS, et al. 2017 ACC/AHA/AAPA/ABC/ACPM/AGS/APhA/ASH/ASPC/NMA/PCNA guideline for the prevention, detection, evaluation, and management of high blood pressure in adults: a report of the American College of Cardiology/American Heart Association Task Force on clinical practice guidelines. J Am Coll Cardiol 2018;71(19):e127–248.

16. Orem C. Epidemiology of pulmonary hypertension in the elderly. J Geriatr Cardiol 2017;14(1):11–6.

17. Lam CS, Borlaug BA, Kane GC, et al. Age-associated increases in pulmonary artery systolic pressure in the general population. Circulation 2009;119(20): 2663–70.

18. Fisher MR, Forfia PR, Chamera E, et al. Accuracy of Doppler echocardiography in the hemodynamic assessment of pulmonary hypertension. Am J Respir Crit Care Med 2009;179(7):615–21.

19. Ahmed I, Hassan Nuri MM, Zakariyya AN, et al. Correlation between Doppler echocardiography and right heart catheterization derived pulmonary artery pressures: impact of right atrial pressures. J Coll Physicians Surg Pak 2016;26(4):255–9.

20. Goldman L, Caldera DL, Nussbaum SR, et al. Multifactorial index of cardiac risk in noncardiac surgical procedures. N Engl J Med 1977;297(16):845–50.

21. Nishimura RA, Otto CM, Bonow RO, et al. 2017 AHA/ACC focused update of the 2014 AHA/ACC guideline for the management of patients with valvular heart disease: a report of the American College of Cardiology/American Heart Association Task Force on clinical practice guidelines. Circulation 2017; 135(25):e1159–95.

22. Fleisher LA, Fleischmann KE, Auerbach AD, et al. 2014 ACC/AHA guideline on perioperative cardiovascular evaluation and management of patients undergoing noncardiac surgery: a report of the American College of Cardiology/American Heart Association task force on practice guidelines. Circulation 2014;130(24):e278–333.

23. Lee TH, Marcantonio ER, Mangione CM, et al. Derivation and prospective validation of a simple index for prediction of cardiac risk of major noncardiac surgery. Circulation 1999;100(10):1043–9.

24. Bilimoria KY, Liu Y, Paruch JL, et al. Development and evaluation of the universal ACS NSQIP surgical risk calculator: a decision aid and informed consent tool for patients and surgeons. J Am Coll Surg 2013; 217(5):833–42.e1-3.

25. Silverton N, Djaiani G. Right ventricular function and perioperative risk assessment: the time has come to stop being sinister. J Cardiothorac Vasc Anesth 2019;33(5):1287–9.

26. Benza RL, Miller DP, Gomberg-Maitland M, et al. Predicting survival in pulmonary arterial hypertension: insights from the Registry to Evaluate Early and Long-Term Pulmonary Arterial Hypertension Disease Management (REVEAL). Circulation 2010; 122(2):164–72.

27. Park YM, Chung WJ, Choi DY, et al. Functional class and targeted therapy are related to the survival in patients with pulmonary arterial hypertension. Yonsei Med J 2014;55(6):1526–32.

28. Amsallem M, Mercier O, Kobayashi Y, et al. Forgotten no more: a focused update on the right ventricle in cardiovascular disease. JACC Heart Fail 2018;6(11):891–903.

29. Tello K, Dalmer A, Axmann J, et al. Reserve of right ventricular-arterial coupling in the setting of chronic overload. Circ Heart Fail 2019;12(1):e005512.

30. Memtsoudis S, Liu SS, Ma Y, et al. Perioperative pulmonary outcomes in patients with sleep apnea after noncardiac surgery. Anesth Analg 2011;112(1): 113–21.

31. Yang EI. Perioperative management of patients with pulmonary hypertension for non-cardiac surgery. Curr Rheumatol Rep 2015;17(3):15.

32. Haddad F, Doyle R, Murphy DJ, et al. Right ventricular function in cardiovascular disease, part II: pathophysiology, clinical importance, and management of right ventricular failure. Circulation 2008;117(13): 1717–31.

33. Cheema A, Ibekwe S, Nyhan D, et al. When your 35-year-old patient has a sternotomy scar: anesthesia for adult patients with congenital heart disease presenting for noncardiac surgery. Int Anesthesiol Clin 2018;56(4):3–20.

34. Goldsmith YB, Ivascu N, McGlothlin D, et al. Perioperative management of pulmonary hypertension. In: Klinger JR, Frantz RP, editors. Diagnosis and management of pulmonary hypertension. New York: Springer New York; 2015. p. 437–64.

35. Studer SM. Preoperative considerations in patients with pulmonary hypertension: your patient needs surgical clearance. Adv Pulm Hypertens 2013;12(1):13–7.

36. Fox DL, Stream AR, Bull T. Perioperative management of the patient with pulmonary hypertension. Semin Cardiothorac Vasc Anesth 2014;18(4):310–8.

37. Tonelli AR, Minai OA. Saudi guidelines on the diagnosis and treatment of pulmonary hypertension: perioperative management in patients with pulmonary hypertension. Ann Thorac Med 2014;9(Suppl 1):S98–107.

38. McGlothlin D, Ivascu N, Heerdt PM. Anesthesia and pulmonary hypertension. Prog Cardiovasc Dis 2012; 55(2):199–217.

39. Memtsoudis SG, Besculides MC, Gaber L, et al. Risk factors for pulmonary embolism after hip and knee arthroplasty: a population-based study. Int Orthop 2009;33(6):1739–45.

40. Kreider ME, Hansen-Flaschen J, Ahmad NN, et al. Complications of video-assisted thoracoscopic lung biopsy in patients with interstitial lung disease. Ann Thorac Surg 2007;83(3):1140–4.

41. Ross AF, Ueda K. Pulmonary hypertension in thoracic surgical patients. Curr Opin Anaesthesiol 2010;23(1):25–33.

42. Lumb AB, Slinger P. Hypoxic pulmonary vasoconstriction: physiology and anesthetic implications. Anesthesiology 2015;122(4):932–46.

43. Gille J, Seyfarth HJ, Gerlach S, et al. Perioperative anesthesiological management of patients with pulmonary hypertension. Anesthesiol Res Pract 2012; 2012:356982.

44. Pilkington SA, Taboada D, Martinez G. Pulmonary hypertension and its management in patients undergoing non-cardiac surgery. Anaesthesia 2015;70(1): 56–70.

45. Hatano S, Keane DM, Boggs RE, et al. Diazepam-ketamine anaesthesia for open heart surgery a "micro-mini" drip administration technique. Can Anaesth Soc J 1976;23(6):648–56.

46. Jackson AP, Dhadphale PR, Callaghan ML, et al. Haemodynamic studies during induction of anaesthesia for open-heart surgery using diazepam and ketamine. Br J Anaesth 1978;50(4):375–8.

47. Friesen RH, Twite MD, Nichols CS, et al. Hemodynamic response to ketamine in children with

pulmonary hypertension. Paediatr Anaesth 2016; 26(1):102–8.

48. Nair AS, Kandukuri B, Gopal TV. Dexmedetomidine in pulmonary hypertension. Acta Anaesthesiol Taiwan 2014;52(3):149.

49. But AK, Ozgul U, Erdil F, et al. The effects of preoperative dexmedetomidine infusion on hemodynamics in patients with pulmonary hypertension undergoing mitral valve replacement surgery. Acta Anaesthesiol Scand 2006;50(10):1207–12.

50. Kwak YL, Lee CS, Park YH, et al. The effect of phenylephrine and norepinephrine in patients with chronic pulmonary hypertension*. Anaesthesia 2002;57(1):9–14.

51. Trempy GA, Nyhan DP, Murray PA. Pulmonary vasoregulation by arginine vasopressin in conscious, halothane-anesthetized, and pentobarbital-anesthetized dogs with increased vasomotor tone. Anesthesiology 1994;81(3):632–40.

52. Evora PR, Pearson PJ, Schaff HV. Arginine vasopressin induces endothelium-dependent vasodilatation of the pulmonary artery. V1-receptor-mediated production of nitric oxide. Chest 1993;103(4): 1241–5.

53. Kerbaul F, Rondelet B, Motte S, et al. Effects of norepinephrine and dobutamine on pressure load-induced right ventricular failure. Crit Care Med 2004;32(4):1035–40.

54. Lahm T, McCaslin CA, Wozniak TC, et al. Medical and surgical treatment of acute right ventricular failure. J Am Coll Cardiol 2010;56(18):1435–46.

55. Rao V, Ghadimi K, Keeyapaj W, et al. Inhaled Nitric Oxide (iNO) and Inhaled Epoprostenol (iPGI2) use in cardiothoracic surgical patients: is there sufficient evidence for evidence-based recommendations? J Cardiothorac Vasc Anesth 2018;32(3):1452–7.

56. Nuttall G, Burckhardt J, Hadley A, et al. Surgical and patient risk factors for severe arterial line complications in adults. Anesthesiology 2016;124(3):590–7.

Advanced Surgical and Percutaneous Approaches to Pulmonary Vascular Disease

Laura M. Piechura, MD[a,b], Daniel E. Rinewalt, MD[a], Hari R. Mallidi, MD[a,b],*

KEYWORDS

- Pulmonary hypertension • Pulmonary vascular disease
- Chronic thromboembolic pulmonary hypertension • Pulmonary thromboendarterectomy
- Atrial septostomy • Potts shunt • Lung transplantation • Ex vivo lung perfusion

KEY POINTS

- Advanced surgical and percutaneous approaches to pulmonary hypertension are undertaken in severe or refractory cases.
- Chronic thromboembolic pulmonary hypertension is a pulmonary vascular disease that can be cured by pulmonary thromboendarterectomy; balloon pulmonary angioplasty is an alternative approach for patients unable to undergo surgery.
- Atrial septostomy and Potts shunt establish right-to-left shunting to reduce right ventricular overload, although at the expense of hypoxemia. These procedures can bridge a patient to transplantation.
- Bilateral lung transplantation is the last resort treatment option for patients with pulmonary hypertension, although its use remains limited by a scarcity of suitable donor organs.
- Ex vivo lung perfusion is a platform for increasing donor lung use by extending the evaluation of marginal donor lungs to establish their suitability for transplant.

INTRODUCTION

Pulmonary vascular disease describes an array of diagnoses that culminate in pulmonary hypertension (PH). Once PH is severe or refractory to medical therapy, procedural interventions may be necessary to extend a patient's course. Herein, we review advanced surgical and percutaneous approaches for the treatment of pulmonary vascular disease (**Fig. 1**).

INTERVENTIONS FOR CHRONIC THROMBOEMBOLIC PULMONARY HYPERTENSION

Chronic thromboembolic PH (CTEPH) develops from incomplete resolution of acute pulmonary emboli. The persistent clot becomes a chronic, fibrotic thrombus that limits flow within the pulmonary vasculature, resulting in obstructive vasculopathy and PH.[1] CTEPH is rare, estimated to occur in 0.1% to 9.1% of cases.[2–4] Although lung ventilation–perfusion scintigraphy is a useful screening test, pulmonary angiography is the gold standard modality. However, computed tomography pulmonary angiography and MRI are options[5–7] (**Fig. 2A–D**).

The recommended treatment for CTEPH is pulmonary thromboendarterectomy (PTE) to remove the organized thrombus[8] (**Fig. 2E, F**). Balloon pulmonary angioplasty (BPA) is a potential treatment option for patients who cannot tolerate PTE. Patients who cannot undergo either modality can be managed with optimal medical therapy.[9,10]

[a] Division of Cardiac Surgery, Brigham and Women's Hospital, 75 Francis Street, Boston, MA 02115, USA;
[b] Division of Thoracic Surgery, Brigham and Women's Hospital, 75 Francis Street, Boston, MA 02115, USA
* Corresponding author. Division of Cardiac Surgery, Brigham and Women's Hospital, 75 Francis Street, Boston, MA 02115.
E-mail address: hmallidi@bwh.harvard.edu

Clin Chest Med 42 (2021) 143–154
https://doi.org/10.1016/j.ccm.2020.10.003

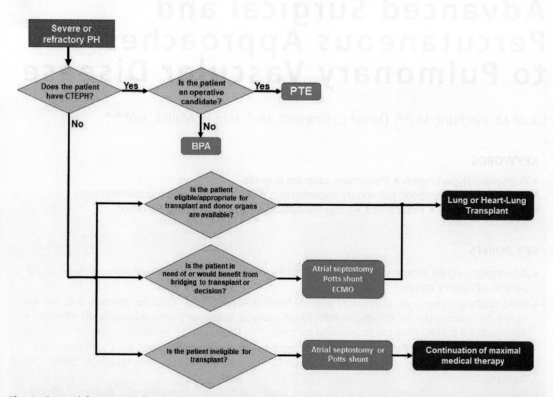

Fig. 1. General framework for the implementation of advanced surgical and percutaneous approaches for PH management. BPA, balloon pulmonary angioplasty; CTEPH, chronic thromboembolic PH; ECMO, extracorporeal membrane oxygenation; PTE, pulmonary thromboendarterectomy.

For patients with incomplete resolution of CTEPH after PTE, options include BPA, medical management, and transplantation.

Pulmonary Thromboendarterectomy

Symptomatic patients with surgically-accessible disease that correlates with their degree of PH and right ventricular (RV) dysfunction should be offered PTE.[11] To date, there are no defined hemodynamic criteria for preoperative risk stratification. A retrospective analysis of 1500 cases performed by the University of California–San Diego group demonstrated that the majority of their patients had preoperative mean pulmonary artery pressure of greater than 30 mm Hg, pulmonary vascular resistance (PVR) of greater than 300 dyne·s·cm^{-5}, and New York Heart Association functional class III or IV symptoms.[12] Patients who may not benefit from the operation include those with life-limiting comorbidities such as advanced malignancy, left-sided heart failure that would be intolerant to increased flow, and parenchymal lung disease with compromised ventilation that would not improve despite restored perfusion.[11]

PTE is performed via median sternotomy with cardiopulmonary bypass and deep hypothermic circulatory arrest.[13] The right pulmonary artery is incised longitudinally. The plane of the endarterectomy is carefully developed around the lumen circumference to encompass the intima, inner media, and entirety of the thromboembolic cast. The dissection can be gently extended into the segmental and subsegmental vessels via an eversion technique. A bloodless field is essential for adequate visualization during the distal portion of the endarterectomy, thus necessitating deep hypothermic circulatory arrest. Usually, 20 minutes of circulatory arrest is sufficient for unilateral endarterectomy.[14] Thereafter, the left-sided endarterectomy is completed in similar fashion. The patient is rewarmed to normothermia and gradually weaned from cardiopulmonary bypass to allow optimization of RV filling and function.

Today, perioperative mortality for PTE is less than 5%. The most common causes of death perioperatively are RV failure owing to persistent PH and reperfusion pulmonary edema (RPE).[15] Published rates of 5-year and 10-year survival range from 75% to 90% and 72% to 75%, respectively.[16,17] When evaluating the outcomes of 550

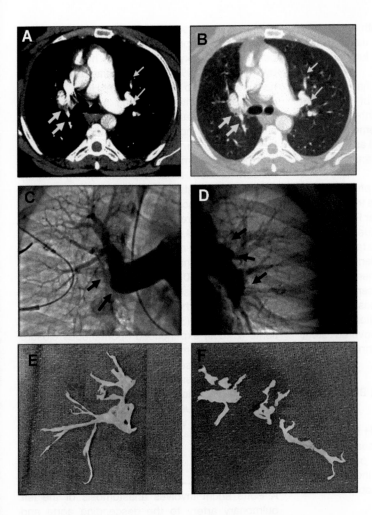

Fig. 2. Representative images from a case of CTEPH. (*A, B*) Transverse sections from computed tomography pulmonary angiography. *Thick yellow arrows* denote significant thromboembolic burden in the proximal branches of the right pulmonary artery. *Thin yellow arrows* denote lesions within the proximal left pulmonary artery. (*C, D*) Images from pulmonary angiography of the right and left lungs, respectively. *Black arrows* indicate proximal filling defects. (*E, F*) Operative specimens after pulmonary thromboendarterectomy of the right and left pulmonary arterial tree.

patients offered PTE at a single institution, those who underwent surgery (49%) had a better 5-year survival than those who were offered but declined surgery (32%), at 83 versus 53% (*P*<.001).[18] After PTE, improvements in hemodynamics can be immediate and profound. Auger and Fedullo[19] describe a mean decrease in PVR of 70% and postoperative PVR generally within 200 to 350 dyne·s·cm^{-5}. This result is persistent out to at least 12 months. Most patients also experience improvement in functional status, RV remodeling, and ejection fraction.[20,21]

Surgical complications unique to PTE include pulmonary artery steal and RPE. Pulmonary artery steal refers to a redistribution of the blood flow from segments previously well perfused to newly-opened segments, resulting in ventilation–perfusion mismatching and hypoxemia; it occurs in about 70% of patients.[22] Most cases resolve with supportive care.[23] RPE develops in areas of the lung previously affected by thromboembolic lesions, and occurs in 9% to 30% of cases.[24]

Manifestations vary from mild hypoxemia to pulmonary hemorrhage and death. Nitric oxide may be beneficial, though at times venovenous extracorporeal membrane oxygenation (ECMO) is required for support.[25,26] Patients with high preoperative and residual postoperative PH are at highest risk for RPE.[27]

Balloon Pulmonary Angioplasty

BPA was initially described for the treatment of congenital pulmonary artery stenosis, but has been implemented for patients with CTEPH who cannot undergo PTE, who have residual disease after PTE, or who require rapid intervention for acute compromise before PTE.[28,29] In general, distal segmental and subsegmental disease may be more amenable to BPA than PTE.

BPA generally entails multiple sessions over a period of weeks. Femoral access is achieved, and individual pulmonary segments are investigated via segmental pulmonary angiography.

Target lesions are serially dilated with undersized balloons (2.0–4.0 mm). Treatment is usually localized to 1 to 2 lobes within the same lung during a session.[30]

Periprocedural mortality for BPA has been reported at 0% to 10%.[30] Resolution of PH occurs gradually over weeks after the intervention.[31] Overall, patients experience improvements in cardiopulmonary hemodynamics as well as functional status, 6-minute walk distances, and exercise tolerance.[32,33]

The most common complications after BPA are RPE and pulmonary vessel injury. The frequency of RPE after BPA is higher than that after PTE at 53% to 60%.[34,35] Combining Pulmonary Edema Predictive Scoring Index results with distal pressure measurements can lower the incidence of RPE and vessel injury while maintaining hemodynamic improvement.[27] Pulmonary artery perforation or rupture occurs in 0% to 7% of cases.[36] Balloon tamponade, reversal of anticoagulation, Gelfoam injection, coil embolization, and covered stent placement may temporize pulmonary artery hemorrhage.[37]

INTERVENTIONS FOR RESCUE OR BRIDGING TO TRANSPLANTATION

Although the overall trajectory of PH is progressive, the rate of change in the disease course can be unpredictable. Options for patients not immediately eligible for transplant include atrial septostomy, Potts shunt, and extracorporeal life support (ECLS) (see **Fig. 1**).

Atrial Septostomy

Atrial septostomy is the recommended shunting procedure for patients with severe or refractory PH.[8] The optimal patient population and timing of implementation are unknown owing to insufficient data. Syncopal episodes (50.6%) and right heart failure (53.4%) were the most commonly documented indications in a recent meta-analysis.[38] A right atrial pressure of greater than 20 mm Hg or preprocedural arterial oxygen saturation of less than 90% may be contraindications, because these conditions may predispose to excessive right-to-left shunting, pulmonary edema, and significant hypoxemia.[38] A baseline right atrial pressure of greater than 20 mm Hg has been associated with increased mortality.[39]

This technique relieves the overloaded RV and mimics Eisenmenger syndrome; patients with Eisenmenger syndrome and concomitant PH live longer than individuals with a comparable degree of primary PH.[40] In balloon dilation atrial septostomy the atrial septum is punctured with a needle and dilated with sequentially larger noncompliant balloons.[41] The procedure should be concluded before arterial oxygen saturation has decreased by more than 10% or LV end-diastolic pressure has increased to more than 18 mm Hg.[42] Although right-to-left shunting worsens systemic hypoxemia, the resultant increase in cardiac output and a reactive increase in hematocrit can offset this phenomenon.[43]

In a recent meta-analysis of 204 patients, balloon dilation atrial septostomy significantly decreased right atrial pressure and arterial oxygen saturation and increased both cardiac index and left atrial pressure.[38] Periprocedural and 30-day mortality were 4.8% and 14.6%, respectively, and the mortality rate after 30 days (mean follow-up of 46.5 months) was 37.7%. The increase in mortality after 30 days highlights the need for bridging to a destination strategy if possible. In these patients, the most common complication was hypoxemia (3%). Nearly one-quarter of patients (23.8%) experienced spontaneous closure of their septostomy, necessitating a repeat procedure. A larger septostomy minimizes the risk of spontaneous closure but can cause an acute rise in LV end-diastolic pressure and profound hypoxemia.[44] Consequently, methods for controlling septostomy size with fenestrated devices are in development.[45–48]

Potts Shunt

A Potts shunt involves anastomosis of the left pulmonary artery to the descending aorta and was initially described to increase right-sided blood flow in cyanotic congenital cardiac syndromes.[49] It has since been used for children and adults with PH.[50,51] The Potts shunt decompresses the overloaded right heart via right-to-left shunting; flow to the descending aorta avoids hypoxemia in the cerebral and coronary circulations. Simulation studies indicate that preserved RV function is essential for benefit from a Potts shunt.[52] Without sufficient RV function, a Potts shunt may leave the patient susceptible to left-to-right shunting, thereby worsening right-sided overload.

A Potts shunt can be created as a direct side-to-side anastomosis or via conduit, including surgical grafts and percutaneous stents.[28,53] Recently, Rosenzweig and colleagues[54] have described the use of a novel unidirectional shunt that incorporates a 1-way valve. This design prevents shunt reversal when systemic pressures exceed the pulmonary artery pressure; flow back into the right heart can re-elevate pulmonary pressures and predispose to edema or hemorrhage.[50]

In the largest series of pediatric patients (n = 24) in whom a Potts shunt was created, 3 experienced early death owing to low cardiac output (12.5%). Two years into their course, the remaining patients reported persistently improved functional capacity.[55,56] In the first case series of percutaneous, transcatheter Potts shunts, 4 adults with pulmonary artery hypertension underwent the procedure, although one died from massive hemothorax during the procedure and another died on postprocedure day 5 from multisystem organ failure.[28] The 2 surviving patients experienced significant symptomatic relief.[28,42] Although a Potts shunt does not preclude transplantation, limited experience and high periprocedural mortality necessitate scrutiny.

Extracorporeal Life Support

ECLS should be considered in patients with PH who present with cardiogenic shock or with ongoing refractory RV failure. ECLS should not be used without a reasonable recovery option, and transplant-ineligible patients may only benefit from ECLS if the aforementioned procedures can facilitate recovery or if their decompensation is reversible.

The primary goal of ECLS for patients with PH is to unload the failing RV and deliver oxygenated blood to the systemic circulation to support end-organ function.[42] The most common strategy is peripheral venoarterial ECMO via percutaneous cannulation of the femoral vessels (**Fig. 3**).[57]

A disadvantage of peripheral femoral cannulation is the potential for North–South or Harlequin syndrome, which occurs when the oxygenated blood returning from the circuit in a retrograde direction competes with the deoxygenated blood being ejected by the LV in an antegrade direction such that oxygenated blood does not reach the coronary circulation or arch vessels, resulting in relative upper body hypoxia.[58] North–South syndrome can be overcome with placement of an additional outflow cannula in the right internal jugular vein, a configuration known as venoarterial–venous ECMO (see **Fig. 3**). In this manner, oxygenated blood from the circuit is delivered to both the femoral artery and right atrium.[59]

Another strategy for ECLS in patients with PH is the use of venovenous ECMO in the presence of an atrial septal defect. In this approach, oxygenated blood returns to the right heart, and right-to-left shunting across the atrial septal defect facilitates systemic oxygenation.[60] This cannulation strategy is most appropriate for patients with peripheral vascular disease and excellent LV function, although it requires the additional step of

septostomy creation in the absence of congenital atrial septal defect.

More recently, the Protek Duo dual lumen cannula (TandemLife, Pittsburgh, PA) has emerged as an additional support modality for patients with right heart failure. Placed in the right internal jugular vein, the inflow lumen of the cannula has multiple ports that drain blood from the right atrium, whereas the outflow lumen has a single drainage port positioned in the main pulmonary artery distal to the pulmonic valve for return of oxygenated blood.[61] When connected to the ECMO circuit, this configuration is termed, Oxy-RVAD. It is ideal for patients with combined RV and respiratory failure.[62]

The use of ECLS for patients with PH has been shown to decrease mortality on the transplant waiting list.[63] In a recent single-center retrospective review of 98 patients with PH (excluding group 2), Rosenzweig and colleagues[64] report an overall 30-day survival of 73.5%, survival to decannulation of 66.3%, and survival to hospital discharge of 54.1%. Of 54 patients cannulated specifically with the intent to bridge to transplantation, 59.3% survived to transplantation. Outcomes related to specific ECLS strategies remain limited to small, single-center studies.[65,66] Although potentially life saving, ECMO does carry risk for frequent and grave complications. Major bleeding affects as many as 81% of patients on ECMO.[67] Neurologic complications include stroke (2%–18%), and serious vascular complications include limb ischemia (4%–50%), thromboembolism (18%), and possible amputation (1%).[68] Sepsis develops in as many as 31% of these patients who remain dependent on mechanical circulatory support, a complication that is often fatal.[68] Although ECLS is a life-saving tool for bridge to recovery or transplant in cases of acute shock, its significant risks reserve it as a last resort modality.

TRANSPLANTATION

Transplantation remains the final treatment alternative for eligible candidates with end-stage disease.[69] Historically heart–lung transplantation was the procdure performed for PH given the associated RV failure; however, we now know that the RV can most often recover after relief of an increased PVR if LV function is suitable.[70,71] The current consensus is that bilateral lung transplantation is the recommended procedure for patients with PH.[72,73]

Lung Transplantation

Current guidelines recommend early consideration of referral to transplant centers for patient

VA   **VAV**

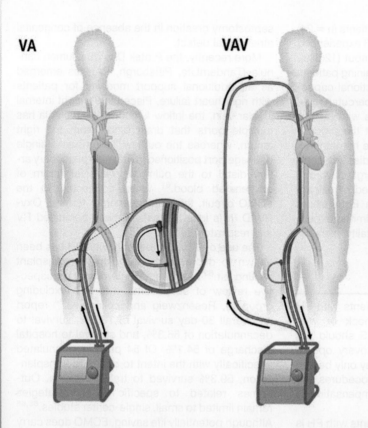

Fig. 3. (*Left*) A peripheral venoarterial ECMO cannulation strategy with arterial outflow cannula in the femoral artery and venous inflow cannula in the femoral vein. Also depicted is an arterial revascularization cannula in the superficial femoral artery to ensure intact perfusion to the lower extremity. (*Right*) Venoarterial venous ECMO cannulation strategy with additional venous outflow cannula in the right internal jugular vein. (*Adapted from* Napp LC, Kühn C, Hoeper MM, et al. Cannulation strategies for percutaneous extracorporeal membrane oxygenation in adults. *Clin Res Cardiol.* 2016;105(4):283-296. https://doi.org/10.1007/s00392-015-0941-1; with permission.)

evaluation.[8,74] Timely assessment in advance of decompensation can allow for pretransplant rehabilitation or reversal of contraindications, although transplant evaluation is not precluded by acute decompensation.[75] Listing for transplantation occurs with New York Heart Association functional class III or IV symptoms.[72] The estimated 1-year mortality of this condition exceeds 10%, which is the estimated 1-year mortality after lung transplantation.[76] Thus, at this disease stage, there is survival benefit to lung transplantation.

Patients who undergo lung transplantation for PH experience similar survival to those who undergo transplantation for parenchymal lung diseases.[73] Patients with PH experienced higher overall survival with bilateral over single lung transplantation. However, patients who undergo lung transplantation for PH experience high rates of early mortality. For adult lung transplant recipients between 1990 and 2015, patients with pulmonary artery hypertension experienced 15.3% mortality before 30 days, compared with 4.5% in patients with chronic obstructive pulmonary disease.[42,77] Causes of death in this patient population included early graft failure (30.7%), multisystem organ failure (15.4%), cardiovascular complications (13.0%), and non-cytomegalovirus infections

(14.2%). The diagnosis of PH was associated with greater risk of mortality at 1-year when compared with chronic obstructive pulmonary disease (hazard ratio, 1.837; P<.0001). For those patients who survive to 1 year, their conditional median survival is 10.0 years.[78] Patients report significant improvement in quality of life and functional status after lung transplantation at least out to 3 years.[79]

Complications common to adult lung transplant recipients include sequelae of chronic immunosuppression including hypertension, renal dysfunction, hyperlipidemia, and diabetes. The factor most limiting of long-term survival continues to be chronic lung allograft dysfunction, which affects 40% to 50% of patients by 5 years after transplantation. Chronic lung allograft dysfunction remains the leading cause of death in lung transplant recipients. Thus, lung transplantation is a successful treatment for mitigating the early mortality of PH, although at the cost of life-long therapy for a new set of chronic, comorbid conditions.[42]

Ex Vivo Lung Perfusion

Although lung transplantation is an effective last resort treatment option, the number of patients on the waitlist outpaces the rate of transplantation owing to a lack of suitable donor lungs.[80] Efforts to improve donor lung use include donation after cardiac death, increased risk donations, and assessment with ex vivo lung perfusion (EVLP) to improve donor lung use by permitting the reevaluation of marginal allografts.[81]

EVLP is a method of ventilating and perfusing lungs in an *ex vivo* setting at normothermic conditions. During EVLP, assessments including oxygenation (Pao_2 to Fio_2 ratio), bronchoscopy, and radiography can be performed to elucidate lung performance and condition. The basic elements of an EVLP circuit include a ventilator, a roller or centrifugal pump, a membrane oxygenator, and a thermoregulatory component (**Fig. 4**).[82] Perfusate is enriched with carbon dioxide via a membrane oxygenator and then pumped through the pulmonary vasculature via a pulmonary artery cannula. The perfusate is collected in a reservoir either by direct return from a pulmonary venous funnel cannula or drainage from an open left atrial cuff. Ventilation is performed via endotracheal tube. Important distinctions between EVLP

protocols include the perfusate, the pulmonary artery pressure parameters, the method of venous outflow, the target flow rate, and the ventilatory settings (**Table 1**).[83]

The use of EVLP in clinical practice is nascent. In 2011, the Toronto group published their landmark report of 20 lung transplants performed after EVLP for allografts initially deemed unsuitable by standard metrics.[84] They described an 86% use rate after EVLP and an equivalent rate of primary graft dysfunction at 72 hours when compared with standard criteria transplants performed over the same time period. From the foundation established by the Lund and Toronto groups, clinical experience in EVLP is now being cultivated globally. Additionally, EVLP has emerged as a powerful basic and translational research platform.[85] To date, results from clinical EVLP differ widely by rates of use for transplant (34%–99%), primary graft dysfunction, and patient survival, highlighting the need to optimize EVLP methodology for maximal clinical benefit.[86–89] Long-term follow-up and upcoming studies will be pivotal for informing future directions in the field.

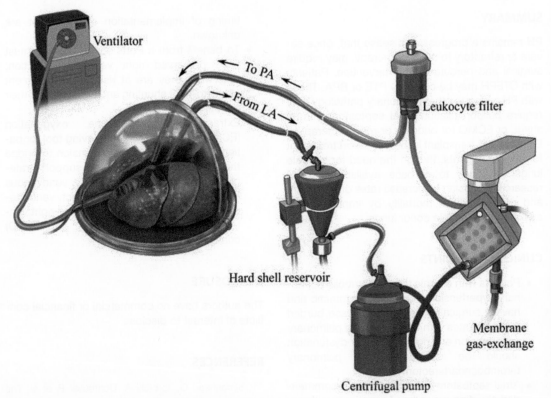

Fig. 4. Typical circuit configuration for EVLP performed via the Toronto protocol. (*From* Cypel M, Keshavjee S. Ex Vivo Lung Perfusion. *Oper Tech Thorac Cardiovasc Surg.* 2014;19(4):433-442. https://doi.org/10.1053/j.optechstcvs.2015.03.001; with permission.)

Table 1
The Toronto and Lund protocols for EVLP

Parameter	Toronto Protocol	Lund Protocol
Perfusion		
Target flow rate	40% cardiac output	100% cardiac output
Pulmonary artery pressure (mm Hg)	≤15	≤20
LA pressure (mm Hg)	3–5	Open
Perfusate	Steen Solution	Steen Solution, Hct 10–15
Ventilation		
Tidal volume (mL/kg)	7	6–8
Respiratory rate	7	10–15
PEEP (cm H_2O)	5	5
Fio_2 (%)	21	50
Temperature (°C)		
At initiation of perfusion	25	15
At initiation of ventilation	32	32
At initiation of evaluation	37	37

The Toronto and Lund protocols are the most widely used methods for EVLP. Key differences in perfusion parameters, ventilation strategy, and temperature management are highlighted.

Abbreviations: Fio_2, fraction of inspired oxygen; Hct, hematocrit; LA, left atrium; PA, pulmonary artery; PEEP, positive end-expiratory pressure.

Adapted from Andreasson AS, Dark JH, Fisher AJ. Ex vivo lung perfusion in clinical lung transplantation–state of the art. Eur J Cardiothorac Surg. 2014;46(5):779-788. https://doi.org/10.1093/ejcts/ezu228; with permission.

SUMMARY

PH remains a progressive disease that, once severe or refractory to medical therapy, may require surgical and percutaneous intervention. Patients with CTEPH may be cured by PTE or BPA. Those with PH owing to other pulmonary pathology may require balloon dilation atrial septostomy, Potts shunt, or ECMO for bridging or rescue therapies. Bilateral lung transplant is the last-resort treatment for eligible patients, though the need for suitable lungs continues to outpace availability. EVLP research is ongoing to increase rates of transplant and reduce waitlist mortality by improving the availability of suitable donor lungs.

CLINICS CARE POINTS

- Patients with chronic thromboembolic pulmonary hypertension who are symptomatic and have a surgically-accessible disease burden that correlates with their degree of pulmonary hypertension and right ventricular dysfunction should be considered for pulmonary thromboendarterectomy.
- Atrial septostomy is currently the recommended shunting procedure for patients with severe or refractory pulmonary hypertension, though the optimal patient population and

timing of implementation of the shunt are unknown.
- To benefit from a Potts shunt, patients must have preserved right ventricular function; otherwise, they are at risk for development of left-to-right shunting and worsening of their condition.
- Extracorporeal membrane oxygenation (ECMO) is a potentially life-saving tool for patients with pulmonary hypertension to bridge them to recovery or transplant; support strategies include venoarterial ECMO, venovenous ECMO with an atrial septal defect, venoarterial-venous ECMO, and oxygenator-right ventricular assist device (oxy-RVAD) configurations.

DISCLOSURE

The authors have no commercial or financial conflicts of interest to disclose.

REFERENCES

1. Simonneau G, Torbicki A, Dorfmüller P, et al. The pathophysiology of chronic thromboembolic pulmonary hypertension. Eur Respir Rev 2017;26(143). https://doi.org/10.1183/16000617.0112-2016.

2. Lang IM, Pesavento R, Bonderman D, et al. Risk factors and basic mechanisms of chronic thromboembolic pulmonary hypertension: a current understanding. Eur Respir J 2013;41(2):462–8.

3. Ende-Verhaar YM, Cannegieter SC, Noordegraaf AV, et al. Incidence of chronic thromboembolic pulmonary hypertension after acute pulmonary embolism: a contemporary view of the published literature. Eur Respir J 2017;49(2). https://doi.org/10.1183/13993003.01792-2016.

4. Pengo V, Lensing AWA, Prins MH, et al. Incidence of chronic thromboembolic pulmonary hypertension after pulmonary embolism. N Engl J Med 2004; 350(22):2257–64.

5. Tunariu N, Gibbs SJR, Win Z, et al. Ventilation-perfusion scintigraphy is more sensitive than multidetector CTPA in detecting chronic thromboembolic pulmonary disease as a treatable cause of pulmonary hypertension. J Nucl Med 2007;48(5):680–4.

6. Kreitner KF, Kunz RP, Ley S, et al. Chronic thromboembolic pulmonary hypertension - assessment by magnetic resonance imaging. Eur Radiol 2007; 17(1):11–21.

7. Kim NH, Delcroix M, Jenkins DP, et al. Chronic thromboembolic pulmonary hypertension. J Am Coll Cardiol 2013;62. https://doi.org/10.1016/j.jacc.2013.10.024.

8. Galiè N, Humbert M, Vachiery JL, et al. 2015 ESC/ERS guidelines for the diagnosis and treatment of pulmonary hypertension: the Joint Task Force for the Diagnosis and Treatment of Pulmonary Hypertension of the European Society of Cardiology (ESC) and the European Respiratory Society (ERS): endorsed by: Association for European Paediatric and Congenital Cardiology (AEPC), International Society for Heart and Lung Transplantation (ISHLT). Russ J Cardiol 2016;133(5):5–64.

9. Simonneau G, D'Armini AM, Ghofrani HA, et al. Predictors of long-term outcomes in patients treated with riociguat for chronic thromboembolic pulmonary hypertension: data from the CHEST-2 open-label, randomised, long-term extension trial. Lancet Respir Med 2016;4(5):372–80.

10. Ghofrani HA, Simonneau G, D'Armini AM, et al. Macitentan for the treatment of inoperable chronic thromboembolic pulmonary hypertension (MERIT-1): results from the multicentre, phase 2, randomised, double-blind, placebo-controlled study. Lancet Respir Med 2017;5(10):785–94.

11. Madani M, Mayer E, Fadel E, et al. Pulmonary endarterectomy: patient selection, technical challenges, and outcomes. Ann Am Thorac Soc 2016;13: S240–7.

12. Jamieson SW, Kapelanski DP, Sakakibara N, et al. Pulmonary endarterectomy: experience and lessons learned in 1,500 cases. Ann Thorac Surg 2003; 76(5):1457–64.

13. Madani MM, Jamieson SW. Technical advances of pulmonary endarterectomy for chronic thromboembolic pulmonary hypertension. Semin Thorac Cardiovasc Surg 2006;18(3):243–9.

14. de Perrot M, Donahoe L. Pulmonary thromboendarterectomy: how I teach it. Ann Thorac Surg 2018; 106(4):945–50.

15. Fedullo P, Kerr KM, Kim NH, et al. Chronic thromboembolic pulmonary hypertension. Am J Respir Crit Care Med 2011;183(12):1605–13.

16. Jamieson SW, Kapelanski DP. Pulmonary endarterectomy. Curr Probl Surg 2000;37(3):165–252.

17. Mahmud E, Madani MM, Kim NH, et al. Chronic thromboembolic pulmonary hypertension: evolving therapeutic approaches for operable and inoperable disease. J Am Coll Cardiol 2018;71(21):2468–86.

18. Quadery SR, Swift AJ, Billings CG, et al. The impact of patient choice on survival in chronic thromboembolic pulmonary hypertension. Eur Respir J 2018; 52(3). https://doi.org/10.1183/13993003.00589-2018.

19. Auger WR, Fedullo PF. Chronic thromboembolic pulmonary hypertension. Semin Respir Crit Care Med 2009;30(4):471–83.

20. Cannon JE, Su L, Kiely DG, et al. Dynamic risk stratification of patient long-term outcome after pulmonary endarterectomy: results from the United Kingdom National Cohort. Circulation 2016; 133(18):1761–71.

21. D'Armini AM, Zanotti G, Ghio S, et al. Reverse right ventricular remodeling after pulmonary endarterectomy. J Thorac Cardiovasc Surg 2007;133(1):162–8.

22. Olman MA, Auger WR, Fedullo PF, et al. Pulmonary vascular steal in chronic thromboembolic pulmonary hypertension. Chest 1990;98:1430–4.

23. Moser KM, Metersky ML, Auger WR, et al. Resolution of vascular steal after pulmonary thromboendarterectomy. Chest 1993;104(5):1441–4.

24. Levinson RM, Shure D, Moser KM. Reperfusion pulmonary edema after pulmonary artery thromboendarterectomy. Am Rev Respir Dis 1986;134(6):1241–5.

25. Lee KC, Cho YL, Lee SY. Reperfusion pulmonary edema after pulmonary endarterectomy. Acta Anaesthesiol Sin 2001;39(2):97–101.

26. Imanaka H, Miyano H, Takeuchi M, et al. Effects of nitric oxide inhalation after pulmonary thromboendarterectomy for chronic pulmonary thromboembolism. Chest 2000;118(1):39–46.

27. Inami T, Kataoka M, Shimura N, et al. Pulmonary edema predictive scoring index (PEPSI), a new index to predict risk of reperfusion pulmonary edema and improvement of hemodynamics in percutaneous transluminal pulmonary angioplasty. JACC Cardiovasc Interv 2013;6(7):725–36.

28. Esch JJ, Shah PB, Cockrill BA, et al. Transcatheter Potts shunt creation in patients with severe pulmonary arterial hypertension: initial clinical experience. J Heart Lung Transplant 2013;32(4):381–7.

29. Elwing JM, Vaidya A, Auger WR. Chronic thrombo-embolic pulmonary hypertension: an update. Clin Chest Med 2018;39(3):605–20.

30. Mahmud E, Behnamfar O, Ang L, et al. Balloon pulmonary angioplasty for chronic thromboembolic pulmonary hypertension. Interv Cardiol Clin 2018;7(1):103–17.

31. Hosokawa K, Abe K, Oi K, et al. Negative acute hemodynamic response to balloon pulmonary angioplasty does not predicate the long-term outcome in patients with chronic thromboembolic pulmonary hypertension. Int J Cardiol 2015;188(1):81–3.

32. Sugimura K, Fukumoto Y, Satoh K, et al. Percutaneous transluminal pulmonary angioplasty markedly improves pulmonary hemodynamics and long-term prognosis in patients with chronic thromboembolic pulmonary hypertension. Circ J 2012;76(2):485–8.

33. Fukui S, Ogo T, Goto Y, et al. Exercise intolerance and ventilatory inefficiency improve early after balloon pulmonary angioplasty in patients with inoperable chronic thromboembolic pulmonary hypertension. Int J Cardiol 2015;180:66–8.

34. Kataoka M, Inami T, Hayashida K, et al. Percutaneous transluminal pulmonary angioplasty for the treatment of chronic thromboembolic pulmonary hypertension. Circ Cardiovasc Interv 2012;5(6):756–62.

35. Mizoguchi H, Ogawa A, Munemasa M, et al. Refined balloon pulmonary angioplasty for inoperable patients with chronic thromboembolic pulmonary hypertension. Circ Cardiovasc Interv 2012;5(6):748–55.

36. Andreassen AK, Ragnarsson A, Gude E, et al. Balloon pulmonary angioplasty in patients with inoperable chronic thromboembolic pulmonary hypertension. Heart 2013;99(19):1415–20.

37. Hosokawa K, Abe K, Oi K, et al. Balloon pulmonary angioplasty-related complications and therapeutic strategy in patients with chronic thromboembolic pulmonary hypertension. Int J Cardiol 2015;197:224–6.

38. Khan MS, Memon MM, Amin E, et al. Use of balloon atrial septostomy in patients with advanced pulmonary arterial hypertension: a systematic review and meta-analysis. Chest 2019;156(1):53–63.

39. Sandoval J, Torbicki A. Atrial septostomy. In: Voelkel N, Schranz D, editors. The right Ventricle in Health and disease. 4th edition. New York: Springer; 2015. p. 419–37.

40. Hopkins WE, Ochoa LL, Richardson GW, et al. Comparison of the hemodynamics and survival of adults with severe primary pulmonary hypertension or Eisenmenger syndrome. J Heart Lung Transplant 1996;15(1 I):100–5.

41. Sandoval J, Gaspar J, Pulido T, et al. Graded balloon dilation atrial septostomy in severe primary pulmonary hypertension: a therapeutic alternative for patients nonresponsive to vasodilator treatment. J Am Coll Cardiol 1998;32(2):297–304.

42. Baillie TJ, Granton JT. Lung transplantation for pulmonary hypertension and strategies to bridge to transplant. Semin Respir Crit Care Med 2017;38(5):701–10.

43. Ciarka A, Vachièry J-L, Houssière A, et al. Atrial septostomy decreases sympathetic overactivity in pulmonary arterial hypertension. Chest 2007;131(6):1831–7.

44. Sandoval J. Interventional therapies in pulmonary hypertension. Rev Esp Cardiol (Engl Ed 2018;71(7):565–74.

45. Lammers AE, Derrick G, Haworth SG, et al. Efficacy and long-term patency of fenestrated Amplatzer devices in children. Catheter Cardiovasc Interv 2007;70(4):578–84.

46. Troost E, Delcroix M, Gewillig M, et al. A modified technique of stent fenestration of the interatrial septum improves patients with pulmonary hypertension. Catheter Cardiovasc Interv 2009;73(2):173–9.

47. Rajeshkumar R, Pavithran S, Sivakumar K, et al. Atrial septostomy with a predefined diameter using a novel occlutech atrial flow regulator improves symptoms and cardiac index in patients with severe pulmonary arterial hypertension. Catheter Cardiovasc Interv 2017;90(7):1145–53.

48. Patel MB, Samuel BP, Girgis RE, et al. Implantable atrial flow regulator for severe, irreversible pulmonary arterial hypertension. Eurointervention 2015;11(6):706–9.

49. Potts WJ, Smith S, Gibson S. Anastomosis of the aorta to a pulmonary artery: certain types in congenital heart disease. J Am Med Assoc 1946;132(11):627–31.

50. Salna M, Van Boxtel B, Rosenzweig EB, et al. Modified Potts shunt in an adult with idiopathic pulmonary arterial hypertension. Ann Am Thorac Soc 2017;14(4):607–9.

51. Keogh AM, Nicholls M, Shaw M, et al. Modified Potts shunt in an adult with pulmonary arterial hypertension and recurrent syncope - three-year follow-up. Int J Cardiol 2015;182:36–7.

52. Delhaas T, Koeken Y, Latus H, et al. Potts Shunt to be preferred above atrial septostomy in pediatric pulmonary arterial hypertension patients: a modeling study. Front Physiol 2018;9. https://doi.org/10.3389/fphys.2018.01252.

53. Boudjemline Y, Sizarov A, Malekzadeh-Milani S, et al. Safety and feasibility of the transcatheter approach to create a reverse Potts shunt in children with idiopathic pulmonary arterial hypertension. Can J Cardiol 2017;33(9):1188–96.

54. Rosenzweig EB, Ankola A, Krishnan U, et al. A novel unidirectional-valved shunt approach for end-stage pulmonary arterial hypertension: early experience in

adolescents and adults. J Thorac Cardiovasc Surg 2019. https://doi.org/10.1016/j.jtcvs.2019.10.149.

55. Baruteau AE, Serraf A, Lévy M, et al. Potts shunt in children with idiopathic pulmonary arterial hypertension: long-term results. Ann Thorac Surg 2012;94(3):817–24.

56. Baruteau A-E, Belli E, Boudjemline Y, et al. Palliative Potts shunt for the treatment of children with drug-refractory pulmonary arterial hypertension: updated data from the first 24 patients. Eur J Cardiothorac Surg 2015;47(3):e105–10.

57. Jayaraman A, Cormican D, Shah P, et al. Cannulation strategies in adult veno-arterial and veno-venous extracorporeal membrane oxygenation: techniques, limitations, and special considerations. Ann Card Anaesth 2017;20(5):11.

58. Rupprecht L, Lunz D, Philipp A, et al. Pitfalls in percutaneous ECMO cannulation. Heart Lung Vessel 2015;7(4):320–6. Available at: http://www.ncbi.nlm.nih.gov/pubmed/26811838. Accessed April 12, 2020.

59. Napp LC, Kühn C, Hoeper MM, et al. Cannulation strategies for percutaneous extracorporeal membrane oxygenation in adults. Clin Res Cardiol 2016;105(4):283–96.

60. Camboni D, Rojas A, Sassalos P, et al. Long-term animal model of venovenous extracorporeal membrane oxygenation with atrial septal defect as a bridge to lung transplantation. ASAIO J 2013;59(6):558–63.

61. Aggarwal V, Einhorn BN, Cohen HA. Current status of percutaneous right ventricular assist devices: first-in-man use of a novel dual lumen cannula. Catheter Cardiovasc Interv 2016;88(3):390–6.

62. Oh DK, Shim TS, Jo K-WJ, et al. Right ventricular assist device with an oxygenator using extracorporeal membrane oxygenation as a bridge to lung transplantation in a patient with severe respiratory failure and right heart decompensation. Acute Crit Care 2019. https://doi.org/10.4266/acc.2018.00416.

63. de Perrot M, Granton JT, McRae K, et al. Impact of extracorporeal life support on outcome in patients with idiopathic pulmonary arterial hypertension awaiting lung transplantation. J Heart Lung Transplant 2011;30(9):997–1002.

64. Rosenzweig EB, Gannon WD, Madahar P, et al. Extracorporeal life support bridge for pulmonary hypertension: a high-volume single-center experience. J Heart Lung Transplant 2019;38(12):1275–85.

65. Hoopes CW, Gurley JC, Zwischenberger JB, et al. Mechanical support for pulmonary veno-occlusive disease: combined atrial septostomy and venovenous extracorporeal membrane oxygenation. Semin Thorac Cardiovasc Surg 2012;24(3):232–4.

66. Bermudez CA, Lagazzi L, Crespo MM. Prolonged support using a percutaneous OxyRVAD in a patient with end-stage lung disease, pulmonary hypertension, and right cardiac failure. ASAIO J 2016;62(4):e37–40.

67. Petricevic M, Milicic D, Boban M, et al. Bleeding and thrombotic events in patients undergoing mechanical circulatory support: a review of literature. Thorac Cardiovasc Surg 2015;63(8):636–46.

68. Subramaniam AV, Barsness GW, Vallabhajosyula S, et al. Complications of temporary percutaneous mechanical circulatory support for cardiogenic shock: an appraisal of contemporary literature. Cardiol Ther 2019;8(2):211–28.

69. McGoon MD, Benza RL, Escribano-Subias P, et al. Pulmonary arterial hypertension: epidemiology and registries. J Am Coll Cardiol 2013;62:D51–9.

70. Gorter TM, Verschuuren EAM, van Veldhuisen DJ, et al. Right ventricular recovery after bilateral lung transplantation for pulmonary arterial hypertension†. Interact Cardiovasc Thorac Surg 2017;24(6):890–7.

71. Schuba B, Michel S, Guenther S, et al. Lung transplantation in patients with severe pulmonary hypertension—Focus on right ventricular remodelling. Clin Transplant 2019;33(6):e13586.

72. Hoeper MM, Benza RL, Corris P, et al. Intensive care, right ventricular support and lung transplantation in patients with pulmonary hypertension. Eur Respir J 2019;53(1). https://doi.org/10.1183/13993003.01906-2018.

73. Yusen RD, Edwards LB, Dipchand AI, et al. The registry of the international society for heart and lung transplantation: thirty-third adult lung and heart–lung transplant report—2016; focus theme: primary diagnostic indications for transplant. J Heart Lung Transplant 2016;35(10):1170–84.

74. Miller DP, Farber HW. "Who'll be the next in line?" The lung allocation score in patients with pulmonary arterial hypertension. J Heart Lung Transplant 2013;32(12):1165–7.

75. Wickerson L, Rozenberg D, Janaudis-Ferreira T, et al. Physical rehabilitation for lung transplant candidates and recipients: an evidence-informed clinical approach. World J Transplant 2016;6(3):517–31.

76. Hoeper MM, Kramer T, Pan Z, et al. Mortality in pulmonary arterial hypertension: prediction by the 2015 European pulmonary hypertension guidelines risk stratification model. Eur Respir J 2017;50(2). https://doi.org/10.1183/13993003.00740-2017.

77. Chambers DC, Yusen RD, Cherikh WS, et al. The registry of the International Society for Heart and Lung Transplantation: Thirty-fourth adult lung and heart-lung transplantation report—2017; focus theme: allograft ischemic time. J Heart Lung Transplant 2017;36(10):1047–59.

78. Yusen RD, Edwards LB, Kucheryavaya AY, et al. The registry of the International Society for Heart and Lung Transplantation: thirty-second official adult lung and heart-lung transplantation report - 2015;

focus theme: early graft failure. J Heart Lung Transplant 2015;34(10):1264–77.

79. Singer JP, Katz PP, Soong A, et al. Effect of lung transplantation on health-related quality of life in the era of the lung allocation score: a U.S. Prospective Cohort Study. Am J Transplant 2017;17(5): 1334–45.

80. Valapour M, Lehr CJ, Skeans MA, et al. OPTN/SRTR 2018 annual data report: lung. Am J Transplant 2020;20(s1):427–508.

81. Cypel M, Keshavjee S. Strategies for safe donor expansion. Curr Opin Organ Transplant 2013; 18(5):513–7.

82. Cypel M, Keshavjee S. Ex vivo lung perfusion. Oper Tech Thorac Cardiovasc Surg 2014;19(4):433–42.

83. Andreasson ASI, Dark JH, Fisher AJ. Ex vivo lung perfusion in clinical lung transplantation–State of the art. Eur J Cardiothorac Surg 2014;46(5):779–88.

84. Cypel M, Yeung JC, Liu M, et al. Normothermic ex vivo lung perfusion in clinical lung transplantation. N Engl J Med 2011;364(15):1431–40.

85. Tane S, Noda K, Shigemura N. Ex vivo lung perfusion: a key tool for translational science in the lungs. Chest 2017;151(6):1220–8.

86. Fisher A, Andreasson A, Chrysos A, et al. An observational study of donor ex vivo lung perfusion in UK lung transplantation: DEVELOP-UK. Health Technol Assess 2016;20(85):1–276.

87. Loor G, Warnecke G, Villavicencio MA, et al. Portable normothermic ex-vivo lung perfusion, ventilation, and functional assessment with the Organ Care System on donor lung use for transplantation from extended-criteria donors (EXPAND): a single-arm, pivotal trial. Lancet Respir Med 2019;7(11):975–84.

88. Sanchez PG, Davis RD, D'Ovidio F, et al. The NOVEL lung trial one-year outcomes. J Heart Lung Transplant 2014;33(4):S71–2.

89. Warnecke G, Van Raemdonck D, Smith MA, et al. Normothermic ex-vivo preservation with the portable Organ Care System Lung device for bilateral lung transplantation (INSPIRE): a randomised, open-label, non-inferiority, phase 3 study. Lancet Respir Med 2018;6(5):357–67.

Critical Care Management of the Patient with Pulmonary Hypertension

Christopher J. Mullin, MD, MHS[a], Corey E. Ventetuolo, MD, MS[a,b],*

KEYWORDS

- Right ventricular failure • Pulmonary hypertension • Pulmonary arterial hypertension
- Extracorporeal membrane oxygenation • Right ventricular assist device

KEY POINTS

- Right ventricular (RV) failure, defined as inadequate cardiac output due to RV dysfunction, is common in patients with pulmonary hypertension (PH) and highly morbid.
- Medical management of critically ill PH patients should include identification and treatment of underlying causes and optimization of RV preload, afterload, and contractility.
- Management of critically ill PH patients is complicated and involvement of PH specialists is advisable, as is transfer to facilities where advanced therapies are available.

INTRODUCTION

Management of a critically ill patient with pulmonary hypertension (PH) is a challenging scenario for clinicians in the intensive care unit (ICU). Despite significant advances in pharmacotherapies for World Symposium on Pulmonary Hypertension group 1 pulmonary arterial hypertension (PAH) (referred to herein as PAH), PAH and all forms of pulmonary vascular disease (referred to herein as PH) remain highly morbid and can be fatal.[1] Nowhere is this more evident than in the ICU. Patients with PAH or inoperable chronic thromboembolic PH (CTEPH) admitted to the ICU have mortality rates estimated at 32% to 41%,[2,3] and the ICU is the most common place of death for PAH patients.[4] In acute illness, PH—regardless of its chronicity or etiology—can lead to rapidly worsening right ventricular (RV) function and result in hemodynamic collapse and death. Advancing pulmonary vascular disease is implicated as the direct or indirect cause of death in a majority of PAH patients; in 1 study, 44% of PAH deaths were attributed directly to RV failure or sudden cardiac death, and another 44% of deaths had progressive disease implicated as a contributing factor.[4] Thus, regardless of the etiology of a PH patient's critical illness, optimal management requires an understanding of RV function, appropriate monitoring and identification of RV failure, and a physiologic approach to the optimization of volume status, RV afterload, and cardiac function.

NORMAL RIGHT VENTRICULAR FUNCTION

The pulmonary circulation is a low-pressure, high-capacitance system that receives almost the entirety of the cardiac output. As cardiac output increases, the pulmonary vascular bed distends, dilates, and recruits previously closed pulmonary vessels. As a result, pulmonary vascular resistance (PVR) decreases, and, under normal conditions, there are only minimal increases in pulmonary arterial (PA) pressure. The RV is designed to function efficiently under these

a Department of Medicine, Brown University, 593 Eddy Street, POB Suite 224, Providence, RI 02903, USA;
b Department of Health Services, Policy, and Practice, Brown University, 593 Eddy Street, POB Suite 224, Providence, RI 02903, USA
* Corresponding author. Department of Medicine, Brown University, 593 Eddy Street, POB Suite 224, Providence, RI 02903.
E-mail address: corey_ventetuolo@brown.edu

Clin Chest Med 42 (2021) 155–165
https://doi.org/10.1016/j.ccm.2020.11.009

circumstances as a compliant chamber able to accommodate large changes in preload. The RV consists of a thin free wall that embraces the more muscular interventricular septum. The RV relies on longitudinal shortening for systolic ejection because it lacks the same circumferential layer of constrictor fibers as the left ventricle (LV) and thus has a bellows-like contraction from the apex toward the RV outflow tract.[5] The RV then can match the cardiac output of the LV with one-fifth the energy expenditure.[5,6] Unlike the LV, where coronary perfusion occurs only during diastole, RV myocardial pressure remains below aortic root pressure throughout the cardiac cycle and allows continuous flow from the right coronary artery.[5,7] Despite many of their physiologic differences, the LV and RV are interdependent in that they share myocardial fibers and the septum,[8] and both are contained within the pericardium.[9] Changes in one ventricle can have a significant impact on the function of the other.[10]

RIGHT VENTRICULAR FAILURE
Definition and Pathophysiology

RV failure, also referred to as right (or right-sided) heart failure, is defined as low cardiac output and/or elevated right-sided filling pressures due to systolic and/or diastolic RV dysfunction.[11] The natural history of RV failure includes systemic hypoperfusion and secondary dysfunction in other organs, including the liver and kidneys. RV failure often begins with a significant increase in RV afterload and/or a decrease in RV contractility, which initiates a cyclical chain of pathophysiologic changes that can result in hemodynamic collapse and death. In response to an abrupt increase in afterload, RV ejection fraction decreases and the RV dilates to increase stroke volume.[12] As the RV progressively dilates, RV end-diastolic volume and pressure increase, which increases RV wall stress, worsens RV performance, and decreases cardiac output.[13] Additionally, RV dilation has detrimental effects on myocardial oxygen delivery and consumption, tricuspid valve function, and systolic and diastolic LV functions. The increase in RV wall stress also increases myocardial oxygen demand and consumption,[14] whereas RV oxygen delivery decreases because blood flow through the right coronary artery to the RV occurs only during diastole.[15] The resulting RV ischemia further decreases RV contractility.[14] Chamber dilation causes widening of the tricuspid valve annulus and increases tricuspid regurgitation that worsens RV loading conditions, ischemia, and performance.[16,17] Lastly, RV dilation and increased RV diastolic pressure cause the interventricular

septum to shift toward the LV; LV filling is reduced and LV stroke volume drops,[18,19] as illustrated in **Fig. 1**. The decline in systemic cardiac output leads to systemic hypotension, which can precipitate further RV ischemia, perpetuating a vicious cycle of biventricular dysfunction, ischemia, and reduced cardiac output. **Fig. 2** illustrates the feed forward nature of the pathophysiologic events seen with progressive RV dysfunction and failure.

The RV can undergo a series of compensatory adaptations in patients who have more chronic and gradual increases in afterload to preserve cardiac function (reviewed elsewhere[20,21]). In most cases, adaptive hypertrophy is insufficient and maladaptive responses, such as fibrosis and inflammation, ensue and lead to decreased contractile reserve and RV failure.[21] Thus, patients with preexisting PH, with or without RV dysfunction, are at high risk for developing RV failure from either progressive pulmonary vascular disease or in the setting of an acute illness.

Precipitants of Right Ventricular Failure

There are many conditions that can cause acute RV failure or precipitate RV failure in patients with underlying PH. These conditions work on 1 or a combination of 5 mechanisms: (1) increased RV afterload, (2) altered RV preload, (3) reduced RV contractility, (4) altered ventricular interdependence, and (5) altered cardiac rhythm.

Acute RV failure without preexisting PH frequently is encountered in the ICU as a complication of some of the most common diseases seen in critical care—namely, acute pulmonary embolism (PE), sepsis, and acute respiratory distress syndrome (ARDS). In acute PE, an abrupt increase in RV afterload frequently causes RV dysfunction,[22] and RV failure is an established mechanism of death in acute PE.[23] In sepsis, PVR can increase and precipitate RV dysfunction.[24] Elevated PVR was present in more than half of patients with severe sepsis or septic shock and was an independent risk factor for death in 1 study.[25] In ARDS, both RV and pulmonary vascular dysfunction are common and associated with increased mortality.[26]

Infection, sepsis, PE, and atrial tachyarrhythmias are some of the typical conditions that can trigger RV failure in patients with chronic PAH or preexisting PH with RV dysfunction. Infections are one of the most common and worrisome triggers for RV decompensation. In a study of 46 patients with PAH or inoperable CTEPH admitted to the ICU, infection was identified as a cause in 11 patients (24%), and infection during ICU hospitalization was associated with worse survival.[2]

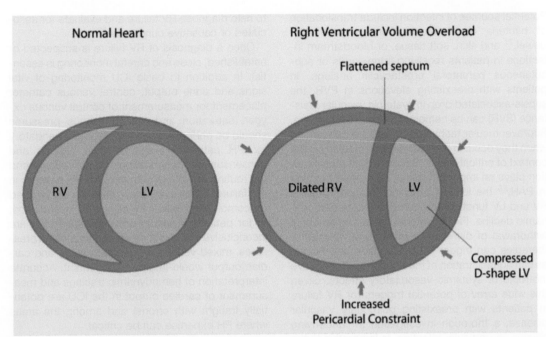

Fig. 1. Ventricular interdependence in RV failure. With progressive RV dilation, the interventricular septum shifts toward the left, creating a D-shaped LV. With constraint from the pericardium, this leads to decreased LV compliance, decreased LV preload, and impaired LV function. (*From* Haddad F, Doyle R, Murphy DJ, Hunt SA. Right ventricular function in cardiovascular disease, part II: pathophysiology, clinical importance, and management of right ventricular failure. Circulation. 2008;117(13):1717-1731).

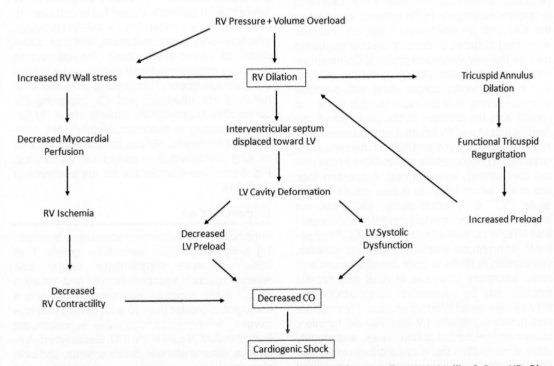

Fig. 2. Pathophysiology of RV failure. CO, cardiac output. (*Adapted from* Pradhan NM, Mullin C, Poor HD. Biomarkers and Right Ventricular Dysfunction. Crit Care Clin. 2020;36(1):141-153).

Potential sources of infection include translocation of bacteria or endotoxin from hypoperfused bowel,[27] and skin, soft tissue, or bloodstream infections in patients receiving intravenous or subcutaneous parenteral prostacyclin analogs. In patients with preexisting elevations in PVR, the sepsis-associated drop in systemic vascular resistance (SVR) can be hemodynamically devastating. Supraventricular tachyarrhythmias are concerning when they occur in PAH patients, particularly in the context of critical illness. Because right atrial function plays an important role in right heart function in PAH,[28] the loss of atrial contraction worsens RV and LV function and can precipitate hemodynamic decline. Finally, intentional or unintentional withdrawal of diuretics or pulmonary vasodilator therapies can trigger RV dysfunction and failure, as can administration of medications with negative inotropic or systemic vasodilatory effects. Given this wide array of potential triggers for RV failure in patients with preexisting pulmonary vascular disease, a thorough investigation for underlying causes, in particular infection, is imperative in the diagnosis and management of RV failure.

Diagnosis and Monitoring of Right Ventricular Failure

Although the symptoms and signs of RV failure can be subtle, intensivists must keep a high degree of suspicion, particularly in PH patients admitted to the ICU with an alternative diagnosis. Fatigue, worsening dyspnea, or even agitation or confusion may be the only symptoms present. On examination, elevated jugular venous pressure, ascites, and lower extremity edema along with cyanosis or cool, clammy skin are more obvious signs and should alert the clinician to the presence of low cardiac output and RV failure. Cardiac biomarkers, in particular troponins and brain natriuretic peptides (BNPs) have various applications in the critical care setting, although data supporting their use in RV failure from PH is less robust than in acute PE.[29] In 1 small study, BNP, but not troponin, predicted mortality in PAH and inoperable CTEPH patients admitted to the ICU.[2] For patients with chronic pulmonary vascular disease, comparison of BNPs to prior baseline values and basic laboratory measures of renal and hepatic function may be informative. Echocardiography may provide useful information about RV structure and function, evaluate LV and valvular function, assess any pericardial abnormalities, and identify other abnormalities that may contribute to RV failure. Bedside cardiac ultrasound is recommended by critical care societies for use in RV dysfunction

to help diagnose RV failure and evaluate for associated or causative conditions.[30]

Once a diagnosis of RV failure is suspected or established, close and careful monitoring is essential. In addition to basic ICU monitoring of vital signs and urine output, central venous catheter placement for measurement of central venous oxygen saturation and central venous pressures should be performed and essentially is mandatory for PH patients in shock. Most experts and consensus recommendations do not recommend the routine use of PA catheters for PH patients in RV failure[11]; however, they often are considered for complicated cases, for severe RV dysfunction, or for patients in whom other available data are inconclusive and direct measurements of PA pressures, mixed venous oxygen saturation, and cardiac output would inform management. Accurate interpretation of hemodynamic tracings and measurement of cardiac output in the ICU are potentially fraught with error(s) and among the areas where PH expertise can be critical.

MANAGEMENT OF RIGHT VENTRICULAR FAILURE

There are no randomized clinical trials or guidelines to inform the management of PH and RV failure in the ICU. Most reviews and consensus statements recommend reliance on PH specialists and expert centers.[11,17,31] After a diagnosis of RV failure in a PH patient is suspected or established, evaluation for an underlying cause—in particular, infection—should be performed, and that cause should be treated appropriately. The approach to RV failure management then should center around 3 physiologic goals: (1) optimizing RV preload, (2) reducing RV afterload, and (3) improving RV contractility. In appropriate patients whose RV failure is refractory to treatment despite these management strategies, RV mechanical support and/or lung transplantation should be considered. **Fig. 3** provides a schematic for the treatment of RV failure.

Supportive Care

Most consensus guidelines recommend maintaining peripheral oxygen saturations greater than 90%,[17] because supplemental oxygen can reverse hypoxic vasoconstriction and improve PVR.[32] Many experts recommend maintaining a hemoglobin greater than 10 g/dL to help optimize oxygen delivery,[17] although this is discordant from standard of care in the ICU. Electrolyte disturbances, other metabolic derangements, and pain also should be managed appropriately. Endotracheal intubation and mechanical ventilation both

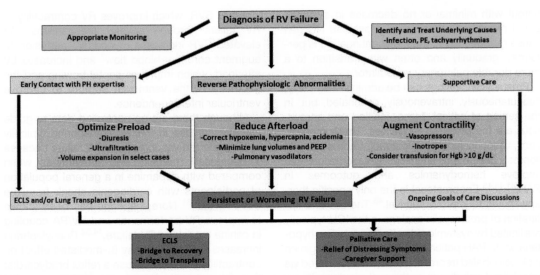

Fig. 3. Scheme for the management of right ventricular failure for the critically ill PH patient. PEEP, positive end-expiratory pressure; Hgb, hemoglobin.

have been associated with poor outcomes in patients with PH and RV failure.[33,34] Induction agents for endotracheal intubation can decrease SVR and arterial blood pressure acutely, which can precipitate cardiac arrest in these patients.[34]

Optimization of Right Ventricular Preload

The RV is designed to accommodate large changes in preload (ie, it is built as a volume chamber), but both hypovolemia and hypervolemia can reduce cardiac output, by mechanisms described previously. There are some rare cases in which PH patients may require volume expansion, but a vast majority of PH patients with RV failure are characterized by high right-sided filling pressures. Volume removal with diuretics or hemofiltration typically is recommended to reduce RV distention and RV wall stress and improve LV filling. The same may be true in RV failure without preexisting PH. In hemodynamically stable patients with acute PE and RV dysfunction, intravenous diuretics led to more rapid improvement in RV function compared with a fluid bolus, although there was no difference in survival.[35] Regardless of the decision to administer or remove volume, this should be done under close monitoring with frequent assessment of hemodynamics and perfusion.[36,37]

Reduction of Right Ventricular Afterload

The reduction of RV afterload is a mainstay of treatment of RV failure in PH. Although pulmonary vasodilators are the primary therapies to achieve this in PAH, it should not be overlooked that hypoxemia, hypercapnia, acidemia, and mechanical

ventilation can contribute to pulmonary afterload and should be addressed as part of basic management. Hypoxic pulmonary vasoconstriction is worsened by acidemia and hypercapnea.[38] Positive pressure ventilation increases intrathoracic pressures and leads to increased PVR and decreased RV and LV preload.[39] Because PVR is lowest around functional residual capacity,[40] mechanical ventilation should be adjusted to avoid high lung volumes and minimize positive end-expiratory pressure. In practice, mechanical ventilation strategies for PH patients attempt to balance potentially negative hemodynamic consequences of positive pressure ventilation against adequate oxygenation and ventilation. Because mechanical ventilation can be devastating for PH patients, there is growing interest in the use of extracorporeal support to avoid intubation in such patients (discussed later).

There are many pharmacotherapies approved to treat PAH.[41] These medications are approved only for group 1 PAH or inoperable or recurrent CTEPH (riociguat). In an ICU setting, inhaled and intravenous pulmonary vasodilators are preferred, because their quick onset and short half-lives allow for rapid initiation and titration based on hemodynamic and clinical response. Inhaled nitric oxide (NO), prostacyclin analogs, and phosphodiesterase (PDE)-5 inhibitors are the agents used most frequently. Inhaled NO (formally Food and Drug Administration approved for neonatal respiratory failure associated with PH) can be administered through nasal cannula, face mask, or a ventilator circuit and has a half-life on the order of seconds. It reduces PVR and increases cardiac output with minimal or no decrease in systemic blood pressure.[42] Withdrawal of inhaled NO can cause rebound PH[43]; thus, discontinuation is performed gradually and often with transition to a more durable pulmonary vasodilator.

Prostacyclin analogs can be administered orally, subcutaneously, intravenously, or inhaled, but, in the setting of critical illness, inhaled and intravenous are the preferred modalities. These medications, which include epoprostenol, treprostinil, and iloprost, are potent, short-acting vasodilators that improve hemodynamics and outcomes in PAH.[41,44,45] Epoprostenol is the only specific therapy shown to improve survival.[46] The use and up-titration of prostacyclin analogs in the ICU typically are limited by systemic side effects, including hypotension. In PAH patients whose outpatient regimen includes inhaled treprostinil or iloprost (delivered via specialized nebulizers) or the oral prostacyclin receptor agonist selexipag, conversion to intravenous or inhaled epoprostenol often is necessary during critical illness, either to escalate treatment or to insure there is no interruption in therapy for patients unable to take nebulized or oral medications. Sildenafil, a PDE-5 inhibitor available in both oral and intravenous formulations, reduces PVR and may augment RV function.[47,48] Data for its use in critical care are limited and its longer half-life and potential for systemic hypotension[49] make it less appealing. Other oral medications commonly used in the management of chronic PAH, such as endothelin receptor antagonists and the soluble guanylate cyclase stimulator riociguat (also approved for nonoperative CTEPH), have not been studied in the ICU setting.

Because these medications are approved only for PAH, caution should be taken with their use in patients with left heart dysfunction or chronic lung disease. Pulmonary vasodilators can precipitate pulmonary edema in patients with LV dysfunction or elevated left heart filling pressures; in patients with parenchymal or obstructive lung disease, they can worsen ventilation-perfusion matching and hypoxemia.[50]

Given the complexities of these medications and their potential for harm when used off-label, the use of pulmonary vasodilators in the ICU should involve PH specialists with experience in their use during critical illness.

Improvement in Right Ventricular Contractility

The contractile function of the RV can be improved by avoiding systemic hypotension with vasopressors, augmenting cardiac output and oxygen delivery with inotropes, and treating inciting factors, namely atrial tachyarrhythmias. Vasopressors

increase SVR, which improves RV contractility in RV failure through several mechanisms. An elevated SVR increases myocardial perfusion to augment coronary blood flow[7] and increases LV afterload, which improves septal bowing and the geometry of the ventricular septum to improve ventricular interdependence.

Although there are no controlled data to guide vasopressor use in PH, norepinephrine typically is the preferred vasopressor in RV failure because it decreased mortality and arrhythmias when compared with dopamine in a general population of participants with cardiogenic shock from the SOAP II trial.[51] Norepinephrine has been shown to improve RV performance and RV/PA coupling in canine models of RV failure.[14,52] Phenylephrine increases PVR without any β_1-mediated effect on contractility[53] and can cause a reflex bradycardia; thus, it is not routinely recommended for use in PH with RV failure. Vasopressin can be used at lower doses (0.01–0.03 U/min), where it causes pulmonary vasodilation via the NO pathway,[54] but higher doses should be used with caution because vasoconstriction can increase PVR.

Each of the inotropes available for use in RV failure has advantages and disadvantages. Dopamine at low or medium doses (<10 µg/kg/min) primarily activates dopaminergic and β_1-receptors and increases cardiac output without a detrimental effect on PVR.[55] Dobutamine primarily activates β_1-receptors at low to medium doses (5–10 µg/kg/min) to improve contractility and PA-RV coupling and reduce PVR. At higher doses, β_2 receptor activation can cause systemic vasodilation and hypotension, which often limits its use at these doses. Dobutamine improves hemodynamics in severe RV infarction and in PH after liver transplantation.[37,56] Milrinone, a selective PDE-3 inhibitor, often is used in pulmonary vascular dysfunction due to LV dysfunction or post–cardiac transplant, because it reduces PA pressures and improves RV function.[57,58] Its use in PAH or isolated RV failure can be limited by systemic hypotension or its effects on an unloaded LV. Dopamine, dobutamine, and milrinone all have a risk of increased tachyarrhythmias, and the latter 2 can cause systemic vasodilation. As such, these medications often are reserved for situations where oxygen delivery remains inadequate despite optimization of RV preload and afterload and after systemic hypotension has been corrected with vasopressors. Levosimendan, a calcium sensitizer that increases the affinity of myocardial troponin C to calcium, is used for acute severe decompensated left heart failure, but data for its use in PH are limited[59] and more studies are needed. Currently, this medication is not available or approved for use in the United States.

Appropriate management of tachyarrhythmias also is necessary to optimize RV contractility. Rate control agents with negative inotropy, such as β-blockers and calcium channel blockers, typically should be avoided, especially in patients with systemic hypotension or shock. Digoxin is an appealing agent for rate control in this scenario, because limited data suggest it may improve cardiac output in PAH.[60] Given the impact of the loss of atrial contraction on RV function, restoration of sinus rhythm, by either chemical or mechanical cardioversion, should be considered.

Mechanical Support and Lung Transplantation

Critically ill PH patients who have evidence of hypoperfusion despite maximal medical therapy should be evaluated for extracorporeal life support (ECLS). Ideally, this should occur in parallel with medical optimization to avoid significant delays and additional end organ dysfunction. The most widely used form of ECLS is extracorporeal membrane oxygenation (ECMO); however, other devices and forms of RV mechanical support have been developed, and there is growing interest in their use. In patients with preexisting PH, ECLS should be viewed as a "bridge to recovery" or a "bridge to transplantation," and the goals of extracorporeal support should be understood before it is offered or initiated. ECLS as a bridge to recovery can be used for PH patients with a potentially reversible cause of acute decompensation—for example, tachyarrhythmia, pneumonia, or need for an operative intervention—or in incident PAH patients to begin or escalate treatment. ECLS as a bridge to transplant typically is reserved for patients with chronic PH who previously have been evaluated for lung transplantation and who can expect to have a favorable outcome after transplant.[61] Consideration and indications for lung transplantation referral and listing for PH are reviewed elsewhere.[11,62]

The use of awake ECMO, or ECMO without mechanical ventilation, has grown in popularity and is appealing because post-transplant survival is worse for pretransplant mechanically ventilated patients[63] and because mechanical ventilation can have deleterious hemodynamic consequences in patients with PH and RV failure. Retrospective single-center studies have reported awake ECMO before lung transplantation for any indication had improved or similar survival compared with lung transplantation without ECMO.[64,65] There are no controlled data and minimal but growing evidence that ECMO as a bridge to recovery or transplantation is an effective strategy specifically in PH patients.[64,66–68] In a single-

center retrospective study of ECMO to support a diverse PH population, survival to hospital discharge was 47% in the 36 patients where ECMO was used as a bridge to recovery or bridge to nontransplant surgery and 53% in the 54 patients bridged to transplant.[67] Additionally, ECMO has been used for cardiopulmonary support during and immediately after lung transplantation for PH,[67,69,70] where it allows for hemodynamic support as the LV adapts to a suddenly normalized preload.[70]

Venoarterial ECMO (VA-ECMO) is the most commonly used mode of ECLS for PH patients. This configuration helps reduce RV preload and afterload, increases systemic blood pressure, and augments cardiac output, reversing many of the pathophysiologic derangements of RV failure. Increased LV afterload, retrograde aortic perfusion, and a cranial-caudal hypoxia gradient are expected potential issues with VA-ECMO in a traditional femoral vessel configuration. Venovenous ECMO (VV-ECMO) can be used in PH patients with only mild disease or RV dysfunction suffering from conditions like ARDS or other forms of severe hypoxemia. Because VV-ECMO provides no direct augmentation of cardiac output, it is not appropriate for frank RV failure and advanced PH. In select cases, a triple cannulation strategy can be used in which extra drainage and return cannulas can be added (eg, VV-arterial and VA-venous) to provide additional hemodynamic unloading or respiratory support, respectively.[71] Further details of cannulation and ECMO strategies for PH patients are available elsewhere.[72,73]

Other ECLS options for PH patients in RV failure include a PA–left atrial approach, where a low resistance membrane oxygenator allows for unloading of the RV and increased LV filling.[74,75] Placement requires a sternotomy—and with that often stabilization on VA-ECMO prior to insertion—but may allow for ambulation and perhaps provides more durable support. RV assist devices (RVADs) have been developed and used in patients with RV failure post-cardiotomy, after LV assist device placement, or secondary to acute myocardial infarction,[76–79] scenarios where PVR is mostly normal. In PAH, pulsatile flow devices can increase PA pressure, worsen pulmonary vascular remodeling, and induce pulmonary edema or hemorrhage.[80,81] There are growing reports of the successful use of RVADs in isolated RV failure from pulmonary vascular disease[81,82] or other etiologies of respiratory failure[83–85]; however, further study and experience are needed before these devices can be recommended for routine use for RV mechanical support in precapillary PH.

Palliative and End-of-Life Care

Cardiopulmonary resuscitation (CPR) in advanced PH usually is unsuccessful. In a multicenter retrospective study of 132 PAH patients who underwent CPR (nearly all were inpatients and most [74%] were in an ICU), only 8 (6%) of patients survived more than 90 days.[86] Because intubation, mechanical ventilation, and CPR have potentially devastating and fatal consequences, it is imperative to assess if these are within the goals of care for PH patients in the ICU. Although there is a relatively large experience and literature about palliative care in the ICU, palliative care in pulmonary vascular disease is both understudied and likely underutilized.[41,87] Key principles of palliative care, such as relief of distressing symptoms, effective communication about goals of care, patient-focused decision making, and caregiver support,[88] are directly applicable to the care of critically ill PH patients. The integration of these palliative care concepts into the care of patients with advanced pulmonary vascular disease and RV failure both before and during ICU admission likely is essential to provide comprehensive care for a patient.

SUMMARY

ICU admission for patients with PH carries a high morbidity and mortality, usually caused by isolated RV failure or RV failure in conjunction with infection, tachyarrhythmias, or other forms of acute illness. Because management for the critically ill PH patient often is complex and challenging, involvement of PH specialists is highly advisable and transfer to ECLS and/or lung transplantation centers in select cases is appropriate. Key management principles of critically ill PH patients should include identification and treatment of underlying causes and an approach cognizant of the pathophysiology of RV failure to optimize RV preload, reduce afterload, and maintain or correct RV contractility.

DISCLOSURE

Dr C.J. Mullin's institution receives clinical trial support from A-Lung Technologies. Dr C.E. Ventetuolo has served as a prior consultant for Acceleron Pharma, Altavant Sciences, and Maquet Cardiovascular. Her institution receives research grants from United Therapeutics and clinical trial support from A-Lung Technologies.

REFERENCES

1. Farber HW, Miller DP, Poms AD, et al. Five-year outcomes of patients enrolled in the REVEAL registry. Chest 2015;148(4):1043–54.
2. Sztrymf B, Souza R, Bertoletti L, et al. Prognostic factors of acute heart failure in patients with pulmonary arterial hypertension. Eur Respir J 2010;35(6):1286–93.
3. Kurzyna M, Zylkowska J, Fijalkowska A, et al. Characteristics and prognosis of patients with decompensated right ventricular failure during the course of pulmonary hypertension. Kardiol Pol 2008;66(10):1033–9 [discussion 1040–31].
4. Tonelli AR, Arelli V, Minai OA, et al. Causes and circumstances of death in pulmonary arterial hypertension. Am J Respir Crit Care Med 2013;188(3):365–9.
5. Sheehan F, Redington A. The right ventricle: anatomy, physiology and clinical imaging. Heart 2008;94(11):1510–5.
6. Redington AN, Rigby ML, Shinebourne EA, et al. Changes in the pressure-volume relation of the right ventricle when its loading conditions are modified. Br Heart J 1990;63(1):45–9.
7. Lowensohn HS, Khouri EM, Gregg DE, et al. Phasic right coronary artery blood flow in conscious dogs with normal and elevated right ventricular pressures. Circ Res 1976;39(6):760–6.
8. Smerup M, Nielsen E, Agger P, et al. The three-dimensional arrangement of the myocytes aggregated together within the mammalian ventricular myocardium. Anat Rec (Hoboken) 2009;292(1):1–11.
9. Kroeker CA, Shrive NG, Belenkie I, et al. Pericardium modulates left and right ventricular stroke volumes to compensate for sudden changes in atrial volume. Am J Physiol Heart Circ Physiol 2003;284(6):H2247–54.
10. Damiano RJ Jr, La Follette P Jr, Cox JL, et al. Significant left ventricular contribution to right ventricular systolic function. Am J Physiol 1991;261(5 Pt 2):H1514–24.
11. Hoeper MM, Benza RL, Corris P, et al. Intensive care, right ventricular support and lung transplantation in patients with pulmonary hypertension. Eur Respir J 2019;53(1):1801906.
12. Greyson CR. Pathophysiology of right ventricular failure. Crit Care Med 2008;36(1 Suppl):S57–65.
13. Guyton AC, Lindsey AW, Gilluly JJ. The limits of right ventricular compensation following acute increase in pulmonary circulatory resistance. Circ Res 1954;2(4):326–32.
14. Kerbaul F, Rondelet B, Motte S, et al. Effects of norepinephrine and dobutamine on pressure load-induced right ventricular failure. Crit Care Med 2004;32(4):1035–40.
15. Gibbons Kroeker CA, Adeeb S, Shrive NG, et al. Compression induced by RV pressure overload decreases regional coronary blood flow in anesthetized dogs. Am J Physiol Heart Circ Physiol 2006;290(6):H2432–8.
16. Chemla D, Castelain V, Herve P, et al. Haemodynamic evaluation of pulmonary hypertension. Eur Respir J 2002;20(5):1314–31.

17. Poor HD, Ventetuolo CE. Pulmonary hypertension in the intensive care unit. Prog Cardiovasc Dis 2012; 55(2):187–98.

18. Gan C, Lankhaar JW, Marcus JT, et al. Impaired left ventricular filling due to right-to-left ventricular interaction in patients with pulmonary arterial hypertension. Am J Physiol Heart Circ Physiol 2006;290(4): H1528–33.

19. Haddad F, Doyle R, Murphy DJ, et al. Right ventricular function in cardiovascular disease, part II: pathophysiology, clinical importance, and management of right ventricular failure. Circulation 2008;117(13): 1717–31.

20. Reddy S, Bernstein D. Molecular mechanisms of right ventricular failure. Circulation 2015;132(18): 1734–42.

21. van der Bruggen CEE, Tedford RJ, Handoko ML, et al. RV pressure overload: from hypertrophy to failure. Cardiovasc Res 2017;113(12):1423–32.

22. Goldhaber SZ, Visani L, De Rosa M. Acute pulmonary embolism: clinical outcomes in the International cooperative pulmonary embolism registry (ICOPER). Lancet 1999;353(9162):1386–9.

23. Konstantinides SV, Meyer G, Becattini C, et al. 2019 ESC Guidelines for the diagnosis and management of acute pulmonary embolism developed in collaboration with the European Respiratory Society (ERS). Eur Heart J 2020;41(4):543–603.

24. Chan CM, Klinger JR. The right ventricle in sepsis. Clin Chest Med 2008;29(4):661–76, ix.

25. Vallabhajosyula S, Kumar M, Pandompatam G, et al. Prognostic impact of isolated right ventricular dysfunction in sepsis and septic shock: an 8-year historical cohort study. Ann Intensive Care 2017; 7(1):94.

26. Bull TM, Clark B, McFann K, et al. National Institutes of Health/National Heart L, blood institute AN. Pulmonary vascular dysfunction is associated with poor outcomes in patients with acute lung injury. Am J Respir Crit Care Med 2010;182(9): 1123–8.

27. Ranchoux B, Bigorgne A, Hautefort A, et al. Gut-lung connection in pulmonary arterial hypertension. Am J Respir Cell Mol Biol 2017;56(3):402–5.

28. Sivak JA, Raina A, Forfia PR. Assessment of the physiologic contribution of right atrial function to total right heart function in patients with and without pulmonary arterial hypertension. Pulm Circ 2016; 6(3):322–8.

29. Pradhan NM, Mullin C, Poor HD. Biomarkers and right ventricular dysfunction. Crit Care Clin 2020; 36(1):141–53.

30. Levitov A, Frankel HL, Blaivas M, et al. Guidelines for the appropriate use of bedside general and cardiac ultrasonography in the evaluation of critically Ill Patients-Part II: cardiac ultrasonography. Crit Care Med 2016;44(6):1206–27.

31. Ventetuolo CE, Klinger JR. Management of acute right ventricular failure in the intensive care unit. Ann Am Thorac Soc 2014;11(5):811–22.

32. Roberts DH, Lepore JJ, Maroo A, et al. Oxygen therapy improves cardiac index and pulmonary vascular resistance in patients with pulmonary hypertension. Chest 2001;120(5):1547–55.

33. Rush B, Biagioni BJ, Berger L, et al. Mechanical ventilation outcomes in patients with pulmonary hypertension in the United States: a national retrospective cohort analysis. J Intensive Care Med 2017; 32(10):588–92.

34. Pritts CD, Pearl RG. Anesthesia for patients with pulmonary hypertension. Curr Opin Anaesthesiol 2010; 23(3):411–6.

35. Schouver ED, Chiche O, Bouvier P, et al. Diuretics versus volume expansion in acute submassive pulmonary embolism. Arch Cardiovasc Dis 2017; 110(11):616–25.

36. Ghignone M, Girling L, Prewitt RM. Volume expansion versus norepinephrine in treatment of a low cardiac output complicating an acute increase in right ventricular afterload in dogs. Anesthesiology 1984; 60(2):132–5.

37. Ferrario M, Poli A, Previtali M, et al. Hemodynamics of volume loading compared with dobutamine in severe right ventricular infarction. Am J Cardiol 1994; 74(4):329–33.

38. Sylvester JT, Shimoda LA, Aaronson PI, et al. Hypoxic pulmonary vasoconstriction. Physiol Rev 2012; 92(1):367–520.

39. Feihl F, Broccard AF. Interactions between respiration and systemic hemodynamics. Part II: practical implications in critical care. Intensive Care Med 2009;35(2):198–205.

40. Howell JB, Permutt S, Proctor DF, et al. Effect of inflation of the lung on different parts of pulmonary vascular bed. J Appl Phys 1961;16:71–6.

41. Klinger JR, Elliott CG, Levine DJ, et al. Therapy for pulmonary arterial hypertension in adults: update of the CHEST guideline and expert panel report. Chest 2019;155(3):565–86.

42. Bhorade S, Christenson J, O'Connor M, et al. Response to inhaled nitric oxide in patients with acute right heart syndrome. Am J Respir Crit Care Med 1999;159(2):571–9.

43. Christenson J, Lavoie A, O'Connor M, et al. The incidence and pathogenesis of cardiopulmonary deterioration after abrupt withdrawal of inhaled nitric oxide. Am J Respir Crit Care Med 2000;161(5): 1443–9.

44. Olschewski H, Simonneau G, Galie N, et al. Inhaled iloprost for severe pulmonary hypertension. N Engl J Med 2002;347(5):322–9.

45. Simonneau G, Barst RJ, Galie N, et al. Continuous subcutaneous infusion of treprostinil, a prostacyclin analogue, in patients with pulmonary arterial

hypertension: a double-blind, randomized, placebo-controlled trial. Am J Respir Crit Care Med 2002; 165(6):800–4.

46. Barst RJ, Rubin LJ, Long WA, et al. A comparison of continuous intravenous epoprostenol (prostacyclin) with conventional therapy for primary pulmonary hypertension. N Engl J Med 1996;334(5):296–301.

47. Nagendran J, Archer SL, Soliman D, et al. Phosphodiesterase type 5 is highly expressed in the hypertrophied human right ventricle, and acute inhibition of phosphodiesterase type 5 improves contractility. Circulation 2007;116(3):238–48.

48. Galie N, Ghofrani HA, Torbicki A, et al. Sildenafil citrate therapy for pulmonary arterial hypertension. N Engl J Med 2005;353(20):2148–57.

49. Vachiery JL, Huez S, Gillies H, et al. Safety, tolerability and pharmacokinetics of an intravenous bolus of sildenafil in patients with pulmonary arterial hypertension. Br J Clin Pharmacol 2011;71(2):289–92.

50. Califf RM, Adams KF, McKenna WJ, et al. A randomized controlled trial of epoprostenol therapy for severe congestive heart failure: the flolan international randomized survival trial (FIRST). Am Heart J 1997;134(1):44–54.

51. De Backer D, Biston P, Devriendt J, et al. Comparison of dopamine and norepinephrine in the treatment of shock. N Engl J Med 2010;362(9):779–89.

52. Ducas J, Duval D, Dasilva H, et al. Treatment of canine pulmonary hypertension: effects of norepinephrine and isoproterenol on pulmonary vascular pressure-flow characteristics. Circulation 1987; 75(1):235–42.

53. Rich S, Gubin S, Hart K. The effects of phenylephrine on right ventricular performance in patients with pulmonary hypertension. Chest 1990;98(5): 1102–6.

54. Evora PR, Pearson PJ, Schaff HV. Arginine vasopressin induces endothelium-dependent vasodilatation of the pulmonary artery. V1-receptor-mediated production of nitric oxide. Chest 1993;103(4): 1241–5.

55. Holloway EL, Polumbo RA, Harrison DC. Acute circulatory effects of dopamine in patients with pulmonary hypertension. Br Heart J 1975;37(5):482–5.

56. Acosta F, Sansano T, Palenciano CG, et al. Effects of dobutamine on right ventricular function and pulmonary circulation in pulmonary hypertension during liver transplantation. Transplant Proc 2005;37(9): 3869–70.

57. Oztekin I, Yazici S, Oztekin DS, et al. Effects of low-dose milrinone on weaning from cardiopulmonary bypass and after in patients with mitral stenosis and pulmonary hypertension. Yakugaku Zasshi 2007;127(2):375–83.

58. Eichhorn EJ, Konstam MA, Weiland DS, et al. Differential effects of milrinone and dobutamine on right ventricular preload, afterload and systolic

performance in congestive heart failure secondary to ischemic or idiopathic dilated cardiomyopathy. Am J Cardiol 1987;60(16):1329–33.

59. Hansen MS, Andersen A, Nielsen-Kudsk JE. Levosimendan in pulmonary hypertension and right heart failure. Pulm Circ 2018;8(3). 2045894018790905.

60. Rich S, Seidlitz M, Dodin E, et al. The short-term effects of digoxin in patients with right ventricular dysfunction from pulmonary hypertension. Chest 1998;114(3):787–92.

61. Rajagopal K, Hoeper MM. State of the art: bridging to lung transplantation using artificial organ support technologies. J Heart Lung Transplant 2016;35(12): 1385–98.

62. Weill D, Benden C, Corris PA, et al. A consensus document for the selection of lung transplant candidates: 2014–an update from the pulmonary transplantation council of the international society for heart and lung transplantation. J Heart Lung Transplant 2015;34(1):1–15.

63. Singer JP, Blanc PD, Hoopes C, et al. The impact of pretransplant mechanical ventilation on short- and long-term survival after lung transplantation. Am J Transplant 2011;11(10):2197–204.

64. Fuehner T, Kuehn C, Hadem J, et al. Extracorporeal membrane oxygenation in awake patients as bridge to lung transplantation. Am J Respir Crit Care Med 2012;185(7):763–8.

65. Ius F, Natanov R, Salman J, et al. Extracorporeal membrane oxygenation as a bridge to lung transplantation may not impact overall mortality risk after transplantation: results from a 7-year single-centre experience. Eur J Cardiothorac Surg 2018;54(2): 334–40.

66. de Perrot M, Granton JT, McRae K, et al. Impact of extracorporeal life support on outcome in patients with idiopathic pulmonary arterial hypertension awaiting lung transplantation. J Heart Lung Transplant 2011;30(9):997–1002.

67. Rosenzweig EB, Gannon WD, Madahar P, et al. Extracorporeal life support bridge for pulmonary hypertension: a high-volume single-center experience. J Heart Lung Transplant 2019;38(12):1275–85.

68. Hoetzenecker K, Donahoe L, Yeung JC, et al. Extracorporeal life support as a bridge to lung transplantation-experience of a high-volume transplant center. J Thorac Cardiovasc Surg 2018; 155(3):1316–1328 e1311.

69. Glorion M, Mercier O, Mitilian D, et al. Central versus peripheral cannulation of extracorporeal membrane oxygenation support during double lung transplant for pulmonary hypertension. Eur J Cardiothorac Surg 2018;54(2):341–7.

70. Tudorache I, Sommer W, Kuhn C, et al. Lung transplantation for severe pulmonary hypertension–awake extracorporeal membrane oxygenation for

postoperative left ventricular remodelling. Transplantation 2015;99(2):451–8.

71. Ius F, Sommer W, Tudorache I, et al. Veno-veno-arterial extracorporeal membrane oxygenation for respiratory failure with severe haemodynamic impairment: technique and early outcomes. Interact Cardiovasc Thorac Surg 2015;20(6):761–7.

72. Napp LC, Kuhn C, Hoeper MM, et al. Cannulation strategies for percutaneous extracorporeal membrane oxygenation in adults. Clin Res Cardiol 2016;105(4):283–96.

73. Grant C Jr, Richards JB, Frakes M, et al. ECMO and right ventricular failure: review of the literature. J Intensive Care Med 2020. https://doi.org/10.1177/0885066619900503. 885066619900503.

74. Schmid C, Philipp A, Hilker M, et al. Bridge to lung transplantation through a pulmonary artery to left atrial oxygenator circuit. Ann Thorac Surg 2008; 85(4):1202–5.

75. Strueber M, Hoeper MM, Fischer S, et al. Bridge to thoracic organ transplantation in patients with pulmonary arterial hypertension using a pumpless lung assist device. Am J Transplant 2009;9(4): 853–7.

76. Aissaoui N, Morshuis M, Schoenbrodt M, et al. Temporary right ventricular mechanical circulatory support for the management of right ventricular failure in critically ill patients. J Thorac Cardiovasc Surg 2013;146(1):186–91.

77. Cheung AW, White CW, Davis MK, et al. Short-term mechanical circulatory support for recovery from acute right ventricular failure: clinical outcomes. J Heart Lung Transplant 2014;33(8):794–9.

78. Anderson M, Morris DL, Tang D, et al. Outcomes of patients with right ventricular failure requiring short-term hemodynamic support with the Impella RP device. J Heart Lung Transplant 2018;37(12):1448–58.

79. Ravichandran AK, Baran DA, Stelling K, et al. Outcomes with the tandem protek duo dual-lumen percutaneous right ventricular assist device. ASAIO J 2018;64(4):570–2.

80. Berman M, Tsui S, Vuylsteke A, et al. Life-threatening right ventricular failure in pulmonary hypertension: RVAD or ECMO? J Heart Lung Transplant 2008; 27(10):1188–9.

81. Rosenzweig EB, Chicotka S, Bacchetta M. Right ventricular assist device use in ventricular failure due to pulmonary arterial hypertension: lessons learned. J Heart Lung Transplant 2016;35(10): 1272–4.

82. Vullaganti S, Tibrewala A, Rich JD, et al. The use of a durable right ventricular assist device for isolated right ventricular failure due to combined pre- and postcapillary pulmonary hypertension. Pulm Circ 2019;9(2). 2045894019831222.

83. Salsano A, Sportelli E, Olivieri GM, et al. RVAD support in the setting of submassive pulmonary embolism. J Extra Corpor Technol 2017;49(4):304–6.

84. Oh DK, Shim TS, Jo KW, et al. Right ventricular assist device with an oxygenator using extracorporeal membrane oxygenation as a bridge to lung transplantation in a patient with severe respiratory failure and right heart decompensation. Acute Crit Care 2020;35(2):117–21.

85. Badu B, Cain MT, Durham LA 3rd, et al. A dual-lumen percutaneous cannula for managing refractory right ventricular failure. ASAIO J 2020;66(8): 915–21.

86. Hoeper MM, Galie N, Murali S, et al. Outcome after cardiopulmonary resuscitation in patients with pulmonary arterial hypertension. Am J Respir Crit Care Med 2002;165(3):341–4.

87. Khirfan G, Tonelli AR, Ramsey J, et al. Palliative care in pulmonary arterial hypertension: an underutilised treatment. Eur Respir Rev 2018;27(150):180069.

88. Edwards JD, Voigt LP, Nelson JE. Ten key points about ICU palliative care. Intensive Care Med 2017;43(1):83–5.

Section V: Advanced Topics

Pulmonary Vascular Disease as a Systemic and Multisystem Disease

Katherine Kearney, MBBS, MMed, FRACP[a,b],
Eugene Kotlyar, MBBS, MD, FRACP[b,c],
Edmund M.T. Lau, BSc, MBBS, PhD, FRACP[d,e,*]

KEYWORDS

- Pulmonary arterial hypertension • Heart failure • Inflammation • Metabolic

KEY POINTS

- Chronic heart failure syndrome is responsible for many of the common manifestations of pulmonary arterial hypertension (PAH), including activation of the sympathetic nervous system and renin-angiotensin-aldosterone system.
- PAH is associated with changes in skeletal and respiratory muscle functions. There is evidence to support exercise training in reversing, to some extent, peripheral muscle dysfunction.
- Markers of systemic inflammation are increased in PAH. Dysregulated immunity and inflammation drive pulmonary vascular remodeling and represent a potential therapeutic target.
- Mitochondrial metabolism is altered in pulmonary vascular cells and right ventricle of patients with PAH. This is characterized by the "Warburg effect" with a shift from mitochondrial oxidation to glycolysis.
- Other systemic manifestations of PAH include endothelial dysfunction, sleep abnormalities, liver and gut dysfunction, and iron deficiency.

INTRODUCTION

Pulmonary arterial hypertension (PAH) is a disease of progressive pulmonary vascular remodeling due to abnormal proliferation of pulmonary vascular endothelial and smooth muscle cells and endothelial dysfunction.[1] The endothelial dysfunction involves dysregulation of vasodilator and vasoconstrictor mediators, with a reduction of vasodilator mediators (prostacyclin and nitric oxide) and upregulation of vasoconstrictor mediators (endothelin-1).[2] These changes raise pulmonary vascular resistance by decreasing the cross-sectional area of the vasculature. PAH is rare with an estimated prevalence of 15 to 50 per million population; however, it portends a poor prognosis, with resultant right heart failure and death.[3] Hemodynamically, PAH is defined by a mean pulmonary artery pressure (mPAP) greater than 20 mm Hg and normal pulmonary artery wedge pressure less than or equal to 15 mm Hg with pulmonary vascular resistance (PVR) greater than 3 Wood Units (WU). Although the underlying disease originates in the pulmonary vasculature, there is accumulating evidence that PAH is a

The authors have no relevant commercial or financial conflicts of interest to declare.
[a] Cardiology Department, St Vincent's Hospital, 394 Victoria Street, Darlinghurst, New South Wales 2010, Australia; [b] St Vincent's Clinical School, University of New South Wales, Sydney, Australia; [c] Heart Transplant Unit, St Vincent's Hospital, 394 Victoria Street, Darlinghurst, New South Wales 2010, Australia; [d] Department of Respiratory Medicine, Royal Prince Alfred Hospital, Missenden Road, Camperdown, New South Wales 2050, Australia; [e] Sydney Medical School, University of Sydney, Camperdown, Australia
* Corresponding author. Department of Respiratory Medicine, Royal Prince Alfred Hospital, Missenden Road, Camperdown, New South Wales 2050, Australia.
E-mail address: edmund.lau@sydney.edu.au

multisystem disease with systemic manifestations and complications.

CHRONIC HEART FAILURE SYNDROME
Systemic Consequence of Right Ventricle-Pulmonary Artery Uncoupling

Elevated pulmonary pressures in PAH create increased afterload for the right ventricle (RV). Adaptation occurs with increased contractility allowing maintenance of normal stroke volume until there is dysfunction of RV-pulmonary arterial coupling. When uncoupling occurs, RV contractility becomes insufficient to match the increased afterload. Impaired coupling may be more pronounced at exercise and contribute to exercise intolerance.[4] Impaired coupling leads to dilatation of the RV via heterometric adaptation. In addition, sarcomere stiffening and myocardial fibrosis contribute to diastolic function. Right ventricular heart failure involves different mechanisms in the acute and chronic phases and are discussed in greater detail elsewhere.

Chronic RV failure is responsible for many of the common manifestations of PAH. The most prominent clinical feature in right-sided heart failure secondary to PAH is peripheral edema but others include cardiohepatic and cardiorenal abnormalities. Signs and symptoms of right-sided heart failure can include elevated jugular venous pressure, liver congestion, hepatomegaly, ascites, bloating, and pleural effusions.

Decreased exercise capacity is one of the defining characteristics of PAH. The major mechanism of exercise limitation in PAH is decreased augmentation of cardiac output with a failing RV. Cardiac output limitation reduces oxygen delivery to exercising muscles as oxygen demands increases, and this is commonly assessed by maximum oxygen uptake, which has a close relationship to morbidity and mortality in patients with chronic heart failure and PAH.[5] **Fig. 1** shows how heart failure causes the resultant multisystem dysfunction that compromises almost every facet of the oxygen transport pathway.

Neurohormonal Activation

The chronic heart failure syndrome of PAH is associated with marked sympathetic nervous system (SNS) activation, as measured by muscle sympathetic nervous system activity. The degree of SNS activation is also correlated with clinical outcomes in patients with PAH.[6] The sympathetic overactivation of the heart failure syndrome is accompanied by autonomic nervous system dysregulation, with spectral analysis of heart rate variability and baroreflex sensitivity showing reductions relative to age- and sex-matched healthy controls,[7] and these changes were correlated with decreased peak oxygen uptake, suggesting correlation with disease severity.

Neurohormonal activation in PAH leads to global vasoconstriction and intravascular water and sodium retention. Decrease in renal blood flow results in activation of the renin-angiotensin-aldosterone system (RAAS).[8] Interestingly, atrial septostomy (a therapeutic procedure for end-stage PAH) has been shown to decrease SNS activation, despite an associated decrease in arterial oxygenation.[9] Relief of right atrial pressure and increase in systemic cardiac output with septostomy seems to downregulate SNS and RAAS.

Autonomic nervous system dysregulation also manifests in increased chemosensitivity to $P_{a}CO_2$ and resultant heightened ventilatory responses both at rest and during exercise. Altered chemosensitivity with lower $Paco_2$ set-point causes ventilatory inefficiency, which becomes more marked during exercise.[10] Thus, patients with PAH hyperventilate both at rest and during exercise, and this is commonly represented by an increase of the VE/VCO_2 slope during cardiopulmonary exercise testing and has been demonstrated to be prognostic in PAH.[11]

It has been shown in experimental animal models that SNS regulation with β-blockers delays progression toward RV failure, improves systolic and diastolic function of the RV[12] and endothelial function.[13] Given this, the role of systemic beta-blockade to mediate the SNS activation has been evaluated but not met with success in PAH. In both portopulmonary hypertension and idiopathic PAH, the use of bisoprolol has been associated with worse hemodynamics and 6-minute walk distance.[14] In patients with portopulmonary hypertension, withdrawal of β-blockers was associated with improvement in exercise tolerance and higher cardiac output.[15]

Direct intervention in the RAAS with aldosterone antagonist,[16] angiotensin-1 receptor blockade,[17] and angiotensin-converting enzyme inhibitor[18] has been shown to reduce development of pulmonary hypertension in animal models. A small pilot study of losartan in patients with pulmonary hypertension secondary to lung disease showed a trend to improvement in the most severe patients.[19] In an animal model of PAH, renal denervation has been shown to reduce disease progression; reduce RV diastolic stiffness, hypertrophy, and fibrosis; and suppress the RAAS.[20] Finally, proof of concept studies using catheter-based denervation of the pulmonary arteries has demonstrated improvements of pulmonary hemodynamics and exercise capacity in human PAH.[21] Further

EFFECTS OF CHF ON O₂ TRANSPORT PATHWAY

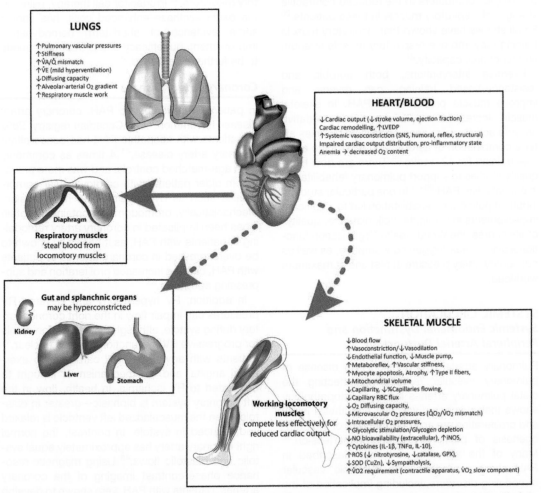

Fig. 1. Impact of heart failure on different aspects of the oxygen transport pathway. (*From* Poole, D. C., Hirai, D. M., Copp, S. W. & Musch, T. I. Muscle oxygen transport and utilization in heart failure: implications for exercise (in)tolerance. Am. J. Physiol. Heart Circ. Physiol. 302, H1050-1063 (2012); with permission.)

multicenter clinical trials are underway for pulmonary artery denervation.

SKELETAL AND RESPIRATORY MUSCLE

Substantial evidence supports findings of skeletal muscle dysfunction in PAH as well as structural changes. Patients with PAH exhibit microcirculation loss and impaired angiogenesis of skeletal muscle.[22] In animal models, these changes were associated with exercise intolerance. Maximal volitional and nonvolitional strength, a metric that does not depend on oxygen supply, is impaired in patients with PAH, indicating derangement of the intrinsic capacity of the skeletal muscle to generate force.[23] The underlying pathophysiology behind this is not clear but may involve atrophy, sarcomere dysfunction, a shift to fast-twitch fibers, and capillary rarefaction.[22] Physical inactivity induces muscle atrophy itself, as well as reduces contractility and causes myocyte fiber transition.[24]

Respiratory muscle dysfunction has also been demonstrated in patients with idiopathic PAH. Patients with PAH have reduced inspiratory and expiratory muscle strength[25] compared with healthy controls, and the respiratory muscle dysfunction seems to be independent of the severity of right heart failure. Patients with chronic thromboembolic pulmonary hypertension (CTEPH) have been found to have reduced force-generating capacity of diaphragmatic slow-twitch fibers and reduced calcium sensitivity in fast-twitch fibers that correlates with maximum inspiratory pressure, suggesting that these are the major pathologic contributors to the reduced contractile strength of inspiratory muscle in these patients.[26] Small studies have shown that inspiratory muscle training may improve respiratory muscle strength and functional capacity.[27]

Exercise interventions, both aerobic and resistance-based training, can reverse and improve muscle properties in PAH. In skeletal muscle, increased capillarization and oxidative enzyme activity were seen on muscle biopsies after a combination of aerobic and resistance exercise training for 12 weeks.[28] There are now high-quality studies to support pulmonary rehabilitation in patients with PAH.[29–31] In one particular study,[29] inpatient pulmonary rehabilitation led to significant improvements in 6-minute walk distance, quality-of-life scores, the World Health Organization functional class, peak oxygen consumption, as well as pulmonary artery pressure at rest and at maximum workload.

SYSTEMIC CIRCULATION
Systemic Endothelial Dysfunction and Peripheral Arterial Dysfunction

Pulmonary arterial hypertension is a disease of pulmonary vascular remodeling, affecting the distal pulmonary arteries initially. Histopathology shows that pulmonary vascular endothelial injury and proliferation are an important part of the pathogenesis of pulmonary arterial hypertension.[32] Many of the signaling pathways described in PAH share similarities with systemic vascular remodeling disorders, including implication of the receptor of advanced glycation end products,[33] the oncoprotein kinase Pim-1,[34] and the transcription factor nuclear factor of activated T cells.[35]

By evaluating endothelial function through forearm blood flow dilatation in response to brachial artery occlusion, it has been shown that peripheral endothelial dysfunction occurs in idiopathic PAH, scleroderma-associated PAH, and CTEPH.[36] The peripheral arterial tone ratio, as measured by this validated technique, was significantly lower than control values in these patients, and this correlates with disease severity.[36,37] Systemic endothelial dysfunction in PAH may have implications for other systemic manifestations of PAH such as coronary artery disease.

Endothelial progenitor cells have been shown to be dysregulated in patients with PAH, specifically in remodeled arteries and plexiform lesions, and dramatically so in patients with BMPR2 mutations.[38] Circulating levels of progenitor cells have also been found to be lower in patients with PAH compared with controls and this correlates to functional class and increased levels of inflammatory mediators.[39] Progenitor cell therapy, using nitric oxide synthase–enhanced cells, has shown some evidence of short-term hemodynamic improvement, but efficacy of this treatment needs to be further established.[40]

Coronary Artery Disease

In patients with idiopathic PAH, coronary artery disease is common.[3] In a Canadian registry, 28% of patients with idiopathic PAH had concomitant coronary artery disease,[41] 4 times as commonly as in age-matched controls, and was more prevalent in older patients with cardiovascular comorbidities such as dyslipidemia and hypertension. Mechanistically, bromodomain-containing protein 4 has been implicated in coronary artery remodeling in patients with PAH, as it has been shown to be overexpressed in coronary arteries of patients with PAH, causing increased proliferation and suppressing apoptosis.[33]

In addition, RV hypertrophy and elevated RV pressures can impair flow in the right coronary artery during systole, although the implication of this for progressive RV dysfunction remains unclear.[42] Patients with advanced PAH can develop exertional angina, and the mechanism is thought to be related to RV ischemia. In health, flow in the left coronary system is biphasic—greater in diastole when the muscularized left ventricle is relaxed and reduced in systole. In contrast, the normal right coronary artery has approximately equal systolic and diastolic flows.[43] Using magnetic resonance phase-contrast imaging of the coronary arteries, patients with PAH were shown to develop biphasic flow in the right coronary artery, in a pattern similar to the left coronary artery, resulting in reduced RV perfusion during systole.[42] **Fig. 2** demonstrates the phasic changes in coronary artery blood flow in health and PAH.

SYSTEMIC INFLAMMATION AND INFECTION

The connection between inflammatory conditions and PAH is well recognized. PAH is a complication of systemic sclerosis,[44] mixed connective tissue disease,[45] and systemic lupus erythematosus.[46] In addition, the risk of developing portopulmonary hypertension is significantly higher with autoimmune hepatitis than with other causes of liver failure.[47]

Schistosomiasis infection causes PAH in 2% to 5% of those infected, after portal hypertension develops, and portocaval shunts develop to create a pathway for eggs to lodge in the pulmonary capillaries—this is the most common cause worldwide for PAH.[48] This damage is irreversible and

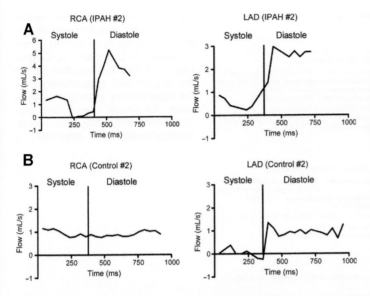

Fig. 2. Coronary artery flow profiles in the right coronary artery (RCA) and left anterior descending (LAD) artery of patients with pulmonary hypertension (PH) and control subjects. Time starts at the ECG R-wave. To average over the groups, time is expressed as percentage of duration of one heartbeat. ECG, electrocardiogram. (*From* van Wolferen SA, Marcus JT, Westerhof N, et al. Right coronary artery flow impairment in patients with pulmonary hypertension. Eur Heart J. 2008 Jan;29(1):120-7. https://doi.org/10.1093/eurheartj/ehm567. Epub 2007 Dec 8. PMID: 18065750; with permission.)

pulmonary vascular damage persists after treatment of schistosomiasis. In patients with human immunodeficiency infection (HIV), PAH can occur in 0.5%.[49] The pathophysiology of HIV-related PAH is incompletely understood but is not attributed to direct viral infection and may relate to increased inflammation.[50]

Systemic inflammation has long been associated with PAH. It is accepted that inflammation contributes to disease susceptibility and progression.[51] A wide array of inflammatory markers is increased in patients with PAH and many correlate with survival or disease severity (**Fig. 3**). Studies have implicated overexpression of cytokines such as interleukin-6 (IL-6) in the pathogenesis of PAH, causing excess cellular proliferation and vascular remodeling in animal models.[52] There is evidence of activation of the innate and adaptive immune systems and subsequent production of cytokines and chemokines that propagate these processes. Dysregulated immunity and altered function of T cells, specifically T-regulatory cells, has been established in PAH.[53]

Efforts at immunomodulation have been attempted to treat PAH. Experimental rat models of pulmonary hypertension have shown reversal of PH, after treatment with IL-6 receptor antagonist.[54] TRANSFORM-UK, an efficacy trial of tocilizumab, an IL-6 receptor antagonist, in patients with PAH has completed recruitment but not reported yet.[38] This important trial provides further information about systemic immunomodulatory therapies. B-cell depletion with rituximab has also been trialed in a small trial that showed safety but was not able to show statistically significant changes in function (6-minue walk test [6MWT])

or hemodynamic parameters.[55] A recent small study of immunomodulation with mercaptopurine in patients with PAH showed a significant decrease in PVR, without significant changes in other hemodynamic and functional parameters.[56] Significant side effects were seen that were limiting for a substantial portion of patients.

ENDOCRINE AND METABOLIC CHANGES
Obesity

Obesity is increasingly prevalent in patients with PAH, with a recent report from the French registry showing 30% were obese[57] and in the large US REVEAL registry, 31% meeting obesity criteria.[58]

The interaction between obesity and pulmonary arterial hypertension is complex. As with other causes of chronic heart failure, it is postulated that there may be some protective effect, often termed the "obesity paradox." The REVEAL registry showed that obesity was an independent predictor of better survival, after adjustment for confounding factors.[59] Interestingly, a reanalysis of the original National Institutes of Health registry found a U-shaped effect of body mass index on mortality, with overweight but not morbidly obese patients having a survival benefit.[60] However, the relationship between obesity and survival in PAH has not been replicated in all registries.[57,61]

Potential mechanisms explaining the protective effect of obesity include obese patients having greater metabolic reserve to meet an increased demand, a reduced response to proinflammatory cytokines such as tumor necrosis factor alpha, or selection bias, in that obese patients may be diagnosed earlier during investigations for dyspnea that may not be strictly related to PAH or heart failure.[62]

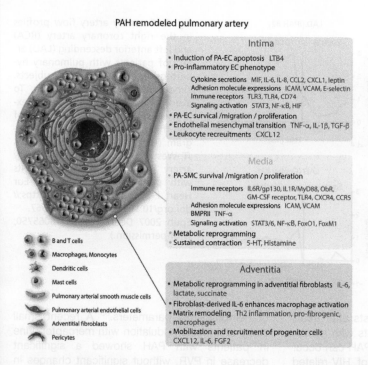

PAH remodeled pulmonary artery

Intima
- Induction of PA-EC apoptosis LTB4
- Pro-inflammatory EC phenotype
  - Cytokine secretions MIF, IL-6, IL-8, CCL2, CXCL1, leptin
  - Adhesion molecule expressions ICAM, VCAM, E-selectin
  - Immune receptors TLR3, TLR4, CD74
  - Signaling activation STAT3, NF-κB, HIF
- PA-EC survival /migration / proliferation
- Endothelial mesenchymal transition TNF-α, IL-1β, TGF-β
- Leukocyte recreuitments CXCL12

Media
- PA-SMC survival /migration / proliferation
  - Immune receptors IL6R/gp130, IL1R/MyD88, ObR,
                     GM-CSF receptor, TLR4, CXCR4, CCR5
  - Adhesion molecule expressions ICAM, VCAM
  - BMPRII TNF-α
  - Signaling activation STAT3/6, NF-κB, FoxO1, FoxM1
- Metabolic reprogramming
- Sustained contraction 5-HT, Histamine

Adventitia
- Metabolic reprogramming in adventitial fibroblasts IL-6, lactate, succinate
- Fibroblast-derived IL-6 enhances macrophage activation
- Matrix remodeling Th2 inflammation, pro-fibrogenic, macrophages
- Mobilization and recruitment of progenitor cells CXCL12, IL-6, FGF2

- B and T cells
- Macrophages, Monocytes
- Dendritic cells
- Mast cells
- Pulmonary arterial smooth muscle cells
- Pulmonary arterial endothelial cells
- Adventitial fibroblasts
- Pericytes

Fig. 3. Chronic inflammation within the 3 vascular compartments in pulmonary arterial hypertension. (*From* Huertas A, Tu L, Humbert M, Guignabert C. Chronic inflammation within the vascular wall in pulmonary arterial hypertension: more than a spectator. Cardiovasc Res. 2020 Apr 1;116(5):885-893. https://doi.org/10.1093/cvr/cvz308. PMID: 31813986.)

Metabolic Dysfunction

Increasing prevalence of obesity portends an increased prevalence of metabolic syndrome, defined as insulin resistance, diabetes, and hyperlipidemia. Glucose intolerance is common in patients with PAH and does not necessarily occur more commonly in obese patients.[63] Frank diabetes mellitus is associated with worse survival in patients with PAH, and in particular, RV stroke work index was lower in patients with diabetes despite no significant difference in mPAP or PVR.[64] A potential mechanism for this has been elucidated from mouse models, where it has been shown that mice with mutated BMPR2 gene develop insulin resistance before the development of PAH.[65] Hyperlipidemia and abnormalities in the metabolism of fatty acids have been demonstrated in both blood and myocardium of patients with PAH, and this is associated with in vivo cardiac steatosis and lipotoxicity.[66]

A recognized downstream target of BMPR2, the most common genetic abnormality in patients with heritable or idiopathic PAH, is PPARγ, a transcription factor with downstream targets involved in both vascular modeling and glucose homeostasis.[67] Low circulating levels of PPARγ, as have been seen in PAH,[68] are associated with a variety of pathologic metabolic states, including obesity, type II diabetes mellitus, and insulin resistance.

The "Warbug effect" describes a metabolic shift toward favoring anaerobic glycolysis in preference to oxidative phosphorylation, even in aerobic conditions. This is most commonly recognized in cancer cells and is the mechanism for the fluorodeoxyglucose (FDG)-PET avidity of malignant cells.[69] This metabolic shift has been seen in pulmonary vascular smooth muscle cells[70] and has been used in experimental animal and clinical contexts to demonstrate PET-FDG avidity in PAH.[71] Abnormalities of glucose metabolism are intrinsically related to abnormalities of lipid metabolism, and given the heart's preference for fatty acid metabolism,[72] these abnormalities have significant implications for RV function; this has been demonstrated in blood and myocardium in patients with PAH and has been associated with in vivo cardiac steatosis and lipotoxicity.[66]

Given this, metformin has shown some promising data in animal models,[73] and in a small clinical study,[74] there are currently clinical trials recruiting for further data on repurposing it. Similarly, PPARγ agonists such as pioglitazone have been shown to reverse PAH in rat models,[75] and although clinical studies have not proceeded due to poor enrollment, this remains a research area of interest.

LIVER AND GUT AXIS
Sick Liver and Portal Hypertension

Portopulmonary hypertension (PoPH) is defined as pulmonary hypertension associated with portal hypertension. PoPH can occur in the absence of liver cirrhosis with extrahepatic causes of portal hypertension.[76] The pathogenesis of pulmonary vascular disease in the setting of portal hypertension remains poorly defined. Postulated pathobiology includes high cardiac output states in chronic liver disease, which could cause shear stress of the arterial wall that triggers a cascade of changes resulting in arterial remodeling.[77] Alternatively or additionally, portosystemic shunts develop that bypass the liver, which may impair phagocytic capacity anyway, and allow the circulation of bacteria and endotoxins to the pulmonary circulation, where deleterious effects occur to the pulmonary vasculature.[76]

These theories would support the role of inflammation in the pathogenesis of PAH. Additional recent published data point to bacterial translocation being involved in the pathogenesis of PAH.[78] This study demonstrated, in a mouse model, the translocation of endotoxin in pulmonary arterial hypertension and suggested toll-like receptor 4 (TLR4) activation and consequently pulmonary vascular remodeling and inflammation. It is postulated that disrupting this gut-lung interaction with TLR4 antagonists may be beneficial in preventing progression of PAH. Recently, bone morphogenic protein 9 (BMP9) has been implicated as a circulating endothelial factor that is protective for PAH. It has been shown that BMP9 is lower in patients with PoPH compared with cirrhosis without PoPH and also other causes of PAH.[79]

Microbiome

A small study has suggested that patients with PAH have a unique gut microbiome profile and that this may offer insight into the contribution of the gut to the pathogenesis of PAH.[80] These data suggest increased gut permeability in patients with PAH, because of decreased beneficial short-chain fatty acid–producing bacteria, as well as increases in bacteria contributing to tryptophan and serotonin biosynthesis, which has previously been linked to the pathogenesis of PAH. It is proposed that the increased gut permeability and altered protein synthesis may contribute to the development of PAH; this is a developing area with a need for further research.

SLEEP

Sleep-disordered breathing is common in patients with PAH, with 82.6% of patients having nocturnal hypoxemia and 89% meeting criteria for sleep apnea on mean apnea-hypopnea index.[81] There is likely to be a bidirectional effect that is operational between sleep-disordered breathing and PAH. Obstructive sleep apnea (OSA) alone can lead to mild elevation in pulmonary artery pressure,[82] and continuous positive airway pressure treatment results in reversal of pulmonary hypertension.[83] On the other hand, OSA can develop or become exacerbated in the setting of fluid overload with rostral fluid shift during sleep to the neck and upper airway.[84] Nocturnal oxygen therapy has been shown to improve 6MWT in patients with both PAH and sleep-disordered breathing.[85]

NEUROLOGIC COMPLICATIONS

Cerebrovascular abnormalities including an impaired cerebral pressure-flow relationship and blunted cerebrovascular reactivity to CO_2 have been shown in patients with PAH.[86] Cognitive sequalae of PAH is evident in patient-reported outcome measure assessments in up to 58% of the patients[25]; this can manifest as worse verbal learning, delayed verbal memory, executive function impairment, and fine motor skills. It is often complicated by depression, anxiety, and decreased quality of life. All of these cognitive challenges affect quality of life. Further research in the area of cognitive mental health and quality of life in patients with PAH is needed to best address these challenges.

SKIN

Microvasculature changes of PAH are evident in nailfold capillary density in patients with scleroderma-associated PAH as well as idiopathic PAH. Although those with scleroderma-associated PAH had the lowest capillary density, there was still a significant difference between those with idiopathic PAH and healthy volunteers.[87] In scleroderma-associated PAH, this capillary density also correlated with severity of PAH.[88] This suggests systemic microvasculature dysfunction, beyond just the pulmonary capillary bed, although it is unknown if this may be related to the cause of PAH or a complication of the disease.

IRON METABOLISM

Iron deficiency is common in patients with PAH[89] and CTEPH[90] and is associated with disease severity and reduced exercise capacity,[91] even in the absence of anemia. This deficiency is associated with inappropriately elevated hepcidin levels[89] and impaired oral absorption.[91] Treatment with iron supplementation has been shown to attenuate the hypoxic vasoconstrictive response.[92,93]

Experimental studies of animal models of PAH and pulmonary artery smooth muscle cells (PASMCs) have shown clinical iron deficiency, as well as iron chelation, enhance the vasoconstrictive response to hypoxia, and endothelin-1 expression in PASMCs was reduced by in vitro iron treatment.[94] Cellular iron homeostasis, regulated by the local hepcidin and ferroportin, if driven to intracellular iron deficiency, can give rise to remodeling of pulmonary arteries and PAH in these models as well.[94]

Diagnosis of iron deficiency in patients with PAH seems best diagnosed with transferrin saturations less than 20%.[89] A small trial of intravenous iron in iron-deficient patients with idiopathic PAH has shown improvement in endurance and aerobic capacity as well as quality of life,[95] but 6MWT did not significantly change. A larger clinical trial of intravenous iron in patients with PAH is completed but results are yet to reported at the time of writing.[96]

SUMMARY

Pulmonary arterial hypertension is a multisystem disease with significant systemic and multiorgan effects. It remains important to understand this complex pathophysiology for both treatment and ongoing research of patients with PAH. Many of the most important breakthroughs in pulmonary hypertension treatment have come from paradigms associated with the systemic manifestations of the disease, and it is hoped that more will eventuate in the near future.

REFERENCES

1. Humbert M, Guignabert C, Bonnet S, et al. Pathology and pathobiology of pulmonary hypertension: state of the art and research perspectives. Eur Respir J 2019;53(1):1801887.
2. Lau EM, Montani D, Jaïs X, et al. Advances in therapeutic interventions for patients with pulmonary arterial hypertension. Circulation 2014;130(24):2189–208.
3. Strange G, Lau EM, Giannoulatou E, et al. Survival of idiopathic pulmonary arterial hypertension patients in the modern era in Australia and New Zealand. Heart Lung Circ 2018;27(11):1368–75.
4. Naeije R, Manes A. The right ventricle in pulmonary arterial hypertension. Eur Respir Rev 2014;23(134):476–87.
5. Weber KT, Kinasewitz GT, Janicki JS, et al. Oxygen utilization and ventilation during exercise in patients with chronic cardiac failure. Circulation 1982;65(6):1213–23.
6. Ciarka A, Doan V, Velez-Roa S, et al. Prognostic significance of sympathetic nervous system activation in pulmonary arterial hypertension. Am J Respir Crit Care Med 2010;181(11):1269–75.
7. Wensel R, Jilek C, Dörr M, et al. Impaired cardiac autonomic control relates to disease severity in pulmonary hypertension. Eur Respir J 2009;34(4):895–901.
8. Hartupee J, Mann DL. Neurohormonal activation in heart failure with reduced ejection fraction. Nat Rev Cardiol 2017;14(1):30–8.
9. Ciarka A, Vachièry JL, Houssière A, et al. Atrial septostomy decreases sympathetic overactivity in pulmonary arterial hypertension. Chest 2007;131(6):1831–7.
10. Weatherald J, Sattler C, Garcia G, et al. Ventilatory response to exercise in cardiopulmonary disease: the role of chemosensitivity and dead space. Eur Respir J 2018;51.
11. Schwaiblmair M, Faul C, von Scheidt W, et al. Ventilatory efficiency testing as prognostic value in patients with pulmonary hypertension. BMC Pulm Med 2012;12:23.
12. de Man FS, Handoko ML, van Ballegoij JJ, et al. Bisoprolol delays progression towards right heart failure in experimental pulmonary hypertension. Circ Heart Fail 2012;5(1):97–105.
13. Perros F, Ranchoux B, Izikki M, et al. Nebivolol for improving endothelial dysfunction, pulmonary vascular remodeling, and right heart function in pulmonary hypertension. J Am Coll Cardiol 2015;65(7):668–80.
14. van Campen JSJA, de Boer K, van de Veerdonk MC, et al. Bisoprolol in idiopathic pulmonary arterial hypertension: an explorative study. Eur Respir J 2016;48:787–96.
15. Provencher S, Herve P, Jais X, et al. Deleterious effects of beta-blockers on exercise capacity and hemodynamics in patients with portopulmonary hypertension. Gastroenterology 2006;130(1):120–6.
16. Boehm M, Arnold N, Braithwaite A, et al. Eplerenone attenuates pathological pulmonary vascular rather than right ventricular remodeling in pulmonary arterial hypertension. BMC Pulm Med 2018;18(1):41.
17. de Man FS, Tu L, Handoko ML, et al. Dysregulated renin-angiotensin-aldosterone system contributes to pulmonary arterial hypertension. Am J Respir Crit Care Med 2012;186(8):780–9.
18. Morrell NW, Morris KG, Stenmark KR. Role of angiotensin-converting enzyme and angiotensin II in development of hypoxic pulmonary hypertension. Am J Physiol 1995;269(4 Pt 2):H1186–94.
19. Morrell NW, Higham MA, Phillips PG, et al. Pilot study of losartan for pulmonary hypertension in chronic obstructive pulmonary disease. Respir Res 2005;6:88.
20. da Silva Gonçalves Bos D, Happé C, Schalij I, et al. Renal denervation reduces pulmonary vascular remodeling and right ventricular diastolic stiffness in experimental pulmonary hypertension. JACC Basic Transl Sci 2017;2(1):22–35.
21. Chen SL, Zhang H, Xie DJ, et al. Hemodynamic, functional, and clinical responses to pulmonary

artery denervation in patients with pulmonary arterial hypertension of different causes: phase II results from the Pulmonary Artery Denervation-1 study. Circ Cardiovasc Interv 2015;8(11):e002837.

22. Potus F, Malenfant S, Graydon C, et al. Impaired angiogenesis and peripheral muscle microcirculation loss contribute to exercise intolerance in pulmonary arterial hypertension. Am J Respir Crit Care Med 2014;190(3):318–28.

23. Manders E, Bogaard HJ, Handoko ML, et al. Contractile dysfunction of left ventricular cardiomyocytes in patients with pulmonary arterial hypertension. J Am Coll Cardiol 2014;64(1):28–37.

24. Jackman RW, Kandarian SC. The molecular basis of skeletal muscle atrophy. Am J Physiol Cell Physiol 2004;287(4):C834–43.

25. White J, Hopkins RO, Glissmeyer EW, et al. Cognitive, emotional, and quality of life outcomes in patients with pulmonary arterial hypertension. Respir Res 2006;7:55.

26. Manders E, Bonta PI, Kloek JJ, et al. Reduced force of diaphragm muscle fibers in patients with chronic thromboembolic pulmonary hypertension. Am J Physiol Lung Cell Mol Physiol 2016;311(1):L20.

27. Saglam M, et al. Inspiratory muscle training in pulmonary hypertension. Eur Respir J 2013;42.

28. Sahni S, Capozzi B, Iftikhar A, et al. Pulmonary rehabilitation and exercise in pulmonary arterial hypertension: an underutilized intervention. J Exerc Rehabil 2015;11(2):74–9.

29. Grünig E, Lichtblau M, Ehlken N, et al. Safety and efficacy of exercise training in various forms of pulmonary hypertension. Eur Respir J 2012;40(1):84–92.

30. Chan L, Chin LMK, Kennedy M, et al. Benefits of intensive treadmill exercise training on cardiorespiratory function and quality of life in patients with pulmonary hypertension. Chest 2013;143(2):333–43.

31. Mereles D, Ehlken N, Kreuscher S, et al. Exercise and respiratory training improve exercise capacity and quality of life in patients with severe chronic pulmonary hypertension. Circulation 2006;114(14):1482–9.

32. Rubin LJ. Primary pulmonary hypertension. N Engl J Med 1997;336(2):111–7.

33. Jolyane M, Lampron MC, Nadeau V, et al. Implication of inflammation and epigenetic readers in coronary artery remodeling in patients with pulmonary arterial hypertension. Arterioscler Thromb Vasc Biol 2017;37(8):1513–23.

34. Roxane P, Courboulin A, Meloche J, et al. Signal transducers and activators of transcription-3/Pim1 axis plays a critical role in the pathogenesis of human pulmonary arterial hypertension. Circulation 2011;123(11):1205–15.

35. Bonnet S, Paulin R, Sutendra G, et al. Dehydroepiandrosterone reverses systemic vascular remodeling through the inhibition of the Akt/GSK3-{beta}/NFAT axis. Circulation 2009;120(13):1231–40.

36. Peled N, Bendayan D, Shitrit D, et al. Peripheral endothelial dysfunction in patients with pulmonary arterial hypertension. Respir Med 2008;102(12):1791–6.

37. Hughes R, Tong J, Oates C, et al. Evidence for systemic endothelial dysfunction in patients and first-order relatives with pulmonary arterial hypertension. Chest 2005;128(6 Suppl):617S.

38. Toshner M, Voswinckel R, Southwood M, et al. Evidence of dysfunction of endothelial progenitors in pulmonary arterial hypertension. Am J Respir Crit Care Med 2009;180(8):780–7.

39. Diller GP, van Eijl S, Okonko DO, et al. Circulating endothelial progenitor cells in patients with Eisenmenger syndrome and idiopathic pulmonary arterial hypertension. Circulation 2008;117(23):3020–30.

40. Granton J, Langleben D, Kutryk MB, et al. Endothelial NO-synthase gene-enhanced progenitor cell therapy for pulmonary arterial hypertension: the PHACeT Trial. Circ Res 2015;117(7):645–54.

41. Shimony A, Eisenberg MJ, Rudski LG, et al. Prevalence and impact of coronary artery disease in patients with pulmonary arterial hypertension. Am J Cardiol 2011;108(3):460–4.

42. van Wolferen SA, Marcus JT, Westerhof N, et al. Right coronary artery flow impairment in patients with pulmonary hypertension. Eur Heart J 2008;29(1):120–7.

43. Wilson RF, Laughlin DE, Ackell PH, et al. Transluminal, subselective measurement of coronary artery blood flow velocity and vasodilator reserve in man. Circulation 1985;72(1):82–92.

44. Hachulla E, Gressin V, Guillevin L, et al. Early detection of pulmonary arterial hypertension in systemic sclerosis: a French nationwide prospective multicenter study. Arthritis Rheum 2005;52(12):3792–800.

45. Fagan KA, Badesch DB. Pulmonary hypertension associated with connective tissue disease. Prog Cardiovasc Dis 2002;45(3):225–34.

46. Asherson RA, Mackworth-Young CG, Boey ML, et al. Pulmonary hypertension in systemic lupus erythematosus. Br Med J Clin Res Ed 1983;287(6398):1024–5.

47. Clinical risk factors for portopulmonary hypertension - Kawut - 2008 - Hepatology - Wiley online Library. Available at: https://aasldpubs.onlinelibrary.wiley.com/doi/full/10.1002/hep.22275.

48. Graham BB, Bandeira AP, Morrell NW, et al. Schistosomiasis-associated pulmonary hypertension: pulmonary vascular disease: the global perspective. Chest 2010;137(6 Suppl):20S–9S.

49. Sitbon O, Lascoux-Combe C, Delfraissy JF, et al. Prevalence of HIV-related pulmonary arterial

hypertension in the current antiretroviral therapy era. Am J Respir Crit Care Med 2008;177(1):108–13.

50. Butrous G. Human immunodeficiency virus-associated pulmonary arterial hypertension: considerations for pulmonary vascular diseases in the developing world. Circulation 2015;131(15): 1361–70.

51. Pathology and pathobiology of pulmonary hypertension: state of the art and research perspectives. Available at: https://www.ncbi.nlm.nih.gov/pmc/articles/PMC6351340/.

52. Huertas A, Tu L, Humbert M, et al. Chronic inflammation within the vascular wall in pulmonary arterial hypertension: more than a spectator. Cardiovasc Res 2020;116(5):885–93.

53. Tamosiuniene R, Tian W, Dhillon G, et al. Regulatory T cells limit vascular endothelial injury and prevent pulmonary hypertension. Circ Res 2011;109(8): 867–79.

54. Tamura Y, Phan C, Tu L, et al. Ectopic upregulation of membrane-bound IL6R drives vascular remodeling in pulmonary arterial hypertension. J Clin Invest 2018;128(5):1956–70.

55. Zamanian R, et al. Late Breaking Abstract - safety and efficacy of B-cell depletion with rituximab for the treatment of systemic sclerosis-associated pulmonary arterial hypertension. Eur Respir J 2019;54.

56. Botros L, Szulcek R, Jansen SMA, et al. The effects of mercaptopurine on pulmonary vascular resistance and BMPR2 expression in pulmonary arterial hypertension. Am J Respir Crit Care Med 2020; 202(2). https://doi.org/10.1164/rccm.202003-0473LE. 296202003-0473LE.

57. Weatherald J, Huertas A, Boucly A, et al. Association between BMI and obesity with survival in pulmonary arterial hypertension. Chest 2018;154(4): 872–81.

58. Farber HW, Miller DP, Poms AD, et al. Five-YEAR OUTCOMES OF PATIENTS ENROLLED in the REVEAL registry. Chest 2015;148(4):1043–54.

59. Poms AD, Turner M, Farber HW, et al. Comorbid conditions and outcomes in patients with pulmonary arterial hypertension: a REVEAL registry analysis. Chest 2013;144(1):169–76.

60. Mazimba S, Holland E, Nagarajan V, et al. Obesity paradox in group 1 pulmonary hypertension: analysis of the NIH-Pulmonary Hypertension registry. Int J Obes (Lond) 2017;41(8):1164–8.

61. McLean LL, Pellino K, Brewis M, et al. The obesity paradox in pulmonary arterial hypertension: the Scottish perspective. ERJ Open Res 2019;5(4): 00241.

62. Arena R, Lavie CJ. The obesity paradox and outcome in heart failure: is excess bodyweight truly protective? Future Cardiol 2009;6(1):1–6.

63. Pugh ME, Robbins IM, Rice TW, et al. Unrecognized glucose intolerance is common in pulmonary arterial hypertension. J Heart Lung Transplant 2011;30(8): 904–11.

64. Benson L, Brittain EL, Pugh ME, et al. Impact of diabetes on survival and right ventricular compensation in pulmonary arterial hypertension. Pulm Circ 2014; 4(2):311–8.

65. West J, Niswender KD, Johnson JA, et al. A potential role for insulin resistance in experimental pulmonary hypertension. Eur Respir J 2013;41(4):861–71.

66. Brittain EL, Talati M, Fessel JP, et al. Fatty acid metabolic defects and right ventricular lipotoxicity in human pulmonary arterial hypertension. Circulation 2016;133(20):1936–44.

67. Assad TR, Hemnes AR. Metabolic dysfunction in pulmonary arterial hypertension. Curr Hypertens Rep 2015;17(3):20.

68. Peroxisome Proliferator-activated receptor Gamma (PPARγ) expression is decreased in pulmonary hypertension and affects endothelial cell Growth | circulation research. Available at: https://www.ahajournals.org/doi/full/10.1161/01.RES.0000073585.50092.14?url_ver=Z39.88-2003&rfr_id=ori:rid:crossref.org&rfr_dat=cr_pub%3dpubmed.

69. Kelloff GJ, Hoffman JM, Johnson B, et al. Progress and promise of FDG-PET imaging for cancer patient management and oncologic drug development. Clin Cancer Res 2005;11(8):2785–808.

70. Archer SL, Gomberg-Maitland M, Maitland ML, et al. Mitochondrial metabolism, redox signaling, and fusion: a mitochondria-ROS-HIF-1alpha-Kv1.5 O2-sensing pathway at the intersection of pulmonary hypertension and cancer. Am J Physiol Heart Circ Physiol 2008;294(2):H570–8.

71. Marsboom G, Wietholt C, Haney CR, et al. Lung F-fluorodeoxyglucose positron emission tomography for diagnosis and monitoring of pulmonary arterial hypertension. Am J Respir Crit Care Med 2012; 185(6):670–9.

72. Opie LH, Knuuti J. The adrenergic-fatty acid load in heart failure. J Am Coll Cardiol 2009;54(18): 1637–46.

73. Dean A, Nilsen M, Loughlin L, et al. Metformin reverses development of pulmonary hypertension via Aromatase inhibition. Hypertension 2016;68(2): 446–54.

74. Liao S, Li D, Hui Z, et al. Metformin added to bosentan therapy in patients with pulmonary arterial hypertension associated with congenital heart defects: a pilot study. ERJ Open Res 2018;4(3). 00060-2018.

75. Legchenko E, Chouvarine P, Borchert P, et al. PPARγ agonist pioglitazone reverses pulmonary hypertension and prevents right heart failure via fatty acid oxidation. Sci Transl Med 2018;10:438.

76. Porres-Aguilar M, Altamirano JT, Torre-Delgadillo A, et al. Portopulmonary hypertension and hepatopulmonary syndrome: a clinician-oriented overview. Eur Respir Rev 2012;21(125):223–33.

77. Herve P, Lebrec D, Brenot F, et al. Pulmonary vascular disorders in portal hypertension. Eur Respir J 1998;11(5):1153–66.

78. Ranchoux B, Bigorgne A, Hautefort A, et al. Gut–lung connection in pulmonary arterial hypertension. Am J Respir Cell Mol Biol 2017;56(3):402–5.

79. Nikolic I, Lai-Ming Y, Peiran Y, et al. Bone morphogenetic protein 9 is a mechanistic biomarker of portopulmonary hypertension. Am J Respir Crit Care Med 2018;199:891–902.

80. Kim S, Rigatto K, Gazzana MB, et al. Altered Gut microbiome profile in patients with pulmonary arterial hypertension. Hypertension 2020;75(4):1063–71.

81. Jilwan FN, Escourrou P, Garcia G, et al. High occurrence of hypoxemic sleep respiratory disorders in precapillary pulmonary hypertension and mechanisms. Chest 2013;143(1):47–55.

82. Sajkov D, Cowie RJ, Thornton AT, et al. Pulmonary hypertension and hypoxemia in obstructive sleep apnea syndrome. Am J Respir Crit Care Med 1994;149(2 Pt 1):416–22.

83. Sajkov D, Wang T, Saunders NA, et al. Continuous positive airway pressure treatment improves pulmonary hemodynamics in patients with obstructive sleep apnea. Am J Respir Crit Care Med 2002; 165(2):152–8.

84. Yumino D, Redolfi S, Ruttanaumpawan P, et al. Nocturnal rostral fluid shift: a unifying concept for the pathogenesis of obstructive and central sleep apnea in men with heart failure. Circulation 2010; 121(14):1598–605.

85. Ulrich S, Keusch S, Hildenbrand FF, et al. Effect of nocturnal oxygen and acetazolamide on exercise performance in patients with pre-capillary pulmonary hypertension and sleep-disturbed breathing: randomized, double-blind, cross-over trial. Eur Heart J 2015;36(10):615–23.

86. Malenfant S, Brassard P, Paquette M, et al. Compromised cerebrovascular regulation and cerebral oxygenation in pulmonary arterial hypertension. J Am Heart Assoc 2017;6(10):e006126.

87. Hofstee HM, Vonk Noordegraaf A, Voskuyl AE, et al. Nailfold capillary density is associated with the presence and severity of pulmonary arterial hypertension in systemic sclerosis. Ann Rheum Dis 2009;68(2): 191–5.

88. Ong YY, Nikoloutsopoulos T, Bond CP, et al. Decreased nailfold capillary density in limited scleroderma with pulmonary hypertension. Asian Pac J Allergy Immunol 1998;16(2–3):81–6.

89. Rhodes CJ, Howard LS, Busbridge M, et al. Iron deficiency and raised hepcidin in idiopathic pulmonary arterial hypertension: clinical prevalence, outcomes, and mechanistic insights. J Am Coll Cardiol 2011;58(3):300–9.

90. Soon E, Treacy CM, Toshner MR, et al. Unexplained iron deficiency in idiopathic and heritable pulmonary arterial hypertension. Thorax 2011;66(4):326–32.

91. Ruiter G, Lankhorst S, Boonstra A, et al. Iron deficiency is common in idiopathic pulmonary arterial hypertension. Eur Respir J 2011;37(6):1386–91.

92. Smith TG, Talbot NP, Privat C, et al. Effects of iron supplementation and depletion on hypoxic pulmonary hypertension: two randomized controlled trials. JAMA 2009;302(13):1444–50.

93. Bart NK, Curtis MK, Cheng HY, et al. Elevation of iron storage in humans attenuates the pulmonary vascular response to hypoxia. J Appl Physiol 1985 2016;121(2):537–44.

94. Lakhal-Littleton S, Crosby A, Frise MC, et al. Intracellular iron deficiency in pulmonary arterial smooth muscle cells induces pulmonary arterial hypertension in mice. Proc Natl Acad Sci U S A 2019; 116(26):13122–30.

95. Ruiter G, Manders E, Happé CM, et al. Intravenous iron therapy in patients with idiopathic pulmonary arterial hypertension and iron deficiency. Pulm Circ 2015;5(3):466–72.

96. Howard LS, Watson GM, Wharton J, et al. Supplementation of iron in pulmonary hypertension: Rationale and design of a phase II clinical trial in idiopathic pulmonary arterial hypertension. Pulm Circ 2013;3(1):100–7.

Adaptation and Maladaptation of the Right Ventricle in Pulmonary Vascular Diseases

Aida Llucià-Valldeperas, PhD, Frances S. de Man, PhD,
Harm J. Bogaard, MD, PhD*

KEYWORDS

- Right ventricle • Right heart failure • Pulmonary vascular diseases • Adaptive remodeling
- Maladaptive remodeling • Right ventricular hypertrophy • Right ventricular dilation

KEY POINTS

- Right ventricle adaptive remodeling to increased afterload is characterized by preserved right ventricle function due to increased contractility and right ventricular hypertrophy.
- Right ventricle maladaptive remodeling to chronic increased afterload is defined by decreased right ventricle function because of an enlarged right ventricle.
- Right heart failure is the result of ventriculoarterial uncoupling.

INTRODUCTION

Pulmonary vascular diseases (PVDs) have significant morbidity and mortality. Patients present with either acute or chronic symptoms resulting from damage to the pulmonary vasculature (eg, hypoxia, hemoptysis) or from the development of right heart failure (eg, exercise intolerance, fluid retention, syncope).[1,2] PVDs embrace a wide and diverse group of underlying pathologies, but this article focuses on right ventricular (RV) adaptation in pulmonary hypertension (PH).

Pulmonary arterial hypertension (PAH) is a vasculopathy that exhibits abnormalities mostly in small pulmonary arteries and arterioles. Excessive pulmonary vascular remodeling and arterial obstruction lead to elevated pulmonary vascular resistance and mean pulmonary artery pressure (mPAP), and consequently increase the RV afterload. Thin walled and crescentic in shape, the RV is highly sensitive to changes in pressure.[3] In PAH, the RV has to adapt to an up to fivefold increase in afterload. Right heart failure (RHF) develops when the RV is unable to cope with the increased demand.[4] As described by the International Right Heart Failure Foundation Scientific Working Group, RHF is *a clinical syndrome due to an alteration of structure and/or function of the right heart circulatory system that leads to suboptimal delivery of blood flow (high or low) to the pulmonary circulation and/or elevated venous pressures—at rest or with exercise.*[5]

In this article, we investigate the changes that the RV undergoes to adapt to the increased afterload and progress to RHF. These changes are comprised in RV (mal)adaptation, and may also be referred as RV remodeling. Thus, cardiac remodeling is an imprecise term that encompasses hypertrophy, fibrosis, and a shape change of the cardiac chambers, depending on the subject. The mechanisms behind cardiac remodeling have been explored extensively in the left ventricle (LV), but not in the RV. There is a thin line between the adaptive and maladaptive phenotypes, as they

Department of Pulmonary Medicine, Amsterdam UMC (Location VUMC), De Boelelaan 1117, Amsterdam 1081 HV, The Netherlands
* Corresponding author.
E-mail address: hj.bogaard@amsterdamumc.nl

Clin Chest Med 42 (2021) 179–194
https://doi.org/10.1016/j.ccm.2020.11.010
0272-5231/21/© 2020 The Authors. Published by Elsevier Inc. This is an open access article under the CC BY license (http://creativecommons.org/licenses/by/4.0/).

are not 2 different responses, but rather a sequence of states of cardiac adaptability.[6] Unfortunately, the mechanisms behind the transition toward RHF remain poorly understood. This article summarizes the current knowledge of both adaptive and maladaptive RV phenotypes linked to PVD, more especially associated to PAH.

THE RIGHT VENTRICLE

To better understand the plasticity of the RV under pathologic conditions, a brief review of its physiologic anatomy and function is necessary.

Right Ventricular Development and Anatomy

The heart is the first organ to develop in the human embryo and starts beating at approximately day 21. All subsequent events depend on the heart's ability to match its output with the demands of oxygen and nutrients; thus, differences among ventricles depend on both the embryologic origin and the hemodynamic environment from the very beginning, even though hemodynamic differences are not present until birth.[7]

The heart is assembled in modules, for instance the LV originates first from the heart tube, whereas the RV arises next from the extracardiac mesoderm within the second heart field.[8] Moreover, each compartment is governed by unique genetic programs; thus, the LV and the RV develop independently. Indeed, several genes have been identified in the development of the RV: *ISL1, HAND2, GATA4, NKX2.5, MEF2C, BOP,* and *FGF10*.[9–15] Some of the previously mentioned genes are present in both ventricles; however, few are chamber-restricted, as HAND1 and HAND2 are limited to the LV and RV, respectively.[10] Nonetheless, adult human cardiomyocytes from both ventricles show a great overlap in gene and protein expression.

After birth, the foramen ovale closes and the RV free wall thins in response to the low resistance and low pressure of the pulmonary circulation; thus, under physiologic conditions, the interventricular septum is concave toward the LV. Hence, both ventricles are morphologically and functionally different. The RV is the most anterior cardiac chamber, has a nonspherical crescentic shape, larger volume, smaller mass and fewer cardiomyocytes, higher collagen content, multiple papillary muscles, and uniformly coarse trabeculations, compared with the ellipsoid and stronger LV.[16] In addition, in the myocardial layer of the RV, it is possible to distinguish 2 myofiber orientations:

1. On the epicardial surface mainly circumferential aggregated myofibers are observed, which are

components of myofiber tracts that are shared with the LV.
2. A subendocardial layer with predominantly longitudinal aggregates.

In contrast to the LV, the third mid-layer containing circumferential fibers is absent in physiologic conditions in the RV.[17,18] However, congenital and acquired modifications have been described in which the mid-layer was also observed in the RV.

Right Ventricular Function

The function of the RV depends on multiple factors: the preload, the contractility of the RV free wall and interventricular septum, the afterload, and the pericardial compliance.[19]

The RV contracts in a peristalticlike pattern starting from the inlet portion and finishing at the infundibulum in 3 steps:

1. Longitudinal shortening with traction of the tricuspid annulus toward the apex
2. Inward radial motion of the RV free wall (also known as "bellows effect")
3. Anteroposterior shortening of the chamber by stretching the free wall over the septum during LV contraction.[18]

In PAH, for example, longitudinal function is relatively preserved, while radial and anteroposterior shortening are decreased (**Fig. 1**).[18] Thus, RV radial motion can be used as a prognostic value in PH patients.[20]

The RV and LV are anatomically interconnected through the septum, the epicardium, and the pericardium. Ventricular interdependence occurs when forces are transmitted between ventricles via common myofibers, perivalvular fibrous annulus, and pericardium; and it is independent of neural, humoral, or circulatory systems. In the healthy situation, the influence of the RV on LV function is insignificant. However, during sustained pressure overload, such as observed in PH, there is a significant influence of RV function on the LV through 3 interrelated events:

1. Leftward septal bowing caused by a prolonged RV free wall peak contraction compared with the septum or LV free wall[16] hampering early diastolic LV filling
2. Decreasing LV filling due to low RV stroke volume (SV)[21,22]
3. Diastolic ventricular interaction because both ventricles compete for space within the nondistensible pericardial sac[23]

Due to the underfilling of the LV, atrophy and reduced contractile function of the LV

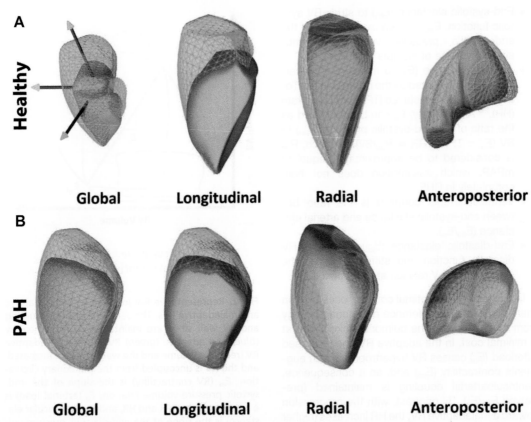

Fig. 1. Global function and decomposed motions of the RV in a healthy subject (*A*) and in a representative patient with PAH (*B*). The green mesh represents end-diastolic RV volume, and the blue surface is the end-systolic RV volume with all motion directions enabled. By decomposing the mechanical pattern of the 3-dimensional RV model, the different anatomically relevant wall motion components can be quantified individually. Each surface represents the volume loss at end systole generated by only the longitudinal (*orange*), radial (*yellow*), or anteroposterior (*gray*) motions, respectively. In (*A*), the relative contribution of each component is approximately 24%. In (*B*), longitudinal function is 17%, whereas radial and anteroposterior shortening decreased to approximately 7%. (*From* Kovacs et al[18]; with permission under the Creative Commons Attribution 4.0 International License (http://creativecommons.org/licenses/by/4.0/).)

cardiomyocytes has been observed in patients with end-stage RHF.[24]

To assess RV function, noninvasive and invasive techniques can be used. Two-dimensional (2D) echocardiography is the most common, and relatively low-cost technique to evaluate RV mechanics and morphology in suspected PH.[25] However, because of the complex anatomy of the RV, RV function cannot be fully explored with 2D echocardiography. Therefore, cardiac MRI is commonly used to assess global RV function (RV volume, mass, and ejection fraction), monitor RV dilatation, estimate transvalvular flow, and detect RV remodeling (myocardial fibrosis and inflammation) in healthy subjects and patients with PVD. Systolic and diastolic RV function can be measured through RV ejection fraction (RVEF) and right atrial pressure,

respectively. Recently developed techniques, such as feature tracking, enable precise strain analyses to assess regional changes in wall motion and contraction patterns.[26] A major advantage of cardiac MRI is that it can provide information on pulmonary vascular dimensions. However, the technique is expensive, requires technical expertise, and is less widely available than echocardiography. In addition, both imaging modalities are highly load-dependent and become less accurate in a pathologic scenario. Thus, to understand ventriculoarterial coupling of the cardiopulmonary unit under physiologic or pathologic conditions, in a load-independent manner, pressure volume (P-V) loops can be used.[27] The main parameters to study RV systolic and diastolic function, as well as the arterial load by P-V loops are as follows:

- End-systolic elastance (E_{es}) to study RV systolic function. E_{es} is given by the slope of the end-systolic pressure versus the end-systolic volume of multiple P-V loops.
- Arterial elastance (E_a) to measure RV afterload. E_a is calculated as the product of the Total Pulmonary Resistance (TPR) and heart rate (HR),[28] Alternatively, E_a can be calculated as the ratio of RV end-systolic pressure (P_{es}) to SV (E_a = TPR · HR = P_{es}/SV). As such, P_{es} is considered to be approximately equal to mPAP, which assumption does not hold completely in RHF.
- Ventriculoarterial coupling is the ratio between end-systolic elastance and arterial elastance (E_{es}/E_a).
- End-diastolic elastance (E_{ed}) to assess RV diastolic function and stiffness. E_{ed} is the slope of the P-V relation at end-diastole.

In the healthy RV, optimal coupling occurs when there is maximal transference of potential energy from the ventricle to the pulmonary circulation at a minimal cost. In the adaptive RV, the increased afterload (E_a) causes RV hypertrophy, which augments contractility (E_{es}) and, as a consequence, ventriculoarterial coupling is maintained (preserved E_{es}/E_a). By contrast, with the progression toward a maladaptive RV, the HR increases (higher E_a) in an attempt to maintain cardiac output and ventriculoarterial uncoupling occurs (decreased E_{es}/E_a)[27,29] (**Fig. 2**). In addition, RV diastolic stiffness (E_{ed}) is related to worse clinical progression in PAH. In patients surviving more than 5 years, the increase in E_{ed} is explained by hypertrophy. However, in patients with poor survival (<5 years), E_{ed} values are not just higher than in controls due to hypertrophy. In fact, in end-stage PAH, other factors (eg, myofibril stiffness, fibrosis) contribute to the increase in RV diastolic stiffness.[30]

As a summary, the RV is coupled to the low pressure and highly compliant pulmonary circulation, which determines its anatomic features and also the energetically efficient way to pump the blood into the pulmonary arteries. During chronic pressure overload, such as in PH, enhancing RV contractility is essential to preserve RV adaptation. Afterward, the gain in ventricular pressures augments the stretch on the RV wall, leading to adaptive hypertrophy. Prolonged increase of RV pressure overload results in RV dilation, maladaptive remodeling, and ventriculoarterial uncoupling.[4] RV dilation may result in tricuspid regurgitation and functional decline. This functional deterioration is characterized by ventricular asynchrony and reduced RV SV, which links to underfilling of the LV.[21]

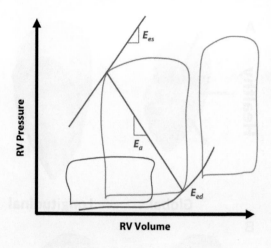

Healthy right ventricle
Adaptive right ventricle
Maladaptive right ventricle

Fig. 2. Representative P-V loops of healthy, adaptive and maladaptive RVs. The ventriculoarterial coupling and RV wall stress are maintained in both healthy (*blue*) and adaptive (*green*) RVs. In the maladaptive RV (*red*), the volume and the wall stress are increased, and the RV is uncoupled from the pulmonary circulation. E_{es} (RV contractility) is the slope of the end-systolic pressure volume relation, E_a (arterial load) is a measure of the TPR and HR, and E_{ed} (ventricular elastance) is the slope of the end-diastolic pressure volume relation.

Several processes have been associated with either adaptive or maladaptive RV phenotypes, such as capillary rarefaction, metabolic shift from oxidative metabolism toward glycolysis, sympathetic hyperactivity, and fibrosis, among others.

In the following sections, we highlight the principal mechanisms involved in RV remodeling to increased pressure overload, from early until late stages of the disease. The progression from initial stages into the uncoupled failing stage is a continuum in which the remodeling events will, eventually, overlap and smoothly transit throughout the stages; it is not a switch on/off process. Notably, the progression from an adaptive to a maladaptive RV with functional loss may take place while the patient is in a stable clinical condition.[31]

EARLY ADAPTIVE MECHANISMS OF THE RIGHT VENTRICLE

RV adaptation to pressure overload is quite variable among patients, and the progression to RHF cannot be predicted currently. Top research priorities are the identification of novel ways to predict and assess RHF, such as new plasma or imaging biomarkers, the generation and optimization of cell/animal models, and the development of innovative therapies. Briefly, the RV adaptive response (homeometric adaptation) is characterized by augmented RV contractility to match the afterload.[32] RV adaptation is illustrated by normal cardiac output, RVEF, and exercise capacity. RV function is maintained through concentric RV hypertrophy (increased mass to volume ratio to reduce wall tension) with minimal dilation and fibrosis. Intracellular mechanisms involved in the RV adaptive phenotype are rarely studied on human samples because of limited availability. Thus, most of the information is obtained from research on the LV and preclinical models such as in vitro cell culture or in vivo animal models. Nevertheless, different mechanisms involved in the adaptive RV remodeling have been proposed, like the regression into a fetal phenotype, increased neurohormonal stimulation, and the hypertrophied RV, all of which are detailed next.

Fetal Phenotype

One of the first mechanisms triggered by pressure overload is a regression toward the fetal phenotype by an upregulation of fetal isogenes and a downregulation of adult isogenes, which remains until end-stage PAH. This fetal regression is described by an altered expression of genes involved in cell metabolism, cardiac contractility, and calcium handling, which may affect the electromechanical conduction system.[7,33]

Cardiac metabolism is determined by energy demand, oxygen delivery, and the availability of substrates. Under physiologic conditions, high glycolytic metabolism occurs in the fetus, whereas oxidative metabolism is predominant in the adult heart.[34] The hypertrophic fetal RV prefers glycolytic metabolism, which maintains ATP production when less oxygen is available.[35] In adult life, hypertrophic cardiomyocytes use a similar transition from oxidative toward glycolytic metabolism. Characteristic of this glycolytic switch is the fact that glucose and not fatty acids become the main substrate for energy production.[36] Increased expression of c-Myc, glycolytic (ie, aldolase, hexokinase, pyruvate kinase, pyruvate dehydrogenase kinase, glucose transporter 1, and glucose-6-phosphate dehydrogenase) and structural (ie, myosin) genes were observed in experimental PH models.[37–40] A shift toward increased glycolysis is observed in the RV of patients with PAH who underwent PET imaging, and the increased glucose uptake correlated with dysfunction and pressure overload.[35,41] Even though the glycolytic adaptation is beneficial in the short-term to

decrease the oxygen demand, it is insufficient to fulfill the demands of the RV and preserve RV function, leading to an energy-starved state and contributing to RHF.[42]

Furthermore, in the RV of subjects with moderate PAH-induced RHF, increased expression of natriuretic peptides and a shift toward the β-myosin heavy chain (β-MHC) isoform is observed. This slower/less active and more efficient β-MHC isoform reduces the ATP demand by cardiomyocytes.[43] The downregulation of α-MHC linked to the upregulation of β-MHC accounts for a reduced shortening velocity and contributes to myocardial dysfunction in PAH.[43] In addition, patients with PAH and patients with chronic thromboembolic PH (CTEPH) present with increased levels of both atrial and brain natriuretic peptides, which are associated with RV hypertrophy and RV dysfunction.[44]

Neurohormonal Activity

The neurohormonal system is involved in cardiovascular homeostasis through the sympathetic nervous system (SNS) and the renin-angiotensin-aldosterone system (RAAS). Pulmonary vascular cells and RV cardiomyocytes express the adrenoceptors β_1 and β_2, evidencing an RV-pulmonary vascular regulation by neurohormonal mechanisms. Patients with PAH present with increased neurohormonal activation. Increased systemic and pulmonary RAAS contributes to pulmonary vascular remodeling.[45] In addition, RV remodeling is regulated by both SNS and RAAS, whereas activation of both systems leads to increased stiffness of the RV and the consequent RV hypertrophy, as well as other molecular changes within the cardiomyocytes.[46,47]

Pressure overload is detected by cardiomyocytes through neurohormonal stimulation and mechanotransduction, which will contribute to RV hypertrophy.[48] Research on the LV showed that circulating and locally produced neurohormones, such as angiotensin II, endothelin-1, and norepinephrine, induce cardiomyocyte hypertrophy through the activation of janus kinase 2 (JAK2) and extracellular signal-regulated kinase, and the subsequent nuclear translocation of NFAT and GATA-4 transcription factors.[49,50] Interestingly, endothelin-1 and its receptor are upregulated in the human hypertrophied RV myocardium in patients with PAH, which might act as an early adaptive mechanism to trigger hypertrophy and maintain RV contractility in the setting of increased RV afterload.[51]

In addition, cardiomyocytes directly sense mechanical stimuli through integrin conformational changes, stretch-activated ion-channels, and sar-comeres[52] (**Fig. 3**). Integrins are transmembrane receptors that connect the extracellular matrix (ECM) to the intracellular cytoskeleton (ie, α-acti-nin and titin) via downstream effectors (ie, focal adhesion kinases) and small GTPases. Titin is a gi-ant sarcomeric protein responsible for the muscle passive stiffness and for keeping myosin mole-cules in place, and so defining the elastic proper-ties of the cardiomyocytes. Actually, mechanical stretch leads to the extension of the unique N2B region in the cardiac titin, thereby revealing new binding places for signaling molecules, such as the Four and a Half LIM domains 2 (FHL2), which modulates titin elasticity and is crucial for cardiac development and hypertrophy signaling.[53]

Right Ventricular Hypertrophy

Pathologic hypertrophy is the consequence of a stressful stimulus on the heart, like an increased he-modynamic load. The hypertrophic growth of the RV in response to hemodynamic stress is a compensa-tory mechanism to reduce both the stress on the RV wall and oxygen consumption, but also to increase the force-generating capacity of the RV up to fivefold to remain coupled to the pulmonary unit.[54]

Adaptive hypertrophy is characterized by an in-crease in cardiomyocyte size through protein synthesis. This results in the addition of sarco-meres in parallel and lateral growth of individual myocytes. Cardiomyocyte hypertrophy occurs in the RV free wall, in muscular bands, and in trabe-culations.[55] Altered myocardial fiber orientation was also described in adaptive hypertrophy. There are different morphologic patterns to describe the hypertrophic phenotype, and the one described in this section matches concentric hypertrophy with increased relative wall thickness and cardiac mass with little or no change in chamber volume.[6]

The hypertrophied RV has increased hypoxia inducible factor-1α (HIF-1α) stabilization, which leads to augmented vascular endothelial growth factor (VEGF) expression and activity as well as enhanced angiogenesis.[56] The hypertrophic response is associated with a proportional in-crease in the number of capillaries to ensure tissue perfusion and preserve RV function. In contrast, incoordinated myofiber growth and vasculariza-tion may lead to RHF. The angiogenic response is regulated by molecular cross-talk between car-diomyocytes and endothelial cells.[57] For example, in the chronic pressure-overload piglet model,

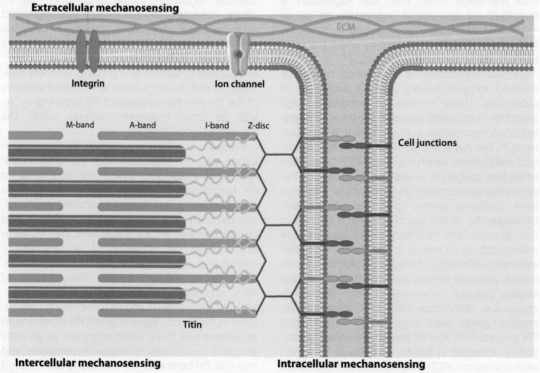

Extracellular mechanosensing

Integrin   Ion channel

M-band   A-band   I-band   Z-disc

ECM

Cell junctions

Titin

Intercellular mechanosensing   **Intracellular mechanosensing**

Fig. 3. Cardiomyocyte mechanosensing mechanisms in PH. Increased pressure overload is sensed by the cardio-myocytes throughout integrin conformational changes, stretch-activated ion-channels, cell junctions, and the sar-comeric titin.

adaptive RV remodeling is associated with an increased capillary density and low degree of fibrosis.[58] Along the same line, in the chronic hypoxia-induced PH murine model, RV angiogenesis is an early adaptive response to ensure a perfect coordination between myocardial capillary growth and cardiomyocyte growth, thereby preserving cardiac function. However, after continued exposure to chronic hypoxia, progressive RV hypertrophy without additional angiogenesis led to the activation of hypoxia-dependent gene expression and RV hypoxia.[59] Insufficient RV angiogenesis is suggested to be a consequence of the VEGF/HIF-1α dysregulation and Akt1 activation, as observed in the Sugen hypoxia model.[60] From the LV of Akt1–transgenic mice, it has been hypothesized that adaptive hypertrophy and appropriate angiogenesis is the result of short-term Akt1 activation; whereas long-term Akt1 activation is linked to maladaptive dilation and capillary rarefaction.[61] A recent study of mice with hypoxia-induced PH demonstrated that Akt signaling is involved in RV remodeling.[62] Therefore, PH experimental models suggest that the maladaptive RV phenotype is the result of a mismatch among RV hypertrophy, metabolism, and angiogenesis that induces myocardial ischemia and subsequent RHF.[60,63]

As Hill and Olson[6] pointed out, the adaptive phenotype observed in patients with PVD is an example of pathologic hypertrophy that, under persistent stress, may lead to heart failure and arrhythmias.

PROLONGED ADAPTATION RESULTS IN THE MALADAPTIVE RIGHT VENTRICLE

The mechanisms behind the transition from RV adaptation to maladaptation and RHF remain elusive. Nevertheless, RHF is characterized by RV dilation, reduced oxygen supply, RV cardiomyocyte growth arrest, RV diastolic stiffness, mitochondrial dysfunction, increased RV inflammation, and pronounced RV fibrosis.

The maladaptive phenotype (heterometric adaptation) appears when the RV experiences irreversible decompensation after a period of immense adaptation. The RV expands to maintain flow output, at the expense of rising filling pressures and systemic congestion.[32] In slowly advancing pressure overload, RV contractility can increase up to fivefold, mitigating RV dilation and the decrease in SV. When RV dilatation becomes inevitable, the septum bows toward the LV, worsening the function of both ventricles. At this time, the RV has progressed into the uncoupled failing stage, characterized by increased tissue stiffness and high metabolic demand.

Interestingly, animal in vivo experimentation supports the idea that chronic pressure overload is responsible for RV hypertrophy, but requires other events, such as myocardial apoptosis, fibrosis, and capillary rarefaction, to promote RV failure.[60]

Right Ventricular Dilation

Sustained and progressive pressure overload during the disease progression will, eventually, limit RV hypertrophy. As an escape mechanism, the RV may dilate to preserve the SV and cardiac output, by means of the Frank-Starling mechanism "increase in SV associated with increased preload." Nevertheless, excessive dilation and overstretching of the RV cardiomyocytes will limit myocardial contractility and ultimately lead to the RV uncoupling from its pulmonary circulation.[27]

RV dilation is associated with (ECM)remodeling and increased collagen turnover.[64] In addition, RV dilation changes the shape of the chamber into a more spherical one, which is associated with functional tricuspid valve regurgitation and elevated right atrial pressure.[65] In fact, significant backward flow into the vena cava during right atrial contraction is associated with RV diastolic stiffness and impaired RV filling in patients with PAH, whereas backward flow due to tricuspid regurgitation was minimal. Consequently, RV SV is reduced because venous return was restricted, and RV volumes may also influence the amount of backflow.[66]

Oxygen Supply-Demand Mismatch

Under physiologic conditions, RV coronary flow is highest in systole; by contrast, LV coronary flow predominantly occurs during diastole. RV perfusion is altered under pathologic conditions, that is, increased in the hypertrophied RV as previously explained, and reduced in maladaptive remodeling. Therefore, progressive blood flow through the coronary system is reduced in advanced PAH, but it is still unclear if it is because of reduced global perfusion due to a lower driving pressure and/or to capillary rarefaction. Regardless, we can appreciate a mismatch at the level of the cardiomyocyte between decreased oxygen supply and increased demand, which could contribute to the development of RHF in PAH.

Reduced coronary flow and capillary rarefaction

The coronary circulation encompasses the blood vessels supplying oxygen and nutrients to the heart muscle. Perfusion abnormalities in the RV were detected in patients with severe PAH with normal coronary angiography.[67,68] Patients with PH with maladaptive RV remodeling have decreased RV systolic coronary flow that is proportional to RV mass and pressure,[68] with reduced myocardial oxygenation.[68,69] An adenosine stress perfusion cardiac MRI study on patients with PAH demonstrated diminished perfusion, which was inversely correlated with RV workload and RVEF.[70] Decreased myocardial perfusion and expression of angiogenic and protective genes and microRNAs may contribute to RV ischemia and RHF, as observed in experimental models of PH.[63,71,72] In addition, higher concentrations of mitochondrial reactive oxygen species (ROS) will, ultimately, suppress angiogenesis, as described in the monocrotaline-induced PAH model.[63]

Capillary rarefaction is characterized by impaired angiogenesis and reduced microvascular density, due to underproliferation of endothelial cells rather than vessel loss, as no apoptosis was observed in RV sections in the Sugen hypoxia rat model.[71] Patients with maladaptive PAH show a decreased capillary density and reduced myoglobin content and activity in the RV.[73] In addition, capillary rarefaction has been described for patients with PAH and linked to RV glutaminolysis.[40] Interestingly, RV capillary density was decreased and morphologically heterogeneous in the Sugen hypoxia rat model, but not significantly altered in the pulmonary artery banding (PAB) model, suggesting that different alterations in the pulmonary vasculature may affect the RV microcirculation.[60]

Mitochondrial dysfunction

The glycolytic shift in the long run induces mitochondrial dysfunction and excessive ROS production, which has been linked to NFAT activation.[74] Both ventricles have similar mitochondrial protein profiles under physiologic conditions; however, under pathologic conditions, the antioxidant response is lower in the RV.[75] In fact, in the monocrotaline rat model, it was shown that antioxidant enzymes were not activated at an early phase, which predisposed the hypertrophied RV to ROS-induced damage (ie, extensive apoptosis) and contributed to RHF.[76] Likewise, in the PAB murine model, earlier downregulation of antioxidant enzymes and increased ROS production was also observed.[42] It has been hypothesized that increased NADPH oxidase and mitochondrial complex II activity leads to enhanced mitochondrial ROS generation.[77]

Interestingly, genes involved in mitochondrial biogenesis and metabolism are altered in the monocrotaline rat model with severe PAH and decompensated RHF, and also in patients with PAH with mutations in the gene encoding for the bone morphogenetic protein receptor type 2 (BMPR2).[78] Excessive ROS production was demonstrated in human PAH-patient derived cells[79] and PH animal models.[75,77,79,80] Indeed, mitochondrial dysfunction is observed in patients with PAH and preliminary results with mitochondria-targeting drugs show hemodynamic improvement in genetically susceptible patients.[81] A recent study with a rat cardiomyocyte cell line carrying common BMPR2 mutations demonstrated reduced mitochondrial respiration with increased mitochondrial superoxide production.[82] Decompensated PAH rats presented with elevated mitochondria-derived ROS levels, reduced HIF-1α and VEGF expression, and capillary rarefaction due to ROS-mediated activation of the pro-oncogenic factor p53.[63] Although little is known about the role of oxidative stress in RV remodeling, in PAH experimental models, oxidative stress has been associated with increased RV apoptosis, fibrosis, and worse RV function.[60,76,78,80]

Neurohormonal Overactivation

The maladaptive phenotype also has been associated with increased chronic sympathetic activation, decreased parasympathetic activity, RV diastolic stiffness, oxidative and nitrosative stress, changes in the β-adrenergic pathway, and decreased activity of the catalytic subunit of adenylate cyclase.[30,83–88]

Increased sympathetic activity, and the subsequent activation of the RAAS, is considered beneficial at early stages of RHF because it offers inotropic support, peripheral vasoconstriction, and salt and water retention to maintain cardiac output and systemic perfusion pressure. However, chronic sympathetic activation is detrimental because it desensitizes β-adrenergic receptors, reduces the chronotropic response, leads to pathologic RV remodeling, impairs the inotropic reserve of the RV, shifts energy metabolism, enhances cardiomyocyte apoptosis, delays HR recovery, and increases mortality.[83,89]

The maladaptive RV in PAH is characterized by increased expression levels of β_2-adrenergic receptors and downregulation of β_1-adrenergic receptors, both associated with systolic dysfunction.[43,83,90,91] β_1-adrenoreceptor downregulation impairs protein kinase A (PKA) activation and subsequent phosphorylation of important proteins involved in calcium handling and sarcomeric function,[92] as explained in the next section.

Diastolic stiffness

Early in the progression of PAH, the RV increases its contractility as a mechanism of adaptation to the augmented afterload. Nevertheless, in advanced stages of the disease, systolic function cannot satisfy the demand and the RV progressively dilates; and diastolic dysfunction becomes impaired. Increased RV diastolic stiffness in patients with PAH is attributed to interstitial and perivascular fibrosis as well as RV cardiomyocyte stiffening.[84] Hypertrophy, fibrosis and sarcomeric disorganization affect cardiomyocyte contractility and increase ventricular stiffness.[93] Myocardial fibrosis and sarcomeric stiffening were reported in patients with PAH and were directly related to increased passive tension of isolated RV cardiomyocytes at different sarcomere lengths. In fact, cardiomyocyte stiffening was associated with decreased titin phosphorylation in the RV, and not to titin isoform composition.[84] Furthermore, 3 main protein modifications contributed to RV diastolic stiffness in PAH. First, decreased PKA-mediated titin phosphorylation increased RV cardiomyocyte stiffness. Second, reduced cardiac troponin I phosphorylation increased calcium sensitivity. And third, altered expression and phosphorylation of calcium-handling proteins, as Sarco/Endoplasmic Reticulum Ca^{2+}-ATPase 2a and phospholamban impaired calcium clearance during diastole.[92]

Fibrosis

Tissue stiffness is directly related to RV fibrosis and cardiomyocyte performance. A recent review from Andersen and colleagues[94] proposed a dual role for RV fibrosis in PVD: (1) an early adaptive response to prevent cardiomyocyte overstretch and ventricular dilatation for optimal function; and (2) a late maladaptive response that augments myocardial stiffness, disturbs cardiomyocyte excitation-contraction coupling, and perturbs the cardiac contraction coordination. Adaptive fibrosis is a compensatory mechanism to support ventricular shape. Ultimately, fibrosis becomes maladaptive because of excessive collagen accumulation and altered collagen structure and organization, damaging the ECM integrity and contributing to cardiac dysfunction.[95]

Cardiac function depends on the contraction and relaxation of the myocardium, which, at the same time, relies on the collagen content in the ECM. Cardiac fibrosis is the result of mechanical stress on both RV interstitium (fibroblasts) and cardiomyocytes. Interstitial fibrosis is characterized by collagen synthesis and deposition by differentiated myofibroblasts, which leads to an increased collagen I/III ratio and augments myocardial stiffness, which has been described in patients with more severe RHF.[84] Little is known of an association between the ECM and the cardiac systole. During systole, the force is transferred throughout the collagen network; thus, fibrosis disrupts the cardiac electromechanical coupling and, subsequently, the synchronized myocardial contraction. A reduced number of gap junctions has been observed in fibrotic tissue, which alters the coordination of the heart contraction because of both deteriorated intercellular coupling and decreased conduction velocity as observed in the PAB rat model.[96] On the other hand, several reports described the contribution of myocardial fibrosis to diastolic dysfunction.[30,97,98] A stiffer myocardium, caused by fibrosis and cardiomyocyte stiffness, is associated with impaired early diastolic filling.[97]

Unfortunately, histologic assessment of RV interstitial fibrosis and collagen composition has been limited to postmortem histomorphometric analyses. Thus, to reveal the importance of RV fibrosis during the progression toward RHF and the eligibility for lung transplantation, new techniques and biomarkers are needed that are sensitive enough to detect interstitial fibrosis. Currently, interstitial fibrosis is also estimated by delayed gadolinium enhancement and T1 mapping cardiac MRI, with limited resolution.[99]

Accordingly, the reversibility of interstitial fibrosis after decreasing the RV afterload has not been studied, even though it has been proposed, opposite to the irreversible replacement fibrosis following cardiomyocyte loss. The RV is able to decrease RV wall thickness and improve RV function after lung transplantation in patients with PAH, and also in patients with CTEPH undergoing pulmonary arterial endarterectomy or balloon angioplasty.[100–104] Despite an immediate reduction in RV size and pulmonary artery pressures, and a normalization of the septal geometry, the functional improvement remains variable and is associated with prior hemodynamics and the duration of disease before lung transplantation.[105]

In summary, regression into a fetal phenotype, the inefficient metabolism and contractility, the altered neurohormonal stimulation, myocardial fibrosis, and the insufficient tissue vascularization, contribute to the deterioration of the RV. Therefore, accumulative and interrelated cell and molecular changes within the RV that start as beneficial adaptations, lead to impaired cardiac function in the long-term, and the consequent maladaptive RV phenotype, as illustrated in **Fig. 4**.

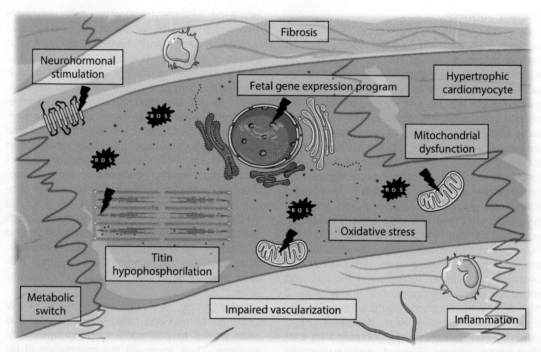

Fig. 4. Pathomechanisms that trigger RV maladaptation. Molecular, cellular, and tissular mechanisms in the cardiomyocyte promote the transition from adaptive to maladaptive RV remodeling in the long run. Image created using Servier Medical Art database under a Creative Commons Attribution 3.0 Unported License.

DISCUSSION

The RHF-specialized research carried out during the past decade evidenced an important role for the RV, and substantial differences between both ventricles regarding their structure, embryologic origin, anatomy, function, and remodeling in response to increased afterload. In the clinical setting, it is easy to observe heterogeneity in the RV response to a given increased afterload, which indicates that some genetic and environmental factors are key and still need to be elucidated. Patients with similar RV afterload can show completely different responses. We speculate in this article that there is a continuum of events of cardiac remodeling. Chronic adaptation processes such as neurohormonal activation, hypertrophy, and reactivation of the fetal gene program will eventually exhaust and result in maladaptation and induce RHF; in some patients, probably at earlier time-points than others.

Another interesting aspect is the role of inflammation in the context of RHF. Except from its contribution to RV fibrosis as previously explained, this subject has been largely ignored. It is well-known that inflammation is involved in pulmonary vascular remodeling.[106] Moreover, patients with PAH have high circulating levels of inflammatory chemokines and cytokines.[107] Whether a high inflammatory milieu contributes to maladaptive RV

remodeling has not been studied. The presence of inflammatory cells and the expression of proinflammatory cytokines and adhesion molecules within the RV have been shown in acute RHF, but not so much in chronic RHF.[108] An original hypothesis to explain the inflammatory role in RV dysfunction is gaining momentum: "a sick pulmonary circulation promotes RV maladaptation." It suggests that proinflammatory mediators released by the altered pulmonary circulation are transported into the coronary circulation and, once there, negatively affect RV function, already challenged by the increased mechanical stress. The harmful influence of the lungs is mediated by immune cells activated within the pulmonary vascular wall, which progressively infiltrate the heart and release chemokines, antibodies, and hormones (ie, angiotensin II and endothelin-1).[108]

Currently, there are no specific therapies to treat RHF, and our knowledge on the mechanisms underlying the adaptive and maladaptive responses of the RV is still under construction. Human tissue is scant and limited to end-stage PAH, and the knowledge on the pathophysiological mechanisms behind PAH and RHF progression are mostly based on studies with animal models. Unfortunately, humans and animals have different physiology and disease progression, and there is no animal model that fully recapitulates the clinical features of PAH. Thus, to move the field forward and to develop RHF-specific therapies, there is a clear need to develop novel strategies to investigate the progression of RV adaptation to RV failure within patients. Advanced imaging techniques and software, interdisciplinary approaches to evaluate multiorgan affectation, as well as development of human cell models are essential.

In conclusion, PVDs result in an excessive increase in RV pressure. To preserve ventriculoarterial coupling, the contractility of the RV increases and RV hypertrophy is induced. Neurohormonal activation and mechanosensing play key roles in this process. In addition, to enhance myocardial efficiency, the fetal gene program is reactivated; however, prolonged activation of these adaptive mechanisms eventually leads to RV diastolic stiffness, ischemia, and mitochondrial dysfunction.

The key questions still under investigation today are as follows: Which mechanisms control RV adaptation in PVD? Can we predict disease progression at early stages? What is the best treatment for both RV and lungs? Unfortunately, research is hampered by limited availability of human samples and the not always successful translation from animal models. Therefore, new strategies and human cell models are fundamental. More information will help to explain disease progression and the succession of RV changes, and will hopefully result in the development of specific treatments to prevent the development of RHF.

CLINICAL CARE POINTS

- Right ventricular function is the major determinant of prognosis in Pulmonary Hypertension.
- Cardiac MRI is the superior method to assess right ventricular adaptation.
- Neurohormonal activation, reduced oxygen delivery and metabolic remodeling are key components of progressive right ventricular dysfunction.
- Given the lack of proven therapies directly improving right ventricular function, symptomatic treatment of right ventricular failure consists of management of preload and afterload.

DISCLOSURE

Research support from private companies (Actelion [Switzerland] and Ferrer [Spain]).

REFERENCES

1. Cummings KW, Bhalla S. Pulmonary vascular diseases. Clin Chest Med 2015;36(2):235–48.

2. Kalva SP. Pulmonary vascular disease: diagnosis and endovascular therapy. Cardiovasc Diagn Ther 2018;8(3):199–200. Available at: https://www.ncbi.nlm.nih.gov/pmc/articles/PMC6039804/.

3. Voelkel NF, Natarajan R, Drake JI, et al. Right ventricle in pulmonary hypertension. Compr Physiol 2011;1(1):525–40.

4. Santos-Ribeiro D, Mendes-Ferreira P, Maia-Rocha C, et al. Pulmonary arterial hypertension: basic knowledge for clinicians. Arch Cardiovasc Dis 2016;109(10):550–61. Available at: https://www.sciencedirect.com/science/article/pii/S1875213616301358?via%3Dihub.

5. Mehra MR, Park MH, Landzberg MJ, et al. Right heart failure: toward a common language. J Heart Lung Transplant 2014;33(2):123–6. Available at: https://www.jhltonline.org/article/S1053-2498(13)01483-6/pdf.

6. Hill JA, Olson EN. Cardiac plasticity. N Engl J Med 2008;358(13):1370–80.

7. Olson EN. A decade of discoveries in cardiac biology. Nat Med 2004;10(5):467–74.

8. Kelly RG, Buckingham ME, Moorman AF. Heart fields and cardiac morphogenesis. Cold Spring Harb Perspect Med 2014;4(10):a015750. Available at: https://www.ncbi.nlm.nih.gov/pmc/articles/PMC4200205/.

9. Bu L, Jiang X, Martin-Puig S, et al. Human ISL1 heart progenitors generate diverse multipotent cardiovascular cell lineages. Nature 2009;460(7251):113–7.

10. Yamagishi H, Yamagishi C, Nakagawa O, et al. The combinatorial activities of Nkx2.5 and dHAND are essential for cardiac ventricle formation. Dev Biol 2001;239(2):190–203. Available at: https://www.sciencedirect.com/science/article/pii/S0012160601904178?via%3Dihub.

11. Zeisberg EM, Ma Q, Juraszek AL, et al. Morphogenesis of the right ventricle requires myocardial expression of Gata4. J Clin Invest 2005;115(6):1522–31. Available at: https://www.ncbi.nlm.nih.gov/pmc/articles/PMC1090473/.

12. Prall OW, Menon MK, Solloway MJ, et al. An Nkx2-5/Bmp2/Smad1 negative feedback loop controls heart progenitor specification and proliferation. Cell 2007;128:947–59. Available at: https://www.cell.com/fulltext/S0092-8674(07)00243-7.

13. Lin Q, Schwarz J, Bucana C, et al. Control of mouse cardiac morphogenesis and myogenesis by transcription factor MEF2C. Science 1997;276(5317):1404–7. Available at: https://www.ncbi.nlm.nih.gov/pmc/articles/PMC4437729/.

14. Phan D, Rasmussen TL, Nakagawa O, et al. BOP, a regulator of right ventricular heart development, is a direct transcriptional target of MEF2C in the developing heart. Development 2005;132(11):2669–78. Available at: https://dev.biologists.org/content/132/11/2669.long.

15. Golzio C, Havis E, Daubas P, et al. ISL1 directly regulates FGF10 transcription during human cardiac outflow formation. PLoS One 2012;7(1): e30677. Available at: https://journals.plos.org/plosone/article?id=10.1371/journal.pone.0030677.

16. Sanz J, Sánchez-Quintana D, Bossone E, et al. Anatomy, function, and dysfunction of the right ventricle: JACC state-of-the-art review. J Am Coll Cardiol 2019;73(12):1463–82.

17. Ozawa K, Funabashi N, Tanabe N, et al. Contribution of myocardial layers of right ventricular free wall to right ventricular function in pulmonary hypertension: analysis using multilayer longitudinal strain by two-dimensional speckle-tracking echocardiography. Int J Cardiol 2016; 215:457–62.

18. Kovács A, Lakatos B, Tokodi M, et al. Right ventricular mechanical pattern in health and disease: beyond longitudinal shortening. Heart Fail Rev 2019;24(4):511–20. Available at: https://link.springer.com/article/10.1007/s10741-019-09778-1.

19. Soliman O, Muslem R, Caliskan K. Right heart failure syndrome. Aging (Albany NY) 2018;11(1): 7–8. Available at: https://www.aging-us.com/full/11/7.

20. Moceri P, Duchateau N, Baudouy D, et al. Three-dimensional right-ventricular regional deformation and survival in pulmonary hypertension. Eur Heart J Cardiovasc Imaging 2018;19(4):450–8. Available at: https://academic.oup.com/ehjcimaging/article/19/4/450/3868545.

21. Gan C, Lankhaar JW, Marcus JT, et al. Impaired left ventricular filling due to right-to-left ventricular interaction in patients with pulmonary arterial hypertension. Am J Physiol Heart Circ Physiol 2006;290: H1528–33. Available at: https://journals.physiology.org/doi/full/10.1152/ajpheart.01031.2005.

22. Marcus JT, Gan CT, Zwanenburg JJ, et al. Interventricular mechanical asynchrony in pulmonary arterial hypertension: left-to-right delay in peak shortening is related to right ventricular overload and left ventricular underfilling. J Am Coll Cardiol 2008;51:750–7. Available at: https://www.sciencedirect.com/science/article/pii/S0735109707037461?via%3Dihub.

23. Lahm T, Douglas IS, Archer SL, et al. Assessment of right ventricular function in the research setting: knowledge gaps and pathways forward. An official American Thoracic Society Research Statement. Am J Respir Crit Care Med 2018;198(4):e15–43. Available at: https://www.atsjournals.org/doi/10.1164/rccm.201806-1160ST.

24. Manders E, Bogaard HJ, Handoko ML, et al. Contractile dysfunction of left ventricular cardiomyocytes in patients with pulmonary arterial hypertension. J Am Coll Cardiol 2014;64(1):28–37.

25. Hur DJ, Sugeng L. Non-invasive multimodality cardiovascular imaging of the right heart and pulmonary circulation in pulmonary hypertension. Front Cardiovasc Med 2019;6:24. Available at: https://www.frontiersin.org/articles/10.3389/fcvm.2019.00024/full#h9.

26. Tao X, Liu M, Liu W, et al. CMR-based heart deformation analysis for quantification of hemodynamics and right ventricular dysfunction in patients with CTEPH. Clin Respir J 2020;14(3):277–84.

27. Vonk Noordegraaf A, Westerhof BE, Westerhof N. The relationship between the right ventricle and its load in pulmonary hypertension. J Am Coll Cardiol 2017;69(2):236–43. Available at: https://www.sciencedirect.com/science/article/pii/S07351097 16369133?via%3Dihub.

28. Sunagawa K, Maughan WL, Sagawa K. Optimal arterial resistance for the maximal stroke work studied in isolated canine left ventricle. Circ Res 1985;56(4):586–95. Available at: https://www.ahajournals.org/doi/10.1161/01.RES.56.4.586.

29. Amsallem M, Mercier O, Kobayashi Y, et al. Forgotten no more: a focused update on the right ventricle in cardiovascular disease. JACC Heart Fail 2018;6(11):891–903. Available at: https://www.sciencedirect.com/science/article/pii/S221317791 830533X?via%3Dihub.

30. Trip P, Rain S, Handoko ML, et al. Clinical relevance of right ventricular diastolic stiffness in pulmonary hypertension. Eur Respir J 2015;45:1603–12. Available at: https://erj.ersjournals.com/content/45/6/1603.long.

31. Van de Veerdonk MC, Bogaard HJ, Voelkel NF. The right ventricle and pulmonary hypertension. Heart Fail Rev 2016;21(3):259–71.

32. Vieillard-Baron A, Naeije R, Haddad F, et al. Diagnostic workup, etiologies and management of acute right ventricle failure : a state-of-the-art paper. Intensive Care Med 2018;44(6): 774–90.

33. Nakao K, Minobe W, Roden R, et al. Myosin heavy chain gene expression in human heart failure. J Clin Invest 1997;100(9):2362–70. Available at: https://www.jci.org/articles/view/119776.

34. Piquereau J, Ventura-Clapier R. Maturation of cardiac energy metabolism during perinatal development. Front Physiol 2018;9:959. Available at: https://www.ncbi.nlm.nih.gov/pmc/articles/PMC6060230/.

35. Ohira H, deKemp R, Pena E, et al. Shifts in myocardial fatty acid and glucose metabolism in pulmonary arterial hypertension: a potential mechanism for a maladaptive right ventricular response. Eur Heart J Cardiovasc Imaging 2016; 17(12):1424–31. Available at: https://academic.oup.com/ehjcimaging/article/17/12/1424/2680062#48627108.

36. Ryan JJ, Archer SL. The right ventricle in pulmonary arterial hypertension: disorders of metabolism, angiogenesis and adrenergic signaling in right ventricular failure. Circ Res 2014;115(1): 176–88. Available at: https://www.ahajournals.org/doi/10.1161/CIRCRESAHA.113.301129.

37. Do E, Baudet S, Verdys M, et al. Energy metabolism in normal and hypertrophied right ventricle of the ferret heart. J Mol Cell Cardiol 1997;29(7): 1903–13.

38. Zhang WH, Qiu MH, Wang XJ, et al. Up-regulation of hexokinase1 in the right ventricle of monocrotaline induced pulmonary hypertension. Respir Res 2014;15(1):119. Available at: https://respiratory-research.biomedcentral.com/articles/10.1186/s12931-014-0119-9.

39. Balestra GM, Mik EG, Eerbeek O, et al. Increased in vivo mitochondrial oxygenation with right ventricular failure induced by pulmonary arterial hypertension: mitochondrial inhibition as driver of cardiac failure? Respir Res 2015;16(1):6. Available at: https://respiratory-research.biomedcentral.com/articles/10.1186/s12931-015-0178-6.

40. Piao L, Fang YH, Parikh K, et al. Cardiac glutaminolysis: a maladaptive cancer metabolism pathway in the right ventricle in pulmonary hypertension. J Mol Med 2013;91(10):1185–97. Available at: https://link.springer.com/article/10.1007/s00109-013-1064-7.

41. Wang L, Li W, Yang Y, et al. Quantitative assessment of right ventricular glucose metabolism in idiopathic pulmonary arterial hypertension patients: a longitudinal study. Eur Heart J Cardiovasc Imaging 2016;17(10):1161–8. Available at: https://academic.oup.com/ehjcimaging/article/17/10/1161/2389097.

42. Reddy S, Bernstein D. Molecular mechanisms of right ventricular failure. Circulation 2015;132(18): 1734–42. Available at: https://www.ahajournals.org/doi/10.1161/CIRCULATIONAHA.114.012975.

43. Lowes BD, Minobe W, Abraham WT, et al. Changes in gene expression in the intact human heart. Downregulation of alpha-myosin heavy chain in hypertrophied, failing ventricular myocardium. J Clin Invest 1997;100:2315–24. Available at: https://www.jci.org/articles/view/119770.

44. Nagaya N, Nishikimi T, Okano Y, et al. Plasma brain natriuretic peptide levels increase in proportion to the extent of right ventricular dysfunction in pulmonary hypertension. J Am Coll Cardiol 1998;31: 202–8.

45. de Man FS, Tu L, Handoko ML, et al. Dysregulated renin-angiotensin-aldosterone system contributes to pulmonary arterial hypertension. Am J Respir Crit Care Med 2012;186(8):780–9.

46. Bogaard HJ, Natarajan R, Mizuno S, et al. Adrenergic receptor blockade reverses right heart remodeling and dysfunction in pulmonary hypertensive rats. Am J Respir Crit Care Med 2010; 182:652–60.

47. Andersen S, Axelsen JB, Ringgaard S, et al. Effects of combined angiotensin II receptor antagonism and neprilysin inhibition in experimental pulmonary hypertension and right ventricular failure. Int J Cardiol 2019;293:203–10.

48. Rain S, Handoko ML, Vonk Noordegraaf A, et al. Pressure-overload-induced right heart failure. Pflugers Arch 2014;466(6):1055–63.

49. Heineke J, Molkentin JD. Regulation of cardiac hypertrophy by intracellular signalling pathways. Nat Rev Mol Cell Biol 2006;7:589–600.

50. Brancaccio M, Fratta L, Notte A, et al. Melusin, a muscle-specific integrin beta1- interacting protein, is required to prevent cardiac failure in response to chronic pressure overload. Nat Med 2003;9:68–75.

51. Nagendran J, Sutendra G, Paterson I, et al. Endothelin axis is upregulated in human and rat right ventricular hypertrophy. Circ Res 2013;112: 347–54. Available at: https://www.ahajournals.org/doi/10.1161/CIRCRESAHA.111.300448.

52. Lyon RC, Zanella F, Omens JH, et al. Mechanotransduction in cardiac hypertrophy and failure. Circ Res 2015;116:1462–76. Available at: https://www.ahajournals.org/doi/10.1161/CIRCRESAHA.116.304937.

53. Radke MH, Peng J, Wu Y, et al. Targeted deletion of titin N2B region leads to diastolic dysfunction and cardiac atrophy. Proc Natl Acad Sci U S A 2007; 104(9):3444–9.

54. de Man FS, Handoko ML, Vonk-Noordegraaf A. The unknown pathophysiological relevance of right ventricular hypertrophy in pulmonary arterial hypertension. Eur Respir J 2019;53(4):1900255. Available at: https://erj.ersjournals.com/content/53/4/1900255.long.

55. Dong Y, Sun J, Yang D, et al. Right ventricular septomarginal trabeculation hypertrophy is associated with disease severity in patients with pulmonary arterial hypertension. Int J Cardiovasc Imaging 2018;34(9):1439–49.

56. Paulin R, Michelakis ED. The metabolic theory of pulmonary arterial hypertension. Circ Res 2014; 115(1):148–64.

57. Oka T, Akazawa H, Naito AT, et al. Angiogenesis and cardiac hypertrophy: maintenance of cardiac function and causative roles in heart failure. Circ Res 2014;114(3):565–71. Available at: https://www.ahajournals.org/doi/10.1161/CIRCRESAHA.114.300507.

58. Noly PE, Haddad F, Arthur-Ataam J, et al. The importance of capillary density-stroke work mismatch for right ventricular adaptation to chronic pressure overload. J Thorac Cardiovasc Surg 2017;154(6):2070–9.

59. Kolb TM, Peabody J, Baddoura P, et al. Right ventricular angiogenesis is an early adaptive response to chronic hypoxia-induced pulmonary hypertension. Microcirculation 2015;22(8):724–36. Available at: https://www.ncbi.nlm.nih.gov/pmc/articles/PMC4715581/.

60. Bogaard HJ, Natarajan R, Henderson SC, et al. Chronic pulmonary artery pressure elevation is insufficient to explain right heart failure. Circulation 2009;120:1951–60. Available at: https://www.ahajournals.org/doi/10.1161/CIRCULATIONAHA.109.883843.

61. Shiojima I, Sato K, Izumiya Y, et al. Disruption of coordinated cardiac hypertrophy and angiogenesis contributes to the transition to heart failure. J Clin Invest 2005;115(8):2108–18. Available at: https://www.ncbi.nlm.nih.gov/pmc/articles/PMC1180541/.

62. Di R, Yang Z, Xu P, et al. Silencing PDK1 limits hypoxia-induced pulmonary arterial hypertension in mice via the Akt/p70S6K signaling pathway. Exp Ther Med 2019;18(1):699–704. Available at: https://www.ncbi.nlm.nih.gov/pmc/articles/PMC6591493/.

63. Sutendra G, Dromparis P, Paulin R, et al. A metabolic remodeling in right ventricular hypertrophy is associated with decreased angiogenesis and a transition from a compensated to a decompensated state in pulmonary hypertension. J Mol Med (Berl) 2013;91:1315–27.

64. Safdar Z, Tamez E, Chan W, et al. Circulating collagen biomarkers as indicators of disease severity in pulmonary arterial hypertension. JACC Heart Fail 2014;2(4):412–21. Available at: https://www.sciencedirect.com/science/article/pii/S2213177914001930?via%3Dihub.

65. Rosenkranz S, Gibbs JS, Wachter R, et al. Left ventricular heart failure and pulmonary hypertension. Eur Heart J 2016;37(12):942–54. Available at: https://academic.oup.com/eurheartj/article/37/12/942/2466016.

66. Marcus JT, Westerhof BE, Groeneveldt JA, et al. Vena cava backflow and right ventricular stiffness in pulmonary arterial hypertension. Eur Respir J 2019;54(4):1900625.

67. Gómez A, Bialostozky D, Zajarias A, et al. Right ventricular ischemia in patients with primary pulmonary hypertension. J Am Coll Cardiol 2001; 38(4):1137–42. Available at: https://www.sciencedirect.com/science/article/pii/S0735109701014966?via%3Dihub.

68. van Wolferen SA, Marcus JT, Westerhof N, et al. Right coronary artery flow impairment in patients with pulmonary hypertension. Eur Heart J 2008; 29(1):120–7. Available at: https://academic.oup.com/eurheartj/article/29/1/120/2398497.

69. Sree Raman K, Stokes M, Walls A, et al. Feasibility of oxygen sensitive cardiac magnetic resonance of the right ventricle in pulmonary artery hypertension. Cardiovasc Diagn Ther 2019; 9(5):502–12.

70. Vogel-Claussen J, Skrok J, Shehata ML, et al. Right and left ventricular myocardial perfusion reserves correlate with right ventricular function and pulmonary hemodynamics in patients with pulmonary arterial hypertension. Radiology 2011;258(1): 119–27. Available at: https://www.ncbi.nlm.nih.gov/pmc/articles/PMC3009386/.

71. Graham BB, Kumar R, Mickael C, et al. Vascular adaptation of the right ventricle in experimental pulmonary hypertension. Am J Respir Cell Mol Biol 2018;59(4):479–89. Available at: https://www.atsjournals.org/doi/10.1165/rcmb.2018-0095OC.

72. Drake JI, Bogaard HJ, Mizuno S, et al. Molecular signature of a right heart failure program in chronic severe pulmonary hypertension. Am J Respir Cell Mol Biol 2011;45:1239–47. Available at: https://www.atsjournals.org/doi/full/10.1165/rcmb.2010-0412OC.

73. Ruiter G, Ying Wong Y, de Man FS, et al. Right ventricular oxygen supply parameters are decreased in human and experimental pulmonary hypertension. J Heart Lung Transplant 2013; 32(2):231–40.

74. Nagendran J, Gurtu V, Fu DZ, et al. A dynamic and chamber-specific mitochondrial remodeling in right ventricular hypertrophy can be therapeutically targeted. J Thorac Cardiovasc Surg 2008;136(1): 168–78.e3. Available at: https://www.jtcvs.org/article/S0022-5223(08)00451-0/fulltext.

75. Gomez-Arroyo J, Mizuno S, Szczepanek K, et al. Metabolic gene remodeling and mitochondrial dysfunction in failing right ventricular hypertrophy secondary to pulmonary arterial hypertension. Circ Heart Fail 2013;6(1):136–44. Available at: https://www.ahajournals.org/doi/10.1161/CIRCHEARTFAILURE.111.966127.

76. Ecarnot-Laubriet A, Rochette L, Vergely C, et al. The activation pattern of the antioxidant enzymes in the right ventricle of rat in response to pressure overload is of heart failure type. Heart Dis 2003; 5(5):308-312.

77. Redout EM, Wagner MJ, Zuidwijk MJ, et al. Right-ventricular failure is associated with increased mitochondrial complex II activity and production of reactive oxygen species. Cardiovasc Res 2007; 75(4):770–81. Available at: https://academic.oup.com/cardiovascres/article/75/4/770/476260#7187441.

78. Potus F, Hindmarch CCT, Dunham-Snary KJ, et al. Transcriptomic signature of right ventricular failure in experimental pulmonary arterial hypertension: deep sequencing demonstrates mitochondrial, fibrotic, inflammatory and angiogenic abnormalities. Int J Mol Sci 2018;19(9):2730. Available at: https://www.mdpi.com/1422-0067/19/9/2730/htm.

79. Bonnet S, Michelakis ED, Porter CJ, et al. An abnormal mitochondrial-hypoxia inducible factor-1alpha-Kv channel pathway disrupts oxygen sensing and triggers pulmonary arterial hypertension in fawn hooded rats: similarities to human pulmonary arterial hypertension. Circulation 2006;113(22):2630–41. Available at: https://www.ahajournals.org/doi/full/10.1161/CIRCULATIONAHA.105.609008.

80. Jernigan NL, Naik JS, Weise-Cross L, et al. Contribution of reactive oxygen species to the pathogenesis of pulmonary arterial hypertension. PLoS One 2017;12:e0180455. Available at: https://journals.plos.org/plosone/article?id=10.1371/journal.pone.0180455.

81. Michelakis ED, Gurtu V, Webster L, et al. Inhibition of pyruvate dehydrogenase kinase improves pulmonary arterial hypertension in genetically susceptible patients. Sci Transl Med 2017;9(413):eaao4583. Available at: https://stm.sciencemag.org/content/9/413/eaao4583.

82. Hemnes AR, Fessel JP, Chen X, et al. BMPR2 dysfunction impairs insulin signaling and glucose homeostasis in cardiomyocytes. Am J Physiol Lung Cell Mol Physiol 2020;318(2):L429–41. Available at: https://journals.physiology.org/doi/full/10.1152/ajplung.00555.2018.

83. Piao L, Fang YH, Parikh KS, et al. GRK2-mediated inhibition of adrenergic and dopaminergic signaling in right ventricular hypertrophy: therapeutic implications in pulmonary hypertension. Circulation 2012;126:2859–69. Available at: https://www.ahajournals.org/doi/10.1161/CIRCULATIONAHA.112.109868.

84. Rain S, Handoko ML, Trip P, et al. Right ventricular diastolic impairment in patients with pulmonary arterial hypertension. Circulation 2013;128:2016–25. Available at: https://www.ahajournals.org/doi/full/10.1161/CIRCULATIONAHA.113.001873.

85. de Man FS, Handoko ML, Guignabert C, et al. Neurohormonal axis in patients with pulmonary arterial hypertension: friend or foe? Am J Respir Crit Care Med 2013;187(1):14–9. Available at: https://www.atsjournals.org/doi/full/10.1164/rccm.201209-1663PP.

86. Velez-Roa S, Ciarka A, Najem B, et al. Increased sympathetic nerve activity in pulmonary artery hypertension. Circulation 2004;110:1308–12. Available at: https://www.ahajournals.org/doi/pdf/10.1161/01.CIR.0000140724.90898.D3.

87. Bristow MR. Why does the myocardium fail? Insights from basic science. Lancet 1998;352(Suppl 1):SI8–14. Available at: https://www.thelancet.com/journals/lancet/article/PIIS0140-6736(98)90311-7/fulltext.

88. da Silva Gonçalves Bós D, Van Der Bruggen CEE, Kurakula K, et al. Contribution of impaired parasympathetic activity to right ventricular dysfunction and pulmonary vascular remodeling in pulmonary arterial hypertension. Circulation 2018;137(9):910–24. Available at: https://www.ahajournals.org/doi/10.1161/CIRCULATIONAHA.117.027451.

89. Kimura K, Ieda M, Kanazawa H, et al. Cardiac sympathetic rejuvenation: a link between nerve function and cardiac hypertrophy. Circ Res 2007;100:1755–64. Available at: https://www.ahajournals.org/doi/full/10.1161/01.res.0000269828.62250.ab.

90. Bristow MR, Ginsburg R, Umans V, et al. Beta 1- and beta 2-adrenergic-receptor subpopulations in nonfailing and failing human ventricular myocardium: coupling of both receptor subtypes to muscle contraction and selective beta 1-receptor down- regulation in heart failure. Circ Res 1986;59:297–309.

91. Bristow MR, Minobe W, Rasmussen R, et al. Beta-adrenergic neuroeffector abnormalities in the failing human heart are produced by local rather than systemic mechanisms. J Clin Invest 1992;89(3):803–15. Available at: https://www.jci.org/articles/view/115659.

92. Rain S, Bos Dda S, Handoko ML, et al. Protein changes contributing to right ventricular cardiomyocyte diastolic dysfunction in pulmonary arterial hypertension. J Am Heart Assoc 2014;3(3):e000716. Available at: https://www.ahajournals.org/doi/full/10.1161/JAHA.113.000716.

93. Hsu S, Kokkonen-Simon KM, Kirk JA, et al. Right ventricular myofilament functional differences in humans with systemic sclerosis-associated versus idiopathic pulmonary arterial hypertension. Circulation 2018;137(22):2360–70. Available at: https://www.ahajournals.org/doi/full/10.1161/CIRCULATIONAHA.117.033147.

94. Andersen S, Nielsen-Kudsk JE, Vonk Noordegraaf A, et al. Right ventricular fibrosis, Circulation 2019;139(2):269–85. Available at: https://www.ahajournals.org/doi/10.1161/CIRCULATIONAHA.118.035326.

95. Polyakova V, Hein S, Kostin S, et al. Matrix metalloproteinases and their tissue inhibitors in pressure-overloaded human myocardium during heart failure progression. J Am Coll Cardiol 2004;44:1609–18. Available at: https://www.sciencedirect.com/science/article/pii/S0735109704015098?via%3Dihub.

96. Kusakari Y, Urashima T, Shimura D, et al. Impairment of excitation contraction coupling in right ventricular hypertrophied muscle with fibrosis induced by pulmonary artery banding. PLoS One 2017;12:e0169564. Available at: https://journals.plos.org/plosone/article?id=10.1371/journal.pone.0169564.

97. Burlew BS, Weber KT. Cardiac fibrosis as a cause of diastolic dysfunction. Herz 2002;27:92–8.

98. Rain S, Andersen S, Najafi A, et al. Right ventricular myocardial stiffness in experimental pulmonary arterial hypertension: relative contribution of fibrosis and myofibril stiffness. Circ Heart Fail 2016; 9:e002636. Available at: https://www.ahajournals.org/doi/10.1161/CIRCHEARTFAILURE.115.002636.

99. Bing R, Dweck MR. Myocardial fibrosis: why image, how to image and clinical implications. Heart 2019;105:1832–40. Available at: https://heart.bmj.com/content/105/23/1832.

100. Kasimir MT, Seebacher G, Jaksch P, et al. Reverse cardiac remodelling in patients with primary pulmonary hypertension after isolated lung transplantation. Eur J Cardiothorac Surg 2004;26:776–81. Available at: https://academic.oup.com/ejcts/article/26/4/776/457495#88649025.

101. Sarashina T, Nakamura K, Akagi S, et al. Reverse right ventricular remodeling after lung transplantation in patients with pulmonary arterial hypertension under combination therapy of targeted medical drugs. Circ J 2017;81:383–90. Available at: https://www.jstage.jst.go.jp/article/circj/81/3/81_CJ-16-0838/_html/-char/en.

102. Gorter TM, Verschuuren EAM, van Veldhuisen DJ, et al. Right ventricular recovery after bilateral lung transplantation for pulmonary arterial hypertension. Interact Cardiovasc Thorac Surg 2017;24:890–7. Available at: https://academic.oup.com/icvts/article/24/6/890/3061410.

103. Berman M, Gopalan D, Sharples L, et al. Right ventricular reverse remodeling after pulmonary endarterectomy: magnetic resonance imaging and clinical and right heart catheterization assessment. Pulm Circ 2014;4:36–44. Available at: https://journals.sagepub.com/doi/full/10.1086/674884.

104. Fukui S, Ogo T, Morita Y, et al. Right ventricular reverse remodelling after balloon pulmonary angioplasty. Eur Respir J 2014;43:1394–402. Available at: https://erj.ersjournals.com/content/43/5/1394.long.

105. Katz WE, Gasior TA, Quinlan JJ, et al. Immediate effects of lung transplantation on right ventricular morphology and function in patients with variable degrees of pulmonary hypertension. J Am Coll Cardiol 1996;27(2):384–91. Available at: https://www.sciencedirect.com/science/article/pii/0735109795005021?via%3Dihub.

106. Tuder RM. Pulmonary vascular remodeling in pulmonary hypertension. Cell Tissue Res 2017;367(3):643–9. Available at: https://www.ncbi.nlm.nih.gov/pmc/articles/PMC5408737/.

107. Humbert M, Monti G, Brenot F, et al. Increased interleukin-1 and interleukin-6 serum concentrations in severe primary pulmonary hypertension. Am J Respir Crit Care Med 1995;151:1628–31.

108. Sun XQ, Abbate A, Bogaard HJ. Role of cardiac inflammation in right ventricular failure. Cardiovasc Res 2017;113(12):1441–52. Available at: https://academic.oup.com/cardiovascres/article/113/12/1441/4082335.

Integrative Omics to Characterize and Classify Pulmonary Vascular Disease

Jane A. Leopold, MD[a],*, Anna R. Hemnes, MD[b]

KEYWORDS

- Genomics • Transcriptomics • Proteomics • Metabolomics • Pulmonary hypertension
- Network analysis • Precision medicine

KEY POINTS

- In patients with pulmonary vascular disease, results from omics studies can be used to understand disease pathobiology, diagnose disease in at-risk patients, select medications and therapeutics, or prognosticate clinical outcomes.
- Most omics studies performed to date in the pulmonary vascular disease field have focused on a single omics platform (ie, genomics, transcriptomics, proteomics, metabolomics) and do not integrate different types of data.
- Newer methodologies to analyze integrated multi-omics big datasets, such as network analysis, have the potential to identify previously unrecognized disease relationships, identify new drug targets, or find targets that can be treated by repurposing approved drugs.

Accumulating evidence supports the utility of omics as a window into disease pathobiology or as an adjunct to aid precision clinical phenotyping.[1] Recent advances in high-throughput biotechnologies and analytical methodologies has enabled widespread utilization of genomics, transcriptomics, proteomics, and metabolomics (collectively referred to as "omics") for deep phenotyping of patients who are at risk for or with established pulmonary vascular disease (**Fig. 1**). Omics analyses are typically performed using blood samples, but the testing platforms may also be used to assay a variety of biospecimens, including disease tissue, urine, and saliva, among others. Results from omics studies collectively have the capacity to provide an all-encompassing view of the molecules important for cellular or tissue structure and function.

The pulmonary vascular disease cohort is particularly amenable to using omics to interrogate disease pathobiology, as pulmonary vascular and right ventricular tissue is not readily available. As symptomatic patients tend to present late in their clinical course, peripheral (or central) circulating omics signatures function as a liquid biopsy of the pulmonary vasculature or right ventricle, and, thereby, can provide a snapshot of a patient's disease status. Furthermore, results from omics studies, when paired with clinical and outcome data, can provide diagnostic as well as prognostic information and identify disease biomarkers.

To date, most defining omics studies in pulmonary vascular disease have been performed in patients with pulmonary arterial hypertension (PAH) and studied a single type of omics. More recently, integrating data across omics platforms has

Funding sources: NHLBI 5U01 HL125215, American Heart Association 19AIML34980000 (J.A. Leopold); NHLBI 5 P01 HL 108800-03, 5 U01 HL 125212-04, 1RO1 HL 142720-01A1 (A.R. Hemnes).

[a] Division of Cardiovascular Medicine, Brigham and Women's Hospital, Harvard Medical School, 77 Avenue Louis Pasteur, NRB0630K, Boston, MA 02115, USA; [b] Division of Allergy, Pulmonary and Critical Care Medicine, Department of Medicine, Vanderbilt University Medical Center, T1218 Medical Center North, 1161 21st Avenue South, Nashville, TN 37232, USA

* Corresponding author.

E-mail address: jleopold@bwh.harvard.edu

Clin Chest Med 42 (2021) 195–205
https://doi.org/10.1016/j.ccm.2020.10.001

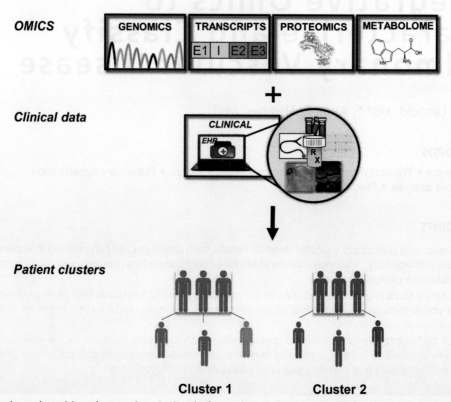

Fig. 1. Omics and precision phenotyping. Omics platforms that analyze genomics, the transcriptome, proteomics, and metabolomics provide information on DNA, RNA, proteins, and metabolites, respectively, at the cellular, tissue, or patient level. When combined with clinical data, omics data allow for precision phenotyping and clustering of patient populations. Even with clustering of like phenotypes, individuals have unique omics signatures and some heterogeneity remains within clusters. E1, exon1; EHR, electronic health record; I, intron; Rx, prescription.

emerged as the next step to inform (endo)phenotyping in pulmonary vascular and other diseases. This, in turn, has created big datasets and a shift to favor analytical methodologies that provide optimal and actionable data outputs. Herein, we discuss omics studies in the context of pulmonary vascular disease and unbiased analytical approaches to illustrate the use of integrated omics datasets to enhance endophenotyping and clinical phenotyping in patients with pulmonary vascular diseases.

GENOMICS AND PULMONARY VASCULAR DISEASE

There was early recognition that PAH was associated occasionally with a strong family history of both PAH and sudden death in young family members, suggesting unrecognized PAH.[2] Concerted international efforts led to the discovery that loss-of-function mutations in the bone morphogenetic protein receptor type 2 (BMPR2) gene, a

member of the transforming growth factor-β (TGFβ) superfamily, underlie approximately 80% of heritable PAH.[3–5] Interestingly, an important feature of this familial form of PAH is incomplete penetrance, such that only ~20% of persons with a BMPR2 mutation ultimately develop the PAH phenotype. Subsequently, it was also recognized that BMPR2 mutations are present in approximately 10% to 15% of patients with idiopathic PAH, perhaps representing de novo mutations in the gene or the first known affected person within a predisposed family.[6] BMPR2 mutations, however, did not account for all heritable PAH, and other early studies identified mutations in the TGFβ signaling pathway such as activin receptorlike kinase (ALK1)[7,8] endoglin (ENG),[9] and SMAD8[10] related to PAH.

Advances in next-generation sequencing have facilitated new discoveries of genetic causes of PAH in more diverse pathways, adding to the concept that there is molecular heterogeneity in the disease. Whole exome and whole genome sequencing have identified mutations in SMAD1, SMAD4, SMAD9, and caveolin 1 (CAV1),[11] as well as several other novel pathways, including the potassium channel Two Pore Domain Channel Subfamily K Member 3 (KCNK3),[12] growth differentiation factor (GDF2),[13] T-box transcription factor 4 (TBX4),[14] ATPase polyamine transporter (ATP13A3),[13] and aquaporin-1 (AQP1).[13] Eukaryotic translation initiation factor-2-α kinase 4 (EIF2AK4) has also recently been associated with pulmonary veno-occlusive disease and pulmonary capillary hemangiomatosis[15,16] (**Fig. 2**). In general, these are rare variants that are inherited in an autosomal recessive fashion. Recent efforts have focused on identification of common genetic variants that confer increased risk for PAH and/or adverse clinical outcomes. These studies identified a locus overlapping the HLA-DPB1 gene[17] and polymorphisms in SOX17[17] and cerebellin (CBLN2)[18] as highly likely candidates.

Despite our understanding of the genetic causes of heritable PAH, in idiopathic PAH, as well as other forms of pulmonary hypertension (PH), most cases are without a clear genetic cause, although these areas continue to be actively investigated. In addition, although the most progress has been made on identifying mutations and rare variants associated with PAH, there is a growing literature on the potential role of epigenetic modifications, such as DNA methylation[19] and chromatin ultrastructural changes[20,21] as mediators of pulmonary vascular disease.

TRANSCRIPTOMICS TO UNDERSTAND PULMONARY VASCULAR DISEASE

With the recognition that gene mutations or modifications may explain only a minority of PH cases, studies have been extended to examine RNA expression patterns and microRNAs in pulmonary vascular disease. A potential challenge to RNA expression studies is, however, the changing nature of RNA patterns. RNA expression, both in blood and tissue, is necessarily dynamic and acutely responsive to exposures and environmental changes. Therefore, findings from analyses of RNA are likely to reflect both the state of pulmonary vascular disease etiology and recent internal and external environmental exposures.

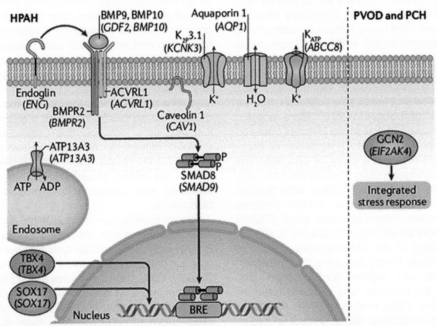

Fig. 2. Genetic causes of PH. Advances in high-throughput sequencing have allowed for new genetic causes of PH to be identified. Beyond bone morphogenetic protein receptor 2 (BMPR2) and related pathway members (endoglin and ACVRL1) and the ligand BMP9, these include mutations in SMAD9, and membrane-related proteins caveolin 1 (CAV1), the potassium channel Two Pore Domain Channel Subfamily K Member 3 (KCNK3), aquaporin-1 (AQP1), and the sulfonylurea receptor 1 protein of the ATP-sensitive potassium channel (ABCC8). Other variants have been identified in the transcription factors T-box transcription factor 4 (TBX4) and SRY-box transcription factor 17 (SOX17), as well as the endosomal ATPase polyamine transporter (ATP13A3). Eukaryotic translation initiation factor-2-α kinase 4 (EIF2AK4) has also recently been associated with pulmonary veno-occlusive disease and pulmonary capillary hemangiomatosis. (*From* Southgate L, Machado RD, Graf S, Morrell NW. Molecular genetic framework underlying pulmonary arterial hypertension. *Nat Rev Cardiol.* 2020;17(2):85-95; with permission.)

Early studies found clear differences in RNA expression patterns between the lungs of patients with PAH compared with controls.[22,23] Similar findings were observed when peripheral blood mononuclear cells were analyzed. The advantage of studying these cells is that they are relatively easy to obtain, offer the convenience of repeated sampling, and potentially reflect the underlying vascular pathology.[24] RNA sequencing has also proven useful to identify novel mechanisms through which endothelial BMPR2 suppression may affect pulmonary vascular disease: when BMPR2 was decreased, there were differences in transcripts related to DNA damage and repair mechanisms, nitric oxide signaling, and growth factor signaling, all of which have been implicated in PAH disease biology.[25] Comparison of lung tissue transcripts from 58 patients with idiopathic PAH and 25 control subjects revealed differential expression of 1140 transcripts. Using gene set enrichment analysis, it was discovered that estrogen receptor 1, interleukin-10 receptor A, tumor necrosis factor-α, and colony-stimulating factor 3 were upstream regulators of the transcripts. Analysis of biological pathways revealed that 16 were significantly "rewired" in PAH as compared with controls, suggesting that in pulmonary vascular disease, there were newly formed or restructured gene interdependencies, which has implications for identifying druggable targets in the disease. Among the interesting findings from these analyses was the identification of negative regulation of WNT-related processes as a potential mediator of sex-based differences in PAH.[26] More recently, RNA sequencing of whole blood samples obtained from patients with idiopathic, heritable, or drug-induced PAH revealed a panel of 25 transcripts that could distinguish patients with PAH from control subjects and was associated with disease severity as well as survival. Further analysis revealed an association between lower SMAD5 levels in whole blood and susceptibility to PAH.[27] This advantage of the aforementioned study is the use of whole blood, indicating that transcriptomics does not require hard-to-obtain biospecimens, for example, lung or heart tissue, to be informative. Other studies of RNAs have also focused on noncoding RNAs, including microRNAs and long noncoding RNAs (reviewed in Ref.[28]), which have been shown to modulate pulmonary vascular disease.

Novel integration of other omics platforms with transcriptomics, such as chromatin and interaction profiling, has also been used to reveal how epigenetic factors affect the pulmonary artery endothelium from patients with PAH. These analyses found that in PAH, there was extensive remodeling of acetylation at H3K27ac, which marks an increase in the activation of transcription, without any evidence of differences in promoters or gene expression. Cell-type–specific gene regulatory network analysis identified transcription factors that were active in PAH compared with controls and regulated 1880 genes in the network. This gene set was enriched for pathways related to endothelial-to-mesenchymal transition and response to growth factors.[29] The value of this integrated omics approach is the additional information revealed by combining data identified a novel endothelial phenotype transition in pulmonary vascular disease, which may have been overlooked had a single omics platform been studied.

PROTEOMIC PROFILING OF PULMONARY VASCULAR DISEASE

Proteomics provides a comprehensive assessment of protein expression, abundance, and post-translational modifications with functional implications. In this manner, proteomics serves as an endophenotypic intermediate between genomics and metabolomics. Over the past 15 years, proteomic studies in pulmonary vascular disease have been performed using varied biospecimens, different disease cohorts and comparator groups, as well as technologies, including mass spectrometry, aptamer-based assay, or antibody-based assays. This has resulted in the identification of many disease-related biomarkers with credible biological relevance, although this heterogeneity has made it difficult to compare between smaller studies, and results from large-scale clinical studies are limited. Nonetheless, proteomics has identified new disease pathways and putative biomarkers.

Results from proteomic studies have implicated inflammation and activation of immune signaling in PH. An early proteomic analysis that used plasma from patients with idiopathic PAH found a fourfold increase in complement 4a des Arg, a component of complement, in patients with PAH compared with healthy controls.[30] The biologic plausibility of complement activation as a biomarker in PH was confirmed recently in preclinical models of PH and the pulmonary vasculature of patients with PAH as well as in patients with congenital heart disease–related PH.[31,32] Another study used unsupervised machine learning to define 4 distinct clusters of immune phenotypes from directed proteomic analysis of chemokines, cytokines, and proinflammatory mediators. These clusters did not segregate by underlying disease etiology, were prognostic, and were associated with 5-year survival rates.[23]

Subsequent proteomic analyses performed using PAH lung tissue explants revealed differences in 25 proteins, including chloride intracellular channel 4, receptor for advanced glycation end products, and periostin. These proteins are related to cell proliferation, migration, and metabolism, all of which are cellular processes that have been linked to PAH.[33] Similar studies performed using blood outgrowth endothelial cells from patients with hereditary PAH identified differences in levels of 22 proteins, including translationally controlled tumor protein, which is related to cell proliferation and apoptosis-resistance in cancer.[34] Global proteomics and posphoproteomics of pulmonary artery endothelial cells isolated from patients with PAH or healthy controls found differential expression of proteins involved in metabolic pathways, nitric oxide generation, and oxidant stress, suggesting mitochondrial dysfunction.[35] Taken together, these studies share common themes that relate pulmonary vascular disease to inflammation and immune-mediated responses, proliferation and apoptosis, and dysregulation of metabolism.

As PH has been associated with exercise intolerance, a proteomic study of skeletal muscle tissue was done to investigate potential etiologies of this phenomenon. This analyses revealed that key proteins related to mitochondrial function and metabolism were downregulated in the skeletal muscle. This finding supported many of the observed abnormalities in the skeletal muscle tissue, including abnormal mitochondrial morphology, decreased oxidative phosphorylation, and increased expression of glycolytic proteins.[36]

Results from proteomic studies have also identified panels of proteins that function as prognostic biomarkers. In one multicenter study, 20 proteins were identified in the plasma proteome of patients with idiopathic or heritable PAH that differentiated survivors from nonsurvivors. A panel of 9 proteins, including proteins related to myocardial stress, vascular remodeling, metabolism, inflammation and immunity, thrombosis, and iron regulation, all mediators of PH that were confirmed in preclinical or clinical studies, was found to be prognostic. Interestingly, this panel was predictive independent of plasma N-terminal pro brain natriuretic protein levels and was shown to improve the prognostic significance of the REVEAL score.[37]

Although most proteomic studies have been performed using biospecimens from patients with PAH, there is emerging evidence from other patient populations at risk for, or with established pulmonary vascular disease. In patients with heart failure with preserved ejection fraction, relevant clinical, laboratory, and echocardiographic data were used to identify 6 distinct clinical phenogroups that differed in all-cause mortality and heart failure hospitalizations at follow-up. Analysis of plasma proteomics found that 15 proteins that included inflammatory and cardiovascular proteins differed between the phenogroups.[38] In a larger study that included 877 individuals in the discovery cohort, proteomics identified 38 proteins that were associated with incident heart failure and replicated in a validation cohort. These proteins collectively identified 4 biologically relevant pathways associated with progression to heart failure: inflammation and apoptosis, extracellular matrix remodeling, blood pressure regulation, and metabolism.[39] Although these studies were not limited to include only patients with left heart failure and pulmonary vascular disease, they identify many of the same pathways implicated in PAH, suggesting commonalities between the underlying diseases and progression to pulmonary vascular disease.

Proteomic studies in chronic thromboembolic pulmonary hypertension (CTEPH) are also limited. To gain insight into pulmonary vascular remodeling in CTEPH, proteomic analysis of endarterectomized samples was compared with a control sample that was a composite of cultured human pulmonary artery endothelial, smooth muscle, and fibroblast cells. The analysis revealed 679 endarterectomy-specific proteins that were related to several key biological processes, including complement and coagulation cascade pathways and extracellular matrix receptor interactions, among others. Although interesting, the control sample was composed of cultured cells and did not include platelets, which make the significance of the findings unclear.[40]

METABOLOMICS AS A SNAPSHOT OF PULMONARY VASCULAR DISEASE AND RIGHT VENTRICULAR DYSFUNCTION

Perturbations in the metabolome has been a central theme in studies of the etiology of PH.[41,42] Modern capacity to study metabolomics more broadly using mass spectrometry, high-performance liquid-phase chromatography, or nuclear magnetic resonance spectroscopy has accelerated recognition of the number of metabolic pathways that are altered in PH. Similar to RNA transcripts, metabolomic profiles are affected by exposures, hormones, fasting, exercise, and circadian rhythms such that the metabolome has the propensity to change rapidly.[43,44]

Studies of endothelial cell metabolomics have identified disruption of several pathways, including an increase in glycolysis, a reduction in glucose oxidation, and a decrease in fatty acid oxidation.[42,45,46] These findings were confirmed in patients with PH who underwent a hyperglycemic clamp. This revealed an impaired insulin response to hyperglycemia in the patients with PH compared with controls with evidence of increased skeletal muscle insulin sensitivity. Metabolomics profiling found elevated ketones and lipid oxidation in PH with fatty acids, acylcarnitines, insulin sensitivity, and ketones correlating with disease severity. Thus, in PH, control of glucose is limited and lipid and ketone metabolism favored.[47] These metabolomic insights are beginning to translate to trials of new therapies for PAH, including dichloroacetate,[48] metformin, and ranolizine.[49,50]

There is also emerging research on metabolomics in other patient populations with or susceptible to pulmonary vascular disease. In patients with heart failure, metabolomics profiling has both diagnostic and prognostic value. Early studies demonstrated that patients with heart failure could be discriminated from healthy controls based on levels of 4 metabolites: histidine, spermidine, phenylalanine, and phosphatidylcholine C34:4.[51] These metabolites, however, were not replicated in another study that identified different metabolites that discriminated heart failure from healthy controls.[52] Other metabolomic studies identified a panel of metabolites, which included increased levels of hydroxyleucine/hydroxyisoleucine and decreased levels of dihydroxy docosatrienoic acid and hydroxyisoleucine as predictors of incident heart failure.[53] Differences in the study design and the populations studied likely contributed to the heterogeneity in the metabolite profiles.

Perhaps one of the most distinct pulmonary vascular disease populations, and, therefore, one that is well suited for metabolomics studies, is CTEPH. Recently, plasma metabolomic profiles comparing CTEPH, idiopathic PAH, and healthy controls found that patients with CTEPH have evidence of aberrant lipid metabolism with increased lipolysis and fatty acid oxidation.[54] In the future, we will likely see metabolomic profiling applied to broader populations of patients with pulmonary vascular disease in which the use of transpulmonary and transcardiac gradients of metabolomics to understand metabolism across these organ systems will have unique value.[55]

Cardiomyocytes are highly metabolically active, and in the normal state prefer fatty acid oxidation to glucose oxidation. In both rodent models and human disease, the failing right ventricle has reduced fatty acid oxidation and enhanced glucose metabolism.[56–60] Although readily demonstrated by PET with 18F-FDG studies,[42] these changes have been demonstrated ex vivo in the right ventricle using metabolomic studies as well.[56,57,61] There have also been studies correlating right ventricle function with less traditionally recognized cardiomyocyte metabolic pathways. For instance, using global metabolomic profiles of pulmonary vascular and right ventricular function at rest and with exercise, indoleamine 2,3-dioxygenase (IDO)-dependent tryptophan metabolites have been shown to correlate well with baseline right ventricular function.[62] Presently, it is unknown how, if at all, to modulate metabolism in the right ventricle to improve outcomes in pulmonary vascular disease.

Perhaps most relevant to clinical care are studies of metabolomic data from plasma to improve clinical predictors of outcomes.[63] For instance, metabolomic profiling identified 20 circulating metabolites that differentiated patients with PAH from both healthy and disease controls as well as 36 metabolites that were confirmed as independent prognostic markers, including transfer RNA-specific modified nucleosides, TCA cycle intermediates, and fatty acid acylcarnitines. Importantly, several of the metabolites tracked with disease severity over time such that correction of metabolite levels correlated with improved clinical outcomes.[63] These data show the potential role of metabolomics in clinical care and assessing risk, as well as response to therapy. Like studies of the plasma transcriptome, the plasma metabolome likely changes in the short and long term, which makes it more suited as an indicator of response to therapy than, for instance, DNA variants that are unchanged over time. Although not ready for clinical use presently, we anticipate that future clinical trials will likely incorporate studies of metabolomics to define treatment responses, particularly in the context of metabolic interventions.

MULTI-OMICS PHENOTYPING, BIG DATA, AND NOVEL METHODOLOGIES FOR INTEGRATING DATA

As multi-omics phenotyping gains traction, consideration of how to approach and analyze these big datasets is warranted. As many prevalent diseases are multifactorial and represent a composite of endophenotypes, it is more likely that results from a multi-omics approach will have broadly applicable prognostic or therapeutic implications in pulmonary vascular disease and PH. Consideration of using a multi-omics study design is especially important when lifestyle or environmental exposures may modify the phenotype, as occurs in in pulmonary vascular disease. For this reason, multi-omics profiling will be pursued to understand all forms of pulmonary vascular disease, as outlined in the omics plan for the National Heart, Lung, and Blood Institute Pulmonary Vascular Disease Phenomics Study (PVDOMICS) study.[64] Other challenges associated with multi-omics phenotyping include defining a relevant sample size, heterogeneity of the disease and control populations studied, significant heterogeneity in the methodologies used to measure and analyze omics that may limit cross-study applicability, and the necessity for a validation cohort or biological confirmation in preclinical models.[65]

Analytical methods for big datasets generated by multi-omics first require data integration at a high level. There are 2 approaches that are often undertaken to analyze the combined outputs from genomics, transcriptomics, proteomic, and metabolomic datasets **Fig 3**. The first method is postanalysis data integration. Here, each of the omics datasets is analyzed individually to generate results and integration of the varied datasets is performed after the initial analysis. This methodology allows for selection of data from each of the platforms that is deemed relevant to pulmonary

vascular disease, which is then integrated or networked together for further analysis. In contrast, the second method uses computational tools to integrate all the omics data into a single big dataset and, once integrated, analysis performed on the entire dataset. This approach has the added advantage of reducing bias.[66]

Analyzing omics big datasets has necessitated the introduction of newer methodologies, such as machine learning and systems or network analysis. Machine learning is a form of artificial intelligence and can be supervised or unsupervised. When machine learning is supervised, the computer algorithm is provided with a training dataset that includes the omics data and how it is linked to an outcome of interest, such as clinical worsening in patients with pulmonary vascular disease or mortality. This allows for the development of a rule that links omics with outcomes and can be used to predict outcomes when a new omics dataset is introduced. In unsupervised machine learning, none of this information is provided, forcing the algorithm to test all possibilities that link the input (omics data) to the output (clinical outcomes).[67] This methodology allows for prediction, prognostication, and clustering to reveal new pulmonary vascular disease phenotypes.

Network analysis is a second newer analytical method that allows for unbiased discovery of

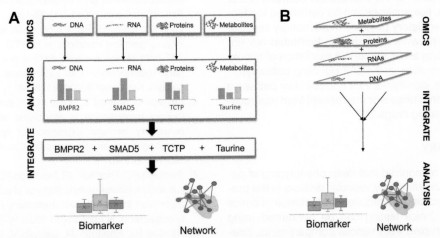

Fig. 3. Approach to integrated data analysis. Multi-omics testing generates big datasets that can be analyzed separately or integrated to create a novel mega dataset. There are 2 approaches that have been used to integrate multi-omics data. (*A*) Initially, results from the omics platforms are analyzed separately. Once the data are available, relevant data from each of the omics platforms can be selected and combined into a new larger dataset for new analyses. In this example, data from each of the omics platforms identifies significant molecules (BMPR2, SMAD5, TCTP, and Taurine). These and other data are then selected and integrated into the new dataset. Analysis may then reveal a new biomarker that was not previously identified in any of the individual omics studies or can be used to generate a network that identifies factors that group together and form a module (red nodes). (*B*) A second method involves integration of the multi-omics data before any analysis. Once combined, the mega dataset is analyzed for discovery of new relevant disease biomarkers as well as diagnostic or prognostic factors.

previously unknown relationships among genes, proteins, and metabolites in an integrated omics dataset. Network analysis maps the components of the integrated omics studies based on known interactions. This creates the network structure in which each component is referred to as a node, connections between nodes are referred to as edges, and highly connected nodes are referred to as hubs. In networks, interactions between nodes are unlikely to occur by chance, suggesting that functional relationships exist among nodes.[68,69] Those genes, proteins, or metabolites that are essential tend to encode hubs that reside at the network's center, whereas disease-related genes, proteins, or metabolites frequently reside at the network's periphery.[68–70] The network architecture may also explain or predict a phenotype. For instance, perturbation of a single node is likely to have many repercussions throughout a network and affect other connected nodes.[68,71] Groups of nodes in the same neighborhood within the network tend to assemble into modules that are identified using unbiased clustering algorithms.[68,70] These modules may contain a group of nodes that share a similar function, or contain disease-related genes. Nodes also can overlap with other modules and reveal novel relationships between disease and nondisease factors that would be important to understand, particularly in the context of druggable targets and potential side effects.[68,69] In some cases, in which the "directionality" of the interactions between nodes is known, flux analyses can be performed to identify key regulatory points.[72] In pulmonary vascular disease, network analysis has facilitated our understanding about microRNA regulation of hypoxia, inflammation, and TGFβ signaling pathways,[73] as well as identify relevant nodes in key pathways that are drug targets or may benefit from repurposing of existing drugs.[65,67]

SUMMARY

It is now recognized that deep phenotyping of patients with pulmonary vascular disease in the precision medicine era requires the inclusion of omics studies. Omics testing can be performed using blood sampled from various compartments, relevant disease tissue if available, or other biospecimens. Omics has the potential to provide a comprehensive assessment of the genes, transcripts, proteins, and metabolites that govern the structure, function, and metabolism of pulmonary vascular cells at timepoints ranging from before disease inception to advanced states of disease. Omics have been used to identify putative biomarkers and have clinical relevance for diagnostic

and prognostic capabilities in PH. More recently, it was realized that it is feasible to integrate multi-omics data across data types and platforms to provide even more granular information about the pulmonary vascular disease phenotype and more robust results. When coupled with clinical data, integrated multi-omics data are the future of precision phenotyping in pulmonary vascular disease.

DISCLOSURE

J.A. Leopold has no disclosures relevant to this publication; A.R. Hemnes has no disclosures relevant to this publication.

REFERENCES

1. Leopold JA, Loscalzo J. Emerging role of precision medicine in cardiovascular disease. Circ Res 2018;122(9):1302–15.
2. Loyd JE, Butler MG, Foroud TM, et al. Genetic anticipation and abnormal gender ratio at birth in familial primary pulmonary hypertension. Am J Respir Crit Care Med 1995;152(1):93–7.
3. Nichols WC, Koller DL, Slovis B, et al. Localization of the gene for familial primary pulmonary hypertension to chromosome 2q31-32. Nat Genet 1997; 15(3):277–80.
4. Machado RD, Pauciulo MW, Thomson JR, et al. BMPR2 haploinsufficiency as the inherited molecular mechanism for primary pulmonary hypertension. Am J Hum Genet 2001;68(1):92–102.
5. Lane KB, Machado RD, Pauciulo MW, et al. Heterozygous germline mutations in BMPR2, encoding a TGF-beta receptor, cause familial primary pulmonary hypertension. The International PPH Consortium. Nat Genet 2000;26(1):81–4.
6. Atkinson C, Stewart S, Upton PD, et al. Primary pulmonary hypertension is associated with reduced pulmonary vascular expression of type II bone morphogenetic protein receptor. Circulation 2002; 105(14):1672–8.
7. Trembath RC, Thomson JR, Machado RD, et al. Clinical and molecular genetic features of pulmonary hypertension in patients with hereditary hemorrhagic telangiectasia. N Engl J Med 2001;345(5):325–34.
8. Harrison RE, Flanagan JA, Sankelo M, et al. Molecular and functional analysis identifies ALK-1 as the predominant cause of pulmonary hypertension related to hereditary haemorrhagic telangiectasia. J Med Genet 2003;40(12):865–71.
9. Chaouat A, Coulet F, Favre C, et al. Endoglin germline mutation in a patient with hereditary haemorrhagic telangiectasia and dexfenfluramine associated pulmonary arterial hypertension. Thorax 2004;59(5):446–8.

10. Shintani M, Yagi H, Nakayama T, et al. A new nonsense mutation of SMAD8 associated with pulmonary arterial hypertension. J Med Genet 2009; 46(5):331–7.

11. Austin ED, Ma L, LeDuc C, et al. Whole exome sequencing to identify a novel gene (caveolin-1) associated with human pulmonary arterial hypertension. Circ Cardiovasc Genet 2012;5(3): 336–43.

12. Ma L, Roman-Campos D, Austin ED, et al. A novel channelopathy in pulmonary arterial hypertension. N Engl J Med 2013;369(4):351–61.

13. Graf S, Haimel M, Bleda M, et al. Identification of rare sequence variation underlying heritable pulmonary arterial hypertension. Nat Commun 2018;9(1): 1416.

14. Zhu N, Gonzaga-Jauregui C, Welch CL, et al. Exome sequencing in children with pulmonary arterial hypertension demonstrates differences compared with adults. Circ Genom Precis Med 2018;11(4): e001887.

15. Eyries M, Montani D, Girerd B, et al. EIF2AK4 mutations cause pulmonary veno-occlusive disease, a recessive form of pulmonary hypertension. Nat Genet 2014;46(1):65–9.

16. Best DH, Sumner KL, Austin ED, et al. EIF2AK4 mutations in pulmonary capillary hemangiomatosis. Chest 2014;145(2):231–6.

17. Rhodes CJ, Batai K, Bleda M, et al. Genetic determinants of risk in pulmonary arterial hypertension: international genome-wide association studies and meta-analysis. Lancet Respir Med 2019;7(3): 227–38.

18. Germain M, Eyries M, Montani D, et al. Genome-wide association analysis identifies a susceptibility locus for pulmonary arterial hypertension. Nat Genet 2013;45(5):518–21.

19. Archer SL, Marsboom G, Kim GH, et al. Epigenetic attenuation of mitochondrial superoxide dismutase 2 in pulmonary arterial hypertension: a basis for excessive cell proliferation and a new therapeutic target. Circulation 2010;121(24):2661–71.

20. Kim GH, Ryan JJ, Marsboom G, et al. Epigenetic mechanisms of pulmonary hypertension. Pulm Circ 2011;1(3):347–56.

21. Meloche J, Potus F, Vaillancourt M, et al. Bromodomain-containing protein 4: the epigenetic origin of pulmonary arterial hypertension. Circ Res 2015; 117(6):525–35.

22. Geraci MW, Moore M, Gesell T, et al. Gene expression patterns in the lungs of patients with primary pulmonary hypertension: a gene microarray analysis. Circ Res 2001;88(6):555–62.

23. Sweatt AJ, Hedlin HK, Balasubramanian V, et al. Discovery of distinct immune phenotypes using machine learning in pulmonary arterial hypertension. Circ Res 2019;124(6):904–19.

24. Bull TM, Coldren CD, Moore M, et al. Gene microarray analysis of peripheral blood cells in pulmonary arterial hypertension. Am J Respir Crit Care Med 2004;170(8):911–9.

25. Rhodes CJ, Im H, Cao A, et al. RNA sequencing analysis detection of a novel pathway of endothelial dysfunction in pulmonary arterial hypertension. Am J Respir Crit Care Med 2015;192(3):356–66.

26. Stearman RS, Bui QM, Speyer G, et al. Systems analysis of the human pulmonary arterial hypertension lung transcriptome. Am J Respir Cell Mol Biol 2019;60(6):637–49.

27. Rhodes CJ, Otero-Nunez P, Wharton J, et al. Whole blood RNA profiles associated with pulmonary arterial hypertension and clinical outcome. Am J Respir Crit Care Med 2020;202(4):586–94.

28. Negi V, Chan SY. Discerning functional hierarchies of microRNAs in pulmonary hypertension. JCI Insight 2017;2(5):e91327.

29. Reyes-Palomares A, Gu M, Grubert F, et al. Remodeling of active endothelial enhancers is associated with aberrant gene-regulatory networks in pulmonary arterial hypertension. Nat Commun 2020; 11(1):1673.

30. Abdul-Salam VB, Paul GA, Ali JO, et al. Identification of plasma protein biomarkers associated with idiopathic pulmonary arterial hypertension. Proteomics 2006;6(7):2286–94.

31. Frid MG, McKeon BA, Thurman JM, et al. Immunoglobulin-driven complement activation regulates proinflammatory remodeling in pulmonary hypertension. Am J Respir Crit Care Med 2020;201(2): 224–39.

32. Zhang X, Hou HT, Wang J, et al. Plasma proteomic study in pulmonary arterial hypertension associated with congenital heart diseases. Sci Rep 2016;6: 36541.

33. Abdul-Salam VB, Wharton J, Cupitt J, et al. Proteomic analysis of lung tissues from patients with pulmonary arterial hypertension. Circulation 2010; 122(20):2058–67.

34. Lavoie JR, Ormiston ML, Perez-Iratxeta C, et al. Proteomic analysis implicates translationally controlled tumor protein as a novel mediator of occlusive vascular remodeling in pulmonary arterial hypertension. Circulation 2014;129(21):2125–35.

35. Xu W, Comhair SAA, Chen R, et al. Integrative proteomics and phosphoproteomics in pulmonary arterial hypertension. Sci Rep 2019;9(1):18623.

36. Malenfant S, Potus F, Fournier F, et al. Skeletal muscle proteomic signature and metabolic impairment in pulmonary hypertension. J Mol Med (Berl) 2015; 93(5):573–84.

37. Rhodes CJ, Wharton J, Ghataorhe P, et al. Plasma proteome analysis in patients with pulmonary arterial hypertension: an observational cohort study. Lancet Respir Med 2017;5(9):717–26.

38. Hedman AK, Hage C, Sharma A, et al. Identification of novel pheno-groups in heart failure with preserved ejection fraction using machine learning. Heart 2020;106(5):342–9.

39. Ferreira JP, Verdonschot J, Collier T, et al. Proteomic bioprofiles and mechanistic pathways of progression to heart failure. Circ Heart Fail 2019;12(5): e005897.

40. Xi Q, Liu Z, Song Y, et al. Proteomic analyses of endarterectomized tissues from patients with chronic thromboembolic pulmonary hypertension. Cardiology 2020;145(1):48–52.

41. Oikawa M, Kagaya Y, Otani H, et al. Increased [18F] fluorodeoxyglucose accumulation in right ventricular free wall in patients with pulmonary hypertension and the effect of epoprostenol. J Am Coll Cardiol 2005;45(11):1849–55.

42. Xu W, Koeck T, Lara AR, et al. Alterations of cellular bioenergetics in pulmonary artery endothelial cells. Proc Natl Acad Sci U S A 2007;104(4):1342–7.

43. Suhre K, Gieger C. Genetic variation in metabolic phenotypes: study designs and applications. Nat Rev Genet 2012;13(11):759–69.

44. Sanders JL, Han Y, Urbina MF, et al. Metabolomics of exercise pulmonary hypertension are intermediate between controls and patients with pulmonary arterial hypertension. Pulm Circ 2019;9(4). 2045894019882623.

45. Fessel JP, Hamid R, Wittmann BM, et al. Metabolomic analysis of bone morphogenetic protein receptor type 2 mutations in human pulmonary endothelium reveals widespread metabolic reprogramming. Pulm Circ 2012;2(2):201–13.

46. Archer SL, Fang YH, Ryan JJ, et al. Metabolism and bioenergetics in the right ventricle and pulmonary vasculature in pulmonary hypertension. Pulm Circ 2013;3(1):144–52.

47. Mey JT, Hari A, Axelrod CL, et al. Lipids and ketones dominate metabolism at the expense of glucose control in pulmonary arterial hypertension: a hyperglycaemic clamp and metabolomics study. Eur Respir J 2020;55(4):1901700.

48. Michelakis ED, Gurtu V, Webster L, et al. Inhibition of pyruvate dehydrogenase kinase improves pulmonary arterial hypertension in genetically susceptible patients. Sci Transl Med 2017;9(413):eaao4583.

49. Khan SS, Cuttica MJ, Beussink-Nelson L, et al. Effects of ranolazine on exercise capacity, right ventricular indices, and hemodynamic characteristics in pulmonary arterial hypertension: a pilot study. Pulm Circ 2015;5(3):547–56.

50. Gomberg-Maitland M, Schilz R, Mediratta A, et al. Phase I safety study of ranolazine in pulmonary arterial hypertension. Pulm Circ 2015;5(4):691–700.

51. Cheng ML, Wang CH, Shiao MS, et al. Metabolic disturbances identified in plasma are associated with outcomes in patients with heart failure: diagnostic and prognostic value of metabolomics. J Am Coll Cardiol 2015;65(15):1509–20.

52. Zordoky BN, Sung MM, Ezekowitz J, et al. Metabolomic fingerprint of heart failure with preserved ejection fraction. PLoS One 2015;10(5):e0124844.

53. Zheng Y, Yu B, Alexander D, et al. Associations between metabolomic compounds and incident heart failure among African Americans: the ARIC Study. Am J Epidemiol 2013;178(4):534–42.

54. Heresi GA, Mey JT, Bartholomew JR, et al. Plasma metabolomic profile in chronic thromboembolic pulmonary hypertension. Pulm Circ 2020;10(1). 2045894019890553.

55. Chouvarine P, Giera M, Kastenmuller G, et al. Transright ventricle and transpulmonary metabolite gradients in human pulmonary arterial hypertension. Heart 2020;106(17):1332–41.

56. Talati MH, Brittain EL, Fessel JP, et al. Mechanisms of lipid accumulation in the bone morphogenic protein receptor 2 mutant right ventricle. Am J Respir Crit Care Med 2016;194(6):719–28.

57. Hemnes AR, Brittain EL, Trammell AW, et al. Evidence for right ventricular lipotoxicity in heritable pulmonary arterial hypertension. Am J Respir Crit Care Med 2014;189(3):325–34.

58. Graham BB, Kumar R, Mickael C, et al. Severe pulmonary hypertension is associated with altered right ventricle metabolic substrate uptake. Am J Physiol Lung Cell Mol Physiol 2015;309(5):L435–40.

59. Piao L, Fang YH, Parikh K, et al. Cardiac glutaminolysis: a maladaptive cancer metabolism pathway in the right ventricle in pulmonary hypertension. J Mol Med (Berl) 2013;91(10):1185–97.

60. Fang YH, Piao L, Hong Z, et al. Therapeutic inhibition of fatty acid oxidation in right ventricular hypertrophy: exploiting Randle's cycle. J Mol Med (Berl) 2012;90(1):31–43.

61. Piao L, Sidhu VK, Fang YH, et al. FOXO1-mediated upregulation of pyruvate dehydrogenase kinase-4 (PDK4) decreases glucose oxidation and impairs right ventricular function in pulmonary hypertension: therapeutic benefits of dichloroacetate. J Mol Med (Berl) 2013;91(3):333–46.

62. Lewis GD, Ngo D, Hemnes AR, et al. Metabolic profiling of right ventricular-pulmonary vascular function reveals circulating biomarkers of pulmonary hypertension. J Am Coll Cardiol 2016;67(2): 174–89.

63. Rhodes CJ, Ghataorhe P, Wharton J, et al. Plasma metabolomics implicates modified transfer RNAs and altered bioenergetics in the outcomes of pulmonary arterial hypertension. Circulation 2017;135(5): 460–75.

64. Hemnes AR, Beck GJ, Newman JH, et al. PVDOMICS: a multi-center study to improve understanding of pulmonary vascular disease through Phenomics. Circ Res 2017;121(10):1136–9.

65. Leopold JA, Maron BA, Loscalzo J. The application of big data to cardiovascular disease: paths to precision medicine. J Clin Invest 2020;130(1): 29–38.

66. Pinu FR, Beale DJ, Paten AM, et al. Systems biology and multi-omics integration: viewpoints from the metabolomics research community. Metabolites 2019; 9(4):76.

67. Perakakis N, Yazdani A, Karniadakis GE, et al. Omics, big data and machine learning as tools to propel understanding of biological mechanisms and to discover novel diagnostics and therapeutics. Metabolism 2018;87:A1–9.

68. Barabasi AL, Gulbahce N, Loscalzo J. Network medicine: a network-based approach to human disease. Nat Rev Genet 2011;12(1):56–68.

69. Goh KI, Cusick ME, Valle D, et al. The human disease network. Proc Natl Acad Sci U S A 2007; 104(21):8685–90.

70. Vidal M, Cusick ME, Barabasi AL. Interactome networks and human disease. Cell 2011;144(6): 986–98.

71. Lusis AJ, Weiss JN. Cardiovascular networks: systems-based approaches to cardiovascular disease. Circulation 2010;121(1):157–70.

72. Chan SY, White K, Loscalzo J. Deciphering the molecular basis of human cardiovascular disease through network biology. Curr Opin Cardiol 2012; 27(3):202–9.

73. Parikh VN, Jin RC, Rabello S, et al. MicroRNA-21 integrates pathogenic signaling to control pulmonary hypertension: results of a network bioinformatics approach. Circulation 2012;125(12):1520–32.

Personalized Medicine for Pulmonary Hypertension:
The Future Management of Pulmonary Hypertension Requires a New Taxonomy

Martin R. Wilkins, MD, FMedSci

KEYWORDS

- Pulmonary hypertension • Precision medicine • Genetics • Endophenotypes • Deep-phenotyping

KEY POINTS

- Pulmonary hypertension is an unmet clinical need that presents late in the natural history of the condition.
- It is a convergent phenotype with a complex molecular pathology.
- The current clinical classification lacks the granularity needed to assist the development and deployment of new treatments.
- The future treatment of pulmonary hypertension depends on the integration of clinical and molecular information to create a new taxonomy that defines patient clusters coupled to druggable targets.

INTRODUCTION

Pulmonary hypertension (PH), whether defined by a resting mean pulmonary artery pressure (mPAP) greater than 20 mm Hg or greater than or equal to 25 mm Hg, is classified into 5 major groups by international consensus[1] (**Box 1**). The classification, first considered in 1973 and revisited at regular intervals since, seeks to include all clinical conditions associated with the development or progression of PH. Patients are assigned to a major group according to whether their PH is judged to be precapillary or postcapillary and the nature of any comorbidities.

Precapillary PH is distributed over Groups 1, 3, 4 and 5 while post-capillary PH is found in Groups 2 and 5.[1] Group 1, labeled pulmonary arterial hypertension (PAH), hosts idiopathic (IPAH), heritable (HPAH), and drug-induced PH, which are diagnoses of exclusion of coexisting diseases, alongside PH caused by congenital heart disease, PH

associated with connective tissue lung disease, and porto-pulmonary PH. Group 3 includes lung disease, including idiopathic pulmonary fibrosis, obstructive sleep apnea and chronic obstructive pulmonary disease, and hypoxia-induced PH. Group 4 is PH caused by chronic thromboembolic disease. Left-sided heart failure from whatever cause is placed in Group 2. Group 5 includes PH from a miscellaneous collection of comorbidities.

This classification is used to develop and assign treatments. There has been some success. Drugs that improve patient symptoms have been licensed for Group 1 and Group 4. Group 1 and Group 4 represent rare conditions with unmet clinical needs and an accelerated route to market. But progress with the development of treatments for PH in Group 2 and Group 3, the most common presentations of PH, has been disappointing. Mortality in these groups remains high, with both elevated pulmonary artery pressure and right

Dr. Wilkins is supported by the British Heart Foundation (RE/18/4/34215).
National Heart and Lung Institute, Imperial College London, Hammersmith Hospital, Du Cane Road, London W12 0NN, UK
E-mail address: m.wilkins@imperial.ac.uk

Clin Chest Med 42 (2021) 207–216
https://doi.org/10.1016/j.ccm.2020.10.004
0272-5231/21/© 2020 The Author. Published by Elsevier Inc.

Box 1
Clinical classification of pulmonary hypertension

Group 1: PAH

Subgroups

- Idiopathic PAH
- Heritable PAH
- Drug- and toxin-induced PAH
- PAH associated with:
  - Connective tissue disease
  - HIV infection
  - Portal hypertension
  - Congenital heart disease
  - Schistosomiasis
- PAH long-term responders to calcium channel blockers
- PAH with overt features of venous/capillaries (pulmonary venous occlusive disease/pulmonary capillary hemangiogenesis) involvement
- Persistent PH of the newborn syndrome

Group 2: PH caused by left heart disease

Subgroups

- PH caused by heart failure with preserved left ventricular ejection fraction (LVEF)
- PH due to heart failure with reduced LVEF
- Valvular heart disease
- Congenital/acquired cardiovascular conditions leading to postcapillary PH

Group 3: PH caused by lung diseases and/or hypoxia

Subgroups

- Obstructive lung disease
- Restrictive lung disease
- Other lung disease with mixed restrictive/obstructive pattern
- Hypoxia without lung disease
- Developmental lung disorders

Group 4: PH caused by pulmonary artery obstructions

Subgroups

- Chronic thromboembolic PH
- Other pulmonary artery obstructions

Group 5: PH with unclear and/or multifactorial mechanisms

Subgroups

- Hematological disorders

- Systemic and metabolic disorders
- Others
- Complex congenital heart disease

Abbreviations: PCH, pulmonary capillary hemangiomatosis; PVOD, pulmonary veno-occlusive disease.
From Simonneau et al. Haemodynamic definitions and updated clinical classification of pulmonary hypertension. European Respiratory Journal 53 (1) 1801913; DOI: 10.1183/13993003.01913-2018 Published 24 January 2019. Reproduced with permission of the © ERS 2020.

ventricular dysfunction representing independent predictors of death.[2–4] Even in Group 1, progress with developing effective therapies is qualified by a lack of impact on disease progression; these drugs, particularly in combination, may slow disease progression but do not arrest or reverse it. This is evident is survival statistics, which show that 5-year mortality is near 50%.[5]

Fortunately, pulmonary vascular disease remains an active area for drug discovery. There is no shortage of potential therapeutic targets, for both new chemical entities and repurposed drugs.[6] To improve success, however, future treatments for PH need to be focused more acutely on the patient as an individual, rather than the patient as part of a group, and this requires a new taxonomy of pulmonary vascular disease.

FIRST, THE PROBLEM WITH AVERAGES

It is widely recognized that patients vary in their response to drugs. This is evident in all studies evaluating treatments for PH. It can be easily overlooked when the data are presented as the mean change in each study group, even when shown with confidence intervals. For example, in a Phase 3 study with imatinib (IMPRES), which investigated the effects of imatinib in patients with Group 1 PAH, the mean placebo-corrected change in 6-minute walk distance (6MWD) after 24 weeks was 32 m (95% confidence interval, 12–52 m; $P=.002$).[7] When the absolute change in 6MWD is plotted as a distribution, the range of responses becomes stark (**Fig. 1**) and difficult to ignore. The fact that more patients improved with active treatment is still evident, but it becomes clear that some patients did not show a beneficial response as judged by the change in their 6MWD.

Various factors, both extrinsic and intrinsic, may influence the outcome measurement. Some, such as concomitant medication, comorbidity, and the genetics of drug transport and metabolism, may

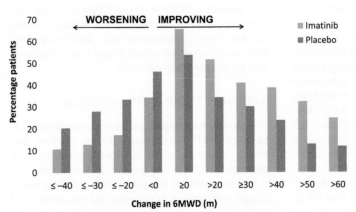

Fig. 1. Distribution of change in 6-minute walk distance after 6 months treatment with either imatinib or placebo. (*Data from* Hoeper MM et al. Imatinib Mesylate as Add-On Therapy for Pulmonary Arterial Hypertension: Results of the Randomized IMPRES Study Circulation. 2013;127:1128-38. https://doi.org/10.1161/CIRCULATIONAHA.112.000765.)

affect the pharmacokinetics of the study medication. Others, such as age, comorbidity, and heritable factors, can affect the pharmacodynamic response.

Prior consideration is given to these in the design of clinical trial protocols, with the aim of minimizing the noise to improve detection of the signal, but pragmatic factors intervene. A consideration of the process around designing a study for Group 1 PAH illustrates this. Because the aim is to find a treatment for pulmonary vascular disease, these studies start out targeting patients with idiopathic, heritable, and drug-induced PAH to reduce the influence of comorbidity. Boundaries are set for age, baseline walk distance, hemodynamics, and licensed therapies. In deciding the inclusion and exclusion criteria, there will be a discussion around whether to enroll patients with connective tissue disease and what constitutes significant parenchymal lung disease. Once the study is started, time pressures on recruitment from a rare patient population mean that trial protocols extend inclusion criteria (or patients are recruited that an adjudication panel might question), and the final study population is not so pure. In the end, patients are recruited from additional subgroups within Group 1, and so trials finish with a cohort of patients with mixed underlying pathology.[7–9]

If the mean response to the study drug is judged to be clinically beneficial in a pivotal trial, the study drug may be licensed for all of Group 1 PAH. The inclusion of small but representative patients from other PAH subgroups in Group 1 is used to justify this. A trivial but enlightening example of

the folly of this approach is to apply it to waist size. No one would take the average waist size of a cohort to design a pair of trousers to fit all. Yet this is what is done for drugs for PAH, driven admittedly by the desire to offer a treatment for a desperate medical condition.

At best, this practice may dilute any signal of efficacy. At worst, the signal may be lost altogether in the average response, and potential therapies may be discarded. A post hoc responder analysis is often used in a successful study to explore whether benefit is observed across all patient groups or, in a less successful trial, to determine whether there is a subgroup that showed some benefit. Unfortunately, the granularity of information available from clinical trials to make this meaningful is poor. Analysts have to rely on a limited clinical vocabulary and range of investigations.

THE LIMITATIONS OF THE CURRENT CLINICAL CLASSIFICATION

The clinical classification of PH was never intended as a guide to drug development.[10] It is understandable that it has been adopted as such, in the absence of anything else, but it was first proposed with the aim of collating the clinical and histologic characteristics of PH.[11] Importantly, it is not based on a deep comprehension of pulmonary vascular disease and plausible drug targets. Iterative revisions have resulted in a few new subgroups or reassigning a patient subgroup to a different major group, but the major categories have remained the same. Simple inspection shows heterogeneity and ambiguity within and between the major groups,[1] a statement to a limited understanding of underlying pathology. In clinical practice, patients can move from one subgroup to another or even a different major group during the course of their illness.

The problem starts with the defining investigation of PH. A key measurement in the diagnostic workup of a patient is the pulmonary artery wedge pressure (PAWP); it influences the group to which a PH patient is assigned. Greater than 15 mm Hg is considered to be raised and indicates a high left-sided filling pressure caused by significant left heart disease; the patient is placed in Group 2 (or in a few cases, Group 5). This is not always an easy measurement to make with confidence,[12,13] and yet a difference of 1 mm Hg can define a patient's diagnostic category and his or her suitability for licensed targeted treatments.

A further complication is that 12% to 38% of patients with PH and a raised PAWP have evidence of a precapillary component to their PH phenotype, based on a diastolic pressure gradient of at least 7 mm Hg or pulmonary vascular resistance (PVR) greater than 3 Wood units.[12] The European Society of Cardiology and European Respiratory Society guidelines recognize these patients as having combined precapillary and postcapillary PH.[14] With an aging population, the number of patients in this category is likely to grow.

The changing demographics of patients also adds complexity to the diagnosis of IPAH. IPAH is now more frequently diagnosed in older (>55 years) patients, but many in the older age group have cardiovascular risk factors (eg, coronary artery disease, systemic hypertension, hyperlipidemia, or diabetes) that predispose to left heart disease. IPAH patients with at least 3 cardiovascular risk factors have been labeled atypical IPAH.[15] The risk profiles and demographic characteristics of patients with atypical IPAH resemble those of PH with heart failure, particularly heart failure with preserved ejection fraction (HFpEF); many of these patients might be regarded as having combined precapillary and postcapillary PH. It has been proposed that typical IPAH, atypical IPAH, and HFpEF might form a disease continuum.[15]

This has implications for clinical trials. Data from patient registries and from clinical trials indicate that patients with PAH and additional cardiovascular risk factors are less responsive to targeted PAH treatments and show higher discontinuation rates.[9,15–17]

The ambiguity extends beyond a discussion of heart failure. Experts frequently have to make an assessment about PH in the context of accompanying lung disease, the size of a septal defect, and the significance of circulating autoantibodies. With the exception of the response to an acute vasodilator challenge, predicting an increased probability of response to calcium channel blockade, there are several additional phenotypes that are not captured in the current classification. These include insulin resistance, iron deficiency, and inflammation, all of which impact on prognosis and so are clinically relevant.

AND THEN THERE IS THE HISTOLOGY

The pioneers struggled with the morphologic features of PH.[11] Fast forward to the present day and the histology of the pulmonary vasculature of patients with PH is still a topic of discussion.

It is clear that the increased PVR in PAH is associated with pronounced vascular remodeling of pulmonary arterioles involving all cellular elements (endothelial cells, vascular smooth muscle cells, and fibroblasts) in the intimal, medial, and adventitial layers of the vessel wall, leading to narrowing of the vessel lumen and increased vascular stiffness.[18,19] The idea that plexiform lesions are pathognomonic of PAH is a misconception. It is also misguided to view structural remodeling of pulmonary arterioles as confined to Group 1. Arteriolar medial hypertrophy and intimal proliferation can occur in patients with pulmonary hypertension that falls into Groups 3 and 4, and have also been described in Group 2 (**Fig. 2**).

The pulmonary veins in PAH patients have been largely ignored, but studies show clear changes including smooth muscle cell hyperplasia and collagen-rich thickening of the intima of pulmonary veins and venules. A recent systematic description of the pulmonary vasculature of patients with Group 2 PH reports changes in the veins and small venules, with similarities to pulmonary venous occlusive disease.[20] In brief, a spectrum of structural changes affecting arterioles through to venules is seen in PH that underscores the difficulty of using hemodynamic measurements to separate disease entities.

INSIGHTS FROM GENETICS

An inevitable conclusion from this discussion is that PH is a convergent phenotype, the end manifestation of several pathologic drivers, and that clinical descriptors are blunt tools for dissecting the late-stage clinical presentation of PH. The development of effective new treatments depends on a better understanding of the pathologic mechanisms operating at a more individual level. Genetics is a good place to start.

Progress with understanding the genetic architecture of PH is most advanced in heritable and

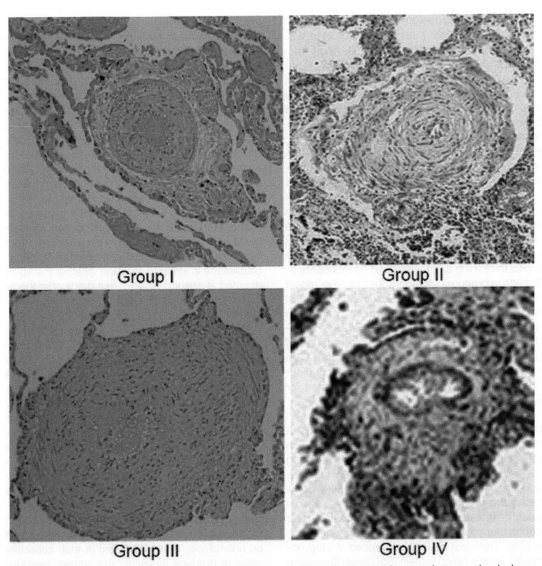

Fig. 2. The pulmonary vasculature in lung tissue from 4 patients with severe pulmonary hypertension is shown. The patients were characterized clinically as Category 1 (IPAH), Category 2 (left ventricular failure), Category 3 (interstitial lung disease), and Category 4 (chronic thromboembolic disease). However, each specimen reveals similar changes in the pulmonary arteriole showing medial hypertrophy and intimal proliferation. Without knowing the clinical phenotype, it would not be possible to distinguish them based on the vascular pathology (*From* Rich S. What is pulmonary arterial hypertension? Pulm Circ. 2012 Jul;2(3):271-2. https://doi.org/10.4103/2045-8932.101388. PMID: 23130095; PMCID: PMC3487295; with permission.)

idiopathic PAH. Pathogenic mutations in *BMPR2*, which encodes bone morphogenetic protein receptor type-2 (BMPR-2), segregate with PAH in families with a history of the condition.[21,22] These mutations predict loss of function. BMPR-2 is a member of the transforming growth factor-β (TGF-β) signaling pathway, and the working hypothesis is that reduced BMPR-2 activity creates an imbalance in bone morphogenetic protein (BMP)–TGF-β, in favor of TGF-β. Rare deleterious variants are now well documented in other genes

in this pathway in PAH patients, emphasizing its significance, notably *GDF-2, ACVRL1, ENG,* and *SMAD8*.[23] Nonetheless, there is a growing list of genes associated with PAH out with those with a direct impact on BMP-TGF-β signaling, including *KCNK3, TBX4, SOX17, ATP13A3, AQP1, ABCC8,* and *KDR*.[23–25] These studies reveal the genetic diversity underlying a clinical diagnosis of PAH.

The obvious question is, "Does this genetic diversity translate into recognizable clinical phenotypes?" This might be demanding, even for rare mutations, which tend to be associated with a larger effect than common variants. Apart from evidence that PAH patients with *BMPR2* mutations have a worse prognosis than patients without documented mutations in this gene,[26] the data are few. But the power of genetics to dissect the PH phenotype and inform clinical management is illustrated by *EIF2AK4*, a gene associated with pulmonary venous occlusive disease (PVOD).[25] In a UK study of 880 patients with IPAH, HPAH, or drug-induced PAH, 9 patients carried biallelic *EIF2AK4* mutations, despite a clinical diagnosis of IPAH made in an expert center.[27] Further investigation of clinical records showed that these patients were younger, had a reduced transfer coefficient for carbon monoxide (Kco), and more interlobular septal thickening and mediastinal lymphadenopathy on computed tomography of the chest compared with patients with PAH without *EIF2AK4* mutations. Radiological assessment alone could not accurately identify the biallelic *EIF2AK4* mutation carriers. Patients with PVOD may not do well if given treatments currently licensed for PAH. The lesson is that young patients with a clinical diagnosis of PAH and low Kco should be tested for *EIF2AK4* mutations.

These genetic insights not only mandate care in patient selection for clinical trials, they also inform drug development. Reviewing the high attrition rate in this space, it is keenly noted that selecting genetically validated drug targets can increase success rates.[28] In consequence, a genetic link between a druggable target and a disease should prioritize that target for further investigation. In that context, targeting BMP-TGF-β signaling deserves priority. The most clinically advanced strategy involves using a fusion protein (Sotatercept) consisting of the extracellular domain of activin receptor IIa (ActRIIa) attached to the Fc portion of human immunoglobulin G1 (IgG1) to sequester TGF-β superfamily ligands, such as activin A and B and growth differentiation factor (GDF)-11, thereby suppressing TGF-β signaling and rebalancing deficient BMPR-2 signaling[29] (ClinicalTrials.gov Identifier: NCT03496207). Early reports from a Phase 2 study are encouraging, and the detail around the data is anticipated with interest. Another approach under early clinical evaluation is directed at improving post-BMPR-2 signaling with tacrolimus.[30] Administering BMP9, a ligand for BMPR-2, is an option in preclinical development, based on the association between *GDF2* mutations and PAH.[31]

Whether these treatments should or could be targeted more accurately is yet unknown, but detailed knowledge of the 300-plus mutations identified in *BMPR2* suggest more selective therapies.[32] Aside from exogenous *BMPR2* gene delivery, still some time away in terms of clinical investigation, there are more immediate options for novel or repurposed drugs. Around 70% of *BMPR2* mutations are nonsense (frame-shift deletions and insertions) mutations.[32] Aminoglycoside antibiotics and drugs such as ataluren permit read-through of premature stop codons and the translation of full-length protein. Around 30% of mutations are missense mutations with single amino acid substitutions, disrupting protein folding and trafficking to the cell surface; chemical chaperones, such as sodium phenyl-butyrate, may rescue BMPR-2 trafficking, while hydroxychloroquine and chloroquine may have a beneficial effect by inhibiting autophagic degradation of BMPR-2. Studies are in setup to examine whether therapies directed at specific *BMPR2* mutations offer therapeutic benefit in PAH, taking personalized medicine to the point of a private medicine.

How far can this be taken? It remains to be established whether other genetically defined targets and their downstream pathways (ie, outside of BMP-TGF-β signaling) are druggable and might permit more precise targeting. Furthermore, the list of genes currently identified accounts for only 25% to 30% of IPAH patients.[24] Additional rare variants that influence thrombosis, inflammation, right ventricular (RV) function and other relevant pathologies may emerge from large-scale international efforts underway, but for most patients with PAH, and certainly PH, there will not be a single major genetic determinant of their phenotype. Common genetic variants, such as those found to influence risk of PAH,[33] have a smaller effect on phenotype. There is interest in their collective value to produce polygenic risk scores. Individually, common variants can provide instruments for Mendelian randomization analysis to define mechanistic pathways and inform druggable targets.[34] But the idea that complex cardiovascular phenotypes, such as PH, can be reduced to a simple genotype-phenotype relationship has been rightfully challenged.[35]

BIG DATA TO THE RESCUE

It has been proposed that complex cardiovascular phenotypes are the clinical manifestation of an interaction of subphenotypes or endo-phenotypes[35] And that these can be resolved by big data.

The importance of accurate phenotyping to the interpretation of genetic data has long been recognized. The value of deep phenotyping, collecting as much information about a patient as possible, has taken on greater significance with the opportunity to use machine learning and network analysis to find clusters that relay clinical information. There are emerging examples of the potential value of this approach.

In a cohort of patients with a clinical diagnosis of HFpEF, a suite of statistical learning algorithms used to analyze phenotype data (67 continuous variables) classified participants into 3 distinct groups that differed markedly in clinical characteristics, cardiac structure and function, invasive hemodynamics, and outcomes.[36] Using data from invasive cardiopulmonary exercise testing (iCPET), network analysis of clinical parameters from 738 patients enabled the development of a novel 10-variable model that defined 4 exercise groups.[37] The patient groups were characterized by exercise profiles drawn from pulmonary function, exercise hemodynamics, and metabolic data and defined differences in rates of hard clinical end points, expanding the range of useful clinical variables beyond peak V_{O_2} that predict hospitalization in patients with exercise intolerance.

Cardiac imaging readily provides high-dimensional data that can be used to better capture the nonlinear motion dynamics of the beating heart. These data can be mined for phenotypes beyond crude measures of global contraction that are only moderately reproducible and insensitive to the underlying disturbances of cardiovascular physiology. In a study of 302 patients with PH, image sequences of the heart acquired using cardiac magnetic resonance imaging (MRI) were used to create time-resolved 3-dimensional segmentations using a fully convolutional network trained on anatomic shape priors.[38] The resulting model was used for survival predictions and outperformed a conventional model based on manually derived volumetric measures.

Advances in technology increase the prospects of collecting more detailed clinical phenotypic information while patients are engaged in activities of daily living. Experience from implanted devices and wearable sensors that permit remote monitoring of electrocardiogram (ECG), blood pressure, oxygen saturation, mobility, and even environment exposure is racing ahead.[39,40] Integrated with electronic patient records, the depth and volume of data will provide a detailed database to identify important phenotypes associated with response to drugs that will inevitably cut across current clinical boundaries.

Add to this a wealth of 'omic' data from noninvasive sampling and cataloging the proteome, transcriptome, metabolome, and microbiome.[41–44] It is now possible to measure thousands of analytes in a small aliquot of plasma or serum. High-throughput platforms for measuring up to 5000 proteins and hundreds of identifiable metabolites (and many thousand unannotated more) and microRNAs in the same sample offer a window on the molecular choreography of PH.

It is still early days, with most 'omic' data from cross-sectional studies comparing PAH, and indeed, more specifically, IPAH and HPAH, with healthy controls. The main aim of these studies has been to identify molecular signatures of disease that might inform prognosis, with some success. Over 1000 proteins have been measured in the plasma proteome of patients with IPAH and HPAH, identifying several that distinguish these patients from healthy controls and around 40 that relate to survival.[41] The transcriptome of circulating white cells and the plasma metabolome can also discriminate IPAH and HPAH from health and categorize patients according to risk.[42,43]

Applied to patients within a larger PH group (as opposed to a clinically defined subgroup) or across currently defined PH groups should bring larger rewards. A panel of 48 circulating cytokines, chemokines, and growth factors has been shown to distinguish immune phenotypes in a population of patients drawn from Group 1 PAH.[45] Unsupervised machine learning (consensus clustering) classified patients into 4 proteomic immune clusters, without guidance from clinical features. The identified clusters were associated with distinctive clinical risk profiles providing information that was not contained in the clinical descriptions of these patients.

These clusters define inflammation endophenotypes. The availability of big data for describing PH sets the scene for describing further endophenotypes, such as thrombosis, fibrosis, cell proliferation, and autophagy. PH might then be regarded as an assembly of these different endophenotypes.[35] Understanding how these are perturbed in each patient who presents with a raised mPAP (or indeed, with breathlessness) offers a more granular view of his or her underlying pathology. This, in turn, can be used to guide targeted intervention(s) to repair the condition. Delivering this requires adopting a more extensive toolset for investigating patients and a different approach to treating them.

TOWARD MECHANISM-BASED THERAPEUTICS

Much has been made of the similarities between PH and cancer, in particular dysregulated cell proliferation and resistance to apoptosis, to the extent that some drugs developed for malignancies are under investigation for PAH.[46] Oncology has begun a transition in treatment strategy toward tumor-agnostic therapies, specifically, the use of drugs based on the genetic and molecular features of the cancer in question without regard to type or primary location.[47] To move to that scenario in PH will require the depth of molecular knowledge about the PH of each patient that oncology currently enjoys.

Oncology has the advantage of tissue biopsies, permitting sequencing for somatic and germline mutations. PH will need to rely more on liquid biopsies, the composition of circulating molecules that report on health. At present, multiplex assays, such as a panel of proteins, are available that improve on single-protein assays (eg, NT-proBNP) and clinical risk scores for defining risk or prognosis.[41] Building on this, combinations of circulating factors (ie, molecular signatures) could be used to define druggable pathologic pathways. For example, further network analysis of a proteome dataset from patients with clinically defined PAH has unmasked increased activity of the complement alternative pathway in some patients.[41,48] A protein cluster was identified that distinguished patients with poor survival, raising interest in trialing intervention with a complement inhibitor (eg, a complement C5a inhibitor) in this group in a biomarker-driven study design. The extent to which the complement alternative pathway is disturbed in other presentations of PH merits investigation.

THE FUTURE OF PULMONARY HYPERTENSION TREATMENT

PH is a global unmet clinical need. It progresses silently and presents late as a convergent phenotype. Dividing PH into broad overlapping clinical categories inhibits rather than assists the

development of new treatments. The early use of dual therapy and even triple therapy in the management plan for PAH has benefited patients, but it is a desperate response to a deeper problem.

The current licensed treatments have been developed on an empiric basis, rather than on an in depth understanding of the underlying pathology. Identifying a therapeutic signal and the patients who may benefit most can be lost in the noise. Without change, the next generation of treatments will be constrained by the same limited vocabulary for categorizing a complex phenotype. The ability to deep-phenotype patients at both the clinical and molecular level and integrate with genetic information opens the door to revisiting how one views and manages this condition (**Fig. 3**). It will require and drive a new taxonomy of PH, one that reduces the reliance on traditional diagnostic criteria alone and incorporates scientific advances in molecular and genetic medicine and innovations in clinical phenotyping, such as advanced imaging and remote sensors.

A major step in this direction has been taken with the National Heart, Lung, and Blood Institute initiative PVDOMICS (Redefining Pulmonary Hypertension through Pulmonary Vascular Disease Phenomics) study[49] (Clinicaltrials.gov NCT02980887). The aim of PVDOMICS is to update the classification of pulmonary vascular disease using a combination of deep clinical phenotyping and 'omic' techniques. It is important to note that 'omic' data are not alternatives to clinical data. Indeed, the project is explicit in requiring in-depth clinical phenotyping using standard operating protocols. The data will be subjected to unbiased network analyses and machine learning to cluster patients according to shared features and identify the molecular basis of these clusters. The expectation is that this will generate new

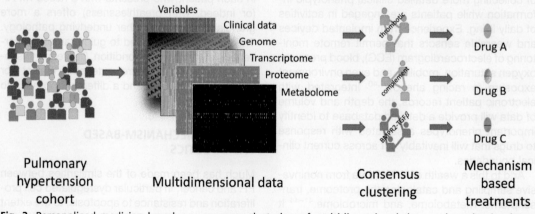

Fig. 3. Personalized medicine based on consensus clustering of multidimensional data and mechanism-based drug treatment.

pulmonary vascular disease ontologies, highlight relevant druggable pathways, and enable targeted mechanism-based treatments.

This is no small task. It will require validation in a separate data set. It will impact on how clinical trials are performed and drugs are licensed. It will need the combined efforts of all interested in improving the management of patients with PH.

REFERENCES

1. Simonneau G, Montani D, Celermajer DS, et al. Haemodynamic definitions and updated clinical classification of pulmonary hypertension. Eur Respir J 2019;53:1801913.
2. Patel NM, Lederer DJ, Borczuk AC, et al. Pulmonary hypertension in idiopathic pulmonary fibrosis. Chest 2007;132:998–1006.
3. Chaouat A, Naeije R, Weitzenblum E. Pulmonary hypertension in COPD. Eur Respir J 2008;32:1371–85.
4. Mejía M, Carrillo G, Rojas-Serrano J, et al. Idiopathic pulmonary fibrosis and emphysema: decreased survival associated with severe pulmonary arterial hypertension. Chest 2009;136:10–5.
5. Available at: https://digital.nhs.uk/data-and-information/publications/statistical/national-pulmonary-hypertension-audit/2019. accessed June17, 2020.
6. Sitbon S, Gomberg-Maitland M, Granton J, et al. Clinical trial design and new therapies for pulmonary arterial hypertension. Eur Respir J 2019;53:1801908.
7. Hoeper MM, Barst RJ, Bourge RC, et al. Imatinib mesylate as add-on therapy for pulmonary arterial hypertension: results of the randomized IMPRES study. Circulation 2013;127:1128–38.
8. Pulido T, Adzerikho I, Channick RN, et al. Macitentan and morbidity and mortality in pulmonary arterial hypertension. N Engl J Med 2013;369:809–18.
9. Galiè N, Barberà JA, Frost AE, et al. Initial use of ambrisentan plus tadalafil in pulmonary arterial hypertension. N Engl J Med 2015;373:834–44.
10. Rich S. What is pulmonary arterial hypertension? Pulm Circ 2012;2:271–2.
11. Hatano S, Strasser Toma, World Health Organization. (1975). Primary pulmonary hypertension : report on a WHO meeting, Geneva, 15-17 October 1973/edited by Shuichi Hatano and Toma Strasser. World Health Organization. Available at: https://apps.who.int/iris/handle/10665/39094. Accessed June 7, 2020.
12. Rosenkranz S, Gibbs JS, Wachter R, et al. Left ventricular heart failure and pulmonary hypertension. Eur Heart J 2016;37:942–54.
13. Johnson SW, Witkin A, Rodriguez-Lopez J, et al. Room for improvement in pulmonary capillary wedge pressure reporting: a review of hemodynamic tracings at a large academic medical center.

Pulm Circ 2020. https://doi.org/10.1177/2045894020929157.
14. Galiè N, Humbert M, Vachiery J-L, et al. 2015 ESC/ERS Guidelines for the diagnosis and treatment of pulmonary hypertension European. Eur Respir J 2015;46:903–75.
15. Opitz CF, Hoeper MM, Gibbs JSR, et al. Pre-capillary, combined, and post-capillary pulmonary hypertension: a pathophysiological continuum. J Am Coll Cardiol 2016;68:368–78.
16. Hoeper MM, Huscher D, Ghofrani HA, et al. Elderly patients diagnosed with idiopathic pulmonary arterial hypertension: results from the COMPERA registry. Int J Cardiol 2013;168:871–80.
17. Charalampopoulos A, Howard LS, Tzoulaki I, et al. Response to pulmonary arterial hypertension drug therapies in patients with pulmonary arterial hypertension and cardiovascular risk factors. Pulm Circ 2014;4:669–78.
18. Stacher E, Graham BB, Hunt JM, et al. Modern age pathology of pulmonary arterial hypertension. Am J Respir Crit Care Med 2012;186:261–72.
19. Humbert M, Guignabert C, Bonnet S, et al. Pathology and pathobiology of pulmonary hypertension: state of the art and research perspectives. Eur Respir J 2019;53:1801887.
20. Fayyaz AU, Edwards WD, Maleszewski JJ, et al. Global pulmonary vascular remodeling in pulmonary hypertension associated with heart failure and preserved or reduced ejection fraction. Circulation 2017;137:1796–810.
21. Deng Z, Haghighi F, Helleby L, et al. Fine mapping of PPH1, a gene for familial primary pulmonary hypertension, to a 3-cM region on chromosome 2q33. Am J Respir Crit Care Med 2000;161:1055–9.
22. International PPHC, Lane KB, Machado RD, et al. Heterozygous germline mutations in BMPR2, encoding a TGF-beta receptor, cause familial primary pulmonary hypertension. Nat Genet 2000; 26:81–4.
23. Gräf S, Haimel M, Bleda M, et al. Identification of rare sequence variation underlying heritable pulmonary arterial hypertension. Nat Commun 2018;9: 1416.
24. Southgate L, Machado RD, Graf S, et al. Molecular genetic framework underlying pulmonary arterial hypertension. Nat Rev Cardiol 2020;17:85–95.
25. Eyries M, Montani D, Girerd B, et al. Familial pulmonary arterial hypertension by KDR heterozygous loss of function. Eur Respir J 2020;55(4):1902165.
26. Evans JD, Girerd B, Montani D, et al. BMPR2 mutations and survival in pulmonary arterial hypertension: an individual participant data meta-analysis. Lancet Respir Med 2016;4:129–37.
27. Hadinnapola C, Bleda M, Haimel M, et al. Phenotypic characterization of EIF2AK4 mutation carriers in a large cohort of patients diagnosed clinically

with pulmonary arterial hypertension. Circulation 2017;136:2022–33.

28. Morgan P, Brown DG, Lennard L, et al. Impact of a five-dimensional framework on R&D productivity at AstraZeneca. Nat Rev Drug Discov 2018;17:167–81.

29. Yung L-M, Yang P, Joshi S, et al. ACTRIIA-Fc rebalances activin/GDF versus BMP signaling in pulmonary hypertension. Sci Transl Med 2020;12(543): eaaz5660.

30. Spiekerkoetter E, Sung YK, Sudheendra D, et al. Randomised placebo-controlled safety and tolerability trial of FK506 (tacrolimus) for pulmonary arterial hypertension. Eur Respir J 2017;50:1602449.

31. Long L, Ormiston ML, Yang X, et al. Selective enhancement of endothelial BMPR-II with BMP9 reverses pulmonary arterial hypertension. Nat Med 2015;21:777–85.

32. Orriols M, Gomez-Puerto MC, Ten Dijke P. BMP Type II receptor as a therapeutic target in pulmonary arterial hypertension. Cell Mol Life Sci 2017;74:2979–95.

33. Rhodes CJ, Batai K, Bleda M, et al. Genetic determinants of risk in pulmonary arterial hypertension: international genome-wide association studies and meta-analysis. Lancet Respir Med 2019;7:227–38.

34. Ulrich A, Wharton J, Thayer TE, et al. Mendelian randomisation analysis of red cell distribution width in pulmonary arterial hypertension. Eur Respir J 2020;55:1901486.

35. Leopold JA, Maron BA, Loscalzo J. The application of big data to cardiovascular disease: paths to precision medicine. J Clin Invest 2020;130:29–38.

36. Shah SJ, Katz DH, Selvaraj S, et al. Phenomapping for novel classification of heart failure with preserved ejection fraction. Circulation 2015;131:269–79.

37. Oldham WM, Oliveira RKF, Wang RS, et al. Network analysis to risk stratify patients with exercise intolerance. Circ Res 2018;122:864–76.

38. Bello GA, Dawes TJW, Duan J, et al. Deep learning cardiac motion analysis for human survival prediction. Nat Mach Intell 2019;1:95–104.

39. Yacoub MH, McLeod C. The expanding role of implantable devices to monitor heart failure and pulmonary hypertension. Nat Rev Cardiol 2018;15:770–9.

40. Soon S, Svavarsdottir H, Downey C, et al. Wearable devices for remote vital signs monitoring in the outpatient setting: an overview of the field. BMJ Innov 2020;6:55–71.

41. Rhodes CJ, Wharton J, Ghataorhe P, et al. Plasma proteome analysis in patients with pulmonary arterial hypertension: an observational cohort study. Lancet Respir Med 2017;5:717–26.

42. Rhodes CJ, Ghataorhe P, Wharton J, et al. Plasma metabolomics implicates modified transfer RNAs and altered bioenergetics in the outcomes of pulmonary arterial hypertension. Circulation 2017;135: 460–75.

43. Rhodes CJ, Otero-Núñez P, Wharton J, et al. Whole blood RNA profiles associated with pulmonary arterial hypertension and clinical outcome. Am J Respir Crit Care Med 2020;202(4):586–94.

44. Thenappan T, Khoruts A, Chen Y, et al. Can intestinal microbiota and circulating microbial products contribute to pulmonary arterial hypertension? Am J Physiol Heart Circ Physiol 2019;317:H1093–101.

45. Sweatt AJ, Hedlin HK, Balasubramanian V, et al. Discovery of distinct immune phenotypes using machine learning in pulmonary arterial hypertension. Circ Res 2019;124:904–19.

46. Cool CD, Kuebler WM, Bogaard HJ, et al. The hallmarks of severe pulmonary arterial hypertension: the cancer hypothesis-ten years later. Am J Physiol Lung Cell Mol Physiol 2020;318:L1115–30.

47. Goldberg KB, Blumenthal GM, McKee AE, et al. The FDA oncology center of excellence and precision medicine. Exp Biol Med (Maywood) 2018;243: 308–12.

48. Frid MG, McKeon BA, Thurman JM, et al. Immunoglobulin-driven complement activation regulates proinflammatory remodeling in pulmonary hypertension. Am J Respir Crit Care Med 2020;201: 224–39.

49. Hemnes AR, Beck GJ, Newman JH, et al. PVDOMICS: a multi-center study to improve understanding of pulmonary vascular disease through phenomics. Circ Res 2017;121:1136–9.

Sex Differences in Pulmonary Hypertension

Hannah Morris, MSc[a,b], Nina Denver, PhD[a], Rosemary Gaw, MSc[a], Hicham Labazi, PhD[a], Kirsty Mair, PhD[a], Margaret R. MacLean, PhD[a,*]

KEYWORDS

- Pulmonary hypertension • Sex • Serotonin • Obesity • Estrogens • BMPR2 • Pulmonary circulation
- Right ventricle

KEY POINTS

- Pulmonary arterial hypertension occurs in women more than men whereas survival in men is worse than in women.
- Estrogens and 16-hydroxyestrogen metabolites are elevated in men and in postmenopausal pulmonary arterial hypertension patients.
- Evidence suggests that estrogens and estrogen metabolites may play a role in the lung pathophysiology of pulmonary arterial hypertension, increase bone morphogenetic protein receptor type II mutation penetrance, and be produced by the lungs and adipose tissue in patients.

INTRODUCTION

Pulmonary hypertension (PH) is defined as a mean pulmonary arterial pressure of greater than 20 mm Hg at rest. It is characterized by a progressive increase in pulmonary arterial pressure, which can be classified into 5 distinct classes of PH set out by the World Health Organization (WHO).[1]

Pulmonary arterial hypertension (PAH) (WHO class I) demonstrates progressive obstruction of distal pulmonary arteries and the development of characteristic plexiform lesions in pulmonary resistance arteries. This results in increased pulmonary arterial pressure and subsequently hypertrophic remodeling of the right heart, before eventual right ventricular (RV) failure and ultimately death.

The pathophysiology of PAH is complex, with multiple mechanisms involved affecting all pulmonary vascular cell types. In addition to an increase in vasoconstriction, pulmonary artery endothelial cell dysfunction, phenotypic switch, metabolic transition, chronic inflammation, and oxidative stress all contribute to a pro-proliferative, apoptotic-resistant phenotype in pulmonary vascular cells.[2] This allows formation of occlusive lesions and increased pulmonary arterial pressure. Further understanding of the etiology of PAH will allow better targeting of its pathologic processes; one area of interest that may develop knowledge and contribute to new therapies is the role of sex in PAH.

THE SEX PARADOX IN PULMONARY ARTERIAL HYPERTENSION

It has been recognized for many years that the incidence of PAH is significantly higher in women than men.[3] The largest PAH registry, the US Registry to Evaluate Early and Long-Term PAH Disease Management (REVEAL), reported 80% of newly diagnosed patients were female.[4] Other more recent PAH registries since have reported a similar bias, with the Spanish, European COMPERA (Comparative Prospective Registry of Newly Initiated Therapies for Pulmonary Hypertension), and Latvian registries reporting a high female-male patient ratio.[5–7] Therefore, female sex

a Strathclyde Institute of Pharmacy and Biomedical Sciences, University of Strathclyde, Glasgow G4 0RE, Scotland; b Institute of Cardiovascular and Medical Sciences, College of Medical Veterinary and Life Sciences, University of Glasgow, Scotland
* Corresponding author. Strathclyde Institute of Pharmacy and Biomedical Sciences, University of Strathclyde, HW406, The Hamnett Wing, 161, Cathedral Street, Glasgow G4 0RE, Scotland.
E-mail address: Mandy.maclean@strath.ac.uk

Clin Chest Med 42 (2021) 217–228
https://doi.org/10.1016/j.ccm.2020.10.005
0272-5231/21/© 2020 Elsevier Inc. All rights reserved.

presents a clinically significant risk factor for the development of PAH. Conversely, despite their lower risk of being diagnosed with the disease, male PAH patients demonstrate significantly poorer outcomes than female patients, with 5-year survival in men with incident PAH at approximately 52% versus 62.5% in women, according to US REVEAL[8]; this observation was replicated in a more recent population of incident patients, at 53% versus 63%, respectively.[9] In addition, PAH progression and outcomes become less pronounced with age. For example, although younger men have exhibited higher right atrial pressures, pulmonary vascular resistance, and mean pulmonary arterial pressures than younger women, this difference was no longer observed after age 45 years old.[6] COMPERA also highlighted a dissipation of female bias after 65 years of age.[10] The general age at which these differences occur coincides with onset of menopause, when ovarian estrogen production in women is diminished.

Given female sex is a risk factor for PAH, the role of sex hormones has become relevant. Studies of sex hormones in both experimental models and patients are complex, with evidence supporting deleterious and protective effects for multiple members of the androgen and estrogen families, suggesting highly context-specific mechanisms.

These issues collectively are referred to as the estrogen, or sex hormone, paradox.

SEX HORMONE SYNTHESIS AND METABOLISM

As **Fig. 1** shows, steroidogenesis begins with derivation from cholesterol. Metabolism starts with translocation of cholesterol to the mitochondrion to form pregnenolone, which is converted to progesterone by 3β-hydroxysteroid dehydrogenase. Both are converted to form androgens; dehydroepiandrosterone (DHEA) and androstenedione (A4) under the action of 17-hydroxylase/17, 20-lyase enzyme. DHEA and A4 conversion continues to androstenediol and testosterone by 17β-hydroxysteroid dehydrogenase (17β-HSDs).[11]

Aromatase (cytochrome P450 [CYP]91A1) is the major enzyme involved in production of the main circulating estrogens estrone (E1) and estradiol (E2). In phase 1 metabolism, E1 and E2 undergo hydroxylation at the C-2 and C-4 positions catalyzed by CYP monooxygenases.[12] CYP1A1, CYP1B1, CYP1A2, and CYP3A4 then permit irreversible conversion to hydroxyestrogens. Of these, the major pathway generates 2-hydroxyestrone (2OHE1) and 2-hydroxyestradiol (2OHE2), whereas the lesser 4-hydroxylation pathway produces 4-hydroxyestrone (4OHE1)

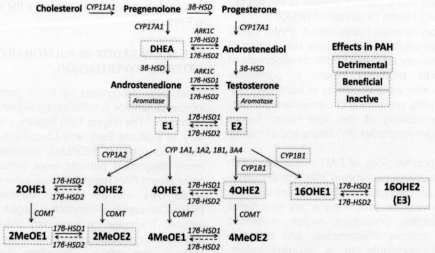

Fig. 1. Sex steroid metabolism pathway. Formation of endogenous estrogen via cholesterol and androgenic substrates DHEA, androstenediol, androstenedione, and testosterone. Aromatization of androstenedione and testosterone generates E1 and E2. Hydroxylation of E1 and E2 occurs at C-2, C-4 and C-16 positions by CYP enzymes (the most prominent being CYP1A1 and CYP1B1, promoting beneficial and detrimental hydroxylation, respectively). Hydroxylation at the C16 of the aliphatic ring generates 16OHE1 and E2 (16OHE2). Alternatively, hydroxylation at C-2 and C-4 produces 2OHE1 and 4OHE1 or E2 (2OHE2 and 4OHE2), known collectively as catechol estrogens. The 2OHE and 4OHE metabolites are rapidly cleared by COMTs to form methoxyestrogens (2MeOE1, 2MeOE2, 4MeOE1, and 4MeOE2). All E1 and E2 metabolites are maintained in equilibrium 17β-HSD1 and 17β-HSD2 enzymes with androgens also regulated by the aldo-keto reductase 1C subfamily (ARK1C) enzyme. The activity of key metabolites is indicated.

and 4-hydroxyestradiol (4OHE2). These catechol estrogens can be methylated rapidly via catechol-O-methyltransferase (COMT) to form methoxyestrogens, including 2-methoxyestradiol (2MeOE2). In addition to catechol metabolism, E1 and E2 may undergo C-16 hydroxylation to form 16-hydroxyestrone (16OHE1) and 16-hydroxyestradiol (16OHE2). E1, E2, and their respective metabolites are maintained in constant equilibrium by dehydrogenation reactions through alcohol reductases (17β-HSD1 and 17β-HSD2).

Premenopause, estrogen synthesis occurs mainly in the ovarian follicles and corpus luteum. In postmenopausal women and in men, estrogen instead is produced by extragonadal sites, where it acts locally in a paracrine fashion. Expression of aromatase in these extragonadal tissues is regulated by tissue-specific promoters so aromatase action can generate high local levels of estrogen with significant biological influence, without significantly affecting circulating levels.[13]

SEX DIFFERENCES AND BONE MORPHOGENETIC PROTEIN RECEPTOR TYPE II

Bone morphogenetic protein receptor type II (BMPR2) mutations are the most common genetic cause of heritable PAH (hPAH). These mutations occur in 75% to 80% of hPAH cases but also in 20% to 25% of idiopathic (iPAH) cases, leading to a loss of BMPR2 function. In BMPR2 mutation carriers, the female penetrance is approximately 40%, whereas male penetrance is approximately 14%.[14] Basal BMPR2 signaling is reduced in female human pulmonary arterial smooth muscle cells (hPASMCs) compared with male hPASMCs and this effect may be estrogen dependent.[15,16] Estrogen itself can decrease the expression of BMPR2 via the ERα receptor.[15,17] The decrease in BMPR2 signaling associates with an increased proliferative phenotype in female hPASMCs due to unopposed and increased phosphoextracellular signal-regulated kinases signaling.[15] In the heart, RV function may be affected more severely in BMPR2 mutation carriers than in noncarriers and further research is required to understand this phenomenon.[18]

The Y chromosome may regulate BMPR2 via the sex-determining region Y transcription factor present on the Y chromosome, which also may contribute to fewer cases of PAH in men.[19] Paradoxically, however, a recent meta-analysis demonstrated in hPAH and iPAH patients that 67% were female whereas the BMPR2 mutation rate is higher in men than women (34.78% vs 29.41%, respectively).[20]

Sex Differences in Animal Models of Pulmonary Arterial Hypertension

There are several commonly used experimental animal models of PAH. Numerous studies on the widely used chronic hypoxia and monocrotaline (MCT) models have demonstrated a more pronounced PH phenotype and worse outcome in male rodents compared with female rodents,[21] whereas ovariectomy in female rodents can induce a more severe PH phenotype.[22] This suggests a protective effect of circulating sex hormones in this context. These models, however, are variable and do not recapitulate many important human characteristics of PH and it generally is conceded they translate poorly to human PH. Research into the female prevalence of PAH had previously been hampered by a lack of appropriate in vivo models, but it is now an area of interest and growth.

More recently, models that replicate human PAH more closely have been developed. The Sugen-hypoxia model mimics the angio-obliterative phenotype of advanced human disease through treatment with vascular endothelial growth factor 2 inhibitor Sugen 5416 in combination with hypoxia.[23] Female Sugen/hypoxia rodents have been reported to develop a more severe disease phenotype than male rodents, which is delayed by ovariectomy; however, hemodynamic alterations and RV dysfunction may be less severe,[24] consistent with the disparity seen between male and female patients. This sex difference, however, not always is observed.[16,25] In addition, estrogen metabolism to mitogenic metabolites may contribute to the pathogenic effects of Sugen because Sugen activates the aryl hydrocarbon receptor causing increased CYP1B1 and CYP1A1 expression.[26]

Many transgenic mouse models of PH display a female bias, suggesting estrogens are an important mediator. These include mice with a mutation in the gene for BMPR2.[27,28] This is associated with proliferation of hPASMCs in PAH.[29,30]

PH occurs spontaneously in female mice heterozygous for BMPR2 signaling target Smad1,[15] mice over-expressing the human serotonin transporter (SERT+)[31,32] or the calcium-binding protein S100A4/MTS (S100A4/MTS+),[33] and rodents treated with dexfenfluramine.[34]

Transgenic mouse models of PH have relatively mild phenotypes, often devoid of RV hypertrophy, suggesting a second hit is required for a robust

PAH phenotype. They have, however, provided other important insights into the role of estrogen in PAH. For example, the PH phenotype observed in female SERT+ mice is removed by ovariectomy and restored on subsequent estrogen replacement.[31] In a mouse model of BMPR2 mutation, inhibition of endogenous estrogen with an inhibitor of estrogen synthesis prevented the onset of PH.[27] Both of these studies implicate estrogen in the development of PH.

AROMATASE AND ESTROGEN SYNTHESIS IN PULMONARY HYPERTENSION

Multiple single-nucleotide polymorphisms (SNPs) in the genes coding for estrogen receptor 1, aromatase, and S100A4/MTS have been associated with the risk of porto-PH (PPHTN). The increased aromatase activity was associated with elevated E2 production in both male and female PPHTN patients and associated with increased risk of PPHTN.[35] Recently this observation has been confirmed and plasma levels of the estrogen metabolite 16OHE2 also accumulates in PPHTN (Kawut SM, unpublished data, 2020).

Aromatase expression has been identified in pulmonary arteries of animal models and in patients with PAH, localized mainly to vascular smooth muscle.[16] Levels of estrogen in hPASMCs derived from PAH patients are high[16] and, therefore, the local concentration of estrogen in the pulmonary artery may exert a powerful influence on pulmonary vasculature. Female patients were found to express significantly higher levels of aromatase in the lungs than male patients, which may contribute to a reduction in BMPR2 signaling through the ERα receptor.[15,17]

Inhibition of estrogen synthesis with anastrozole reduces moderate and severe experimental PH and restores BMPR2 signaling in female animals but not male animals via a reduction in endogenous estrogen.[16] Estrogen inhibition with anastrozole and fulvestrant also has beneficial effects in female BMPR2 mutant mice,[27] and metformin can exert therapeutic effects in females Sugen/hypoxia rats, in part via aromatase inhibition.[36] Clinically, the therapeutic potential of aromatase inhibition also has been demonstrated in a small-scale clinical trial using anastrozole, where it was well tolerated and improved 6-minute walk distance in postmenopausal women and men.[37]

In some patient subgroups where male PAH patients are more prevalent, such as PAH associated with human immunodeficiency (HIV), sleep apnea, and PPHTN,[8] estrogen also may contribute to the disease pathobiology. For instance, in HIV, dysregulation in sex hormone concentrations has been reported in both sexes. In 1 study, E2 was reported to significantly increase over an 18-month period in male patients with HIV.[38] Furthermore, obstructive sleep apnea is most common in obese men,[39] where elevated circulating estrogen levels are higher due to increased expression and activity of aromatase within adipose tissue.[39,40] Consistent with this, endogenous estrogens contribute to experimental PH in obese male mice.[41] Aromatase expression in visceral adipose tissue (VAT) was significantly higher in lean female mice than male mice, but in obese animals a marked increase in aromatase expression in VAT was observed in male mice but not female mice.[41] Obesity may predispose male mice to PAH through VAT dysfunction, resulting in altered estrogen production and metabolism.[41] Thus, changes in aromatase expression and estrogen production clinically and experimentally suggest endogenous estrogen may contribute to the pathobiology of PAH in both male mice and female mice by sexually dimorphic mechanisms.

The implication of estrogen levels in PAH in male animal models is consistent with recent reports that circulating estrogen levels are elevated in men with iPAH as well as postmenopausal women with iPAH.[42,43]

Although evidence suggests that endogenous estrogens are pathogenic in PAH, paradoxically, exogenously administered estrogens or ovarian-derived circulating estrogens have a protective effect on RV hypertrophy and function in experimental animals.[44,45] This suggests that endogenous estrogens produced by the lungs are pathogenic in the pulmonary circulation whereas circulating estrogens in animal models may protect RV function. Evidence suggests it is the metabolism of endogenous estrogens to mitogenic metabolites that exert the pathogenic effects of endogenous estrogen. It is likely that ovarian-derived or exogenously administered estrogen is not metabolized in the same way as endogenous estrogens produced by the pulmonary arteries. This may explain the differential effects of endogenous estrogens and exogenously administered or ovarian-derived estrogens in experimental PH. Clinically, however, there are no reports of RV dysfunction in the millions of women taking anastrozole for breast cancer suggesting endogenous estrogens do not protect RV function in women.

ESTROGEN METABOLISM IN PULMONARY ARTERIAL HYPERTENSION

Because estrogen synthesis and metabolism usually are in a tightly regulated equilibrium, it is intriguing to speculate that PAH may involve dysfunctional estrogen synthesis and metabolism resulting in accumulation of mitogenic estrogen metabolites (**Fig. 2**).

The 16α-hydroxylation pathway forming 16OHE1 and 16OHE2 metabolites is a key estrogen metabolism pathway implicated in PAH. CYP1B1, which mediates their formation, is expressed by all cell types of the pulmonary vascular wall.[25]

CYP1B1 overexpression has been observed in hPASMCs from both idiopathic and hereditary PAH patients, and in chronic-hypoxic and Sugen-hypoxic mice.[25] In addition, various SNPs in CYP1B1 have been associated with increased disease penetrance in hPAH.[14] For example, 4-fold greater penetrance was observed in female *BMPR2* mutation carriers homozygous for the *CYP1B1 N453S* polymorphism.[14] Paradoxically, Epstein-Barr virus (EBV)-immortalized cultured B cells from hPAH patients have 10-fold lower expression of CYP1B1 than control groups in female but not male hPAH patients.[46] This reflects phenotypic difference between these immortalized B cells and primary cultures of hPASMCs. In addition, estrogen influences B cell maturation and selection, permitting B cells to mature to immunocompetence.[47] BMP2 and BMP4 also have roles in the development, growth potential, and apoptosis of B cells.[48] Hence, B cells are likely to be altered phenotypically in hPAH female patients, which may affect estrogen metabolism and explain differential expression of CYP1B1 in EBV-immortalized B cells and hPASMCs.

In African American women, a CYP1B1 SNP rs162561 was associated with RV ejection fraction (RVEF), and, in white subjects, higher E2 metabolite levels were associated with significantly higher RVEF. The CYP1B1 SNP identified is in tight linkage disequilibrium with SNPs associated with oncogenesis and PH, suggesting these pathways may underpin sexual dimorphism in RV failure.[49]

Overexpression of CYP1B1 in the lungs has been demonstrated in the female dexfenfluramine-treated and SERT+ models of PAH.[34,50] In addition, CYP1B1 knockout mice are not susceptible to dexfenfluramine-induced PH, suggesting that CYP1B1 also mediates experimental PH via serotonin signaling.[8] The CYP1B1 antagonist tetramethoxystilbene (TMS) attenuates E2-induced proliferation in hPASMCs[51] and demonstrates therapeutic effects in in vivo models of PAH.[25,50] TMS also can prevent the development of PH in obese mice.[41] Thus, CYP1B1 potentially may provide a valuable novel therapeutic target.

16α-HYDROXYESTROGENS

16OHE1 is a pro-proliferative estrogen metabolite. Importantly, 16OHE1 covalently binds to estrogen receptors with a higher affinity than 2-hydroxy metabolites and 4-hydroxy metabolites. Importantly, circulating 16OHE1 has been shown to increase in PAH patients[52,53] and associate with increased penetrance in female hPAH patients.[14]

16OHE1 is highly proliferative via ERα in hPASMCs, in particular those from female PAH patients,[25,51] resulting in increased oxidative stress.[51] 16OHE1 has been observed to cause experimental PH in mice[25] and suppress beneficial BMP signaling in control mice, while increasing PAH disease penetrance in *BMPR2*-mutant mice via up-regulation of miR-29.[54,55] In obese mice, 16OHE1 also is produced by VAT, where there also is increased CYP1B1 expression.[41] In these obese mice, 16OHE1 contributes to oxidative stress, suggesting estrogen inhibitors may be beneficial in treating obese PAH patients.[41]

A shift from 2-methoxyestrogen to 16-hydroxyestrogen production also may be associated with development of iPAH and penetrance in hPAH.[14]

Higher levels of 16OHE2 were detected in the plasma of PAH patients compared with controls in a recent proof-of-concept study and found to induce proliferation in female PAH patient hPASMCs.[52] The same study showed increased migration of blood outgrowth endothelial cells

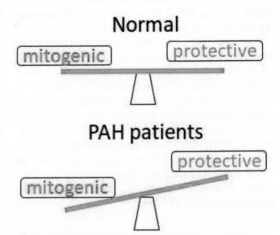

Fig. 2. Estrogen and estrogen metabolites in PAH. Hypothesis: metabolism to mitogenic and protective estrogen metabolites is normally balanced. There is dysfunctional estrogen metabolism in PAH and an accumulation of mitogenic metabolites which contributes to the pathogenesis of PAH.

from male and female PAH patients when stimulated with 16OHE2.[52] Intriguingly, in a small proof-of-concept clinical trial, the ERα inhibitor fulvestrant caused decreased plasma levels of 16OHE2.[56] 16OHE2 levels are high in pregnant women, and pregnancy is a risk factor for PAH. So, although evidence suggests the hypothesis that 16OHE2 may mediate PAH, much research is required to test this hypothesis in vitro and in vivo.

2-HYDROXYLATION/METHYLATION ESTROGEN METABOLITES

E1 and E2 also can undergo hydroxylation by CYP enzymes to produce 2-hydroxyestrogens and 4-hydroxyestrogens. These are metabolized further by COMTs to methoxyestrogens (see **Fig. 2**). Unlike E1/E2 and 16α-hydroxyestrogens, hydroxy metabolites and methoxy metabolites exhibit little estrogenic activity[57] and appear to confer protective effects in PAH.

Studies have identified protective pulmonary vascular effects of 2-hydroxyestrogens and 4-hydroxyestrogens. In animal studies, 2OHE2 was demonstrated to reverse MCT-induced PH parameters in male rats,[58] in bleomycin-induced PH in ovariectomized rats,[59] and in metabolic syndrome–associated PH.[60] Additionally, 4OHE2 has shown antiproliferative effects specifically in hPASMCs derived from male rats but not female rats, postulated to be through increased BMPR2 signaling.[15] The protective effects of hydroxyestrogens, however, now are demonstrated to arise from their COMT-mediated conversion to methoxyestrogens. COMT is influenced by sex; male rats express more COMT than female rats,[61] and E2 down-regulates COMT activity,[62,63] which may contribute to sex disparity.

Methoxyestrogen 2ME2 is the most researched and potentially clinically beneficial estrogen metabolite in PH. Tofovic and colleagues[58,59] have demonstrated 2ME2 can estrogen receptor-independent attenuation of MCT-induced or bleomycin-induced PH. Similarly, 2ME2 reduces chronic hypoxic PH progression alongside reduction in oxidative stress[64] and hypoxia inducible factor-1α levels.[65] Highly potent 2ME2 analog 2-ethoxyestradiol also improves experimental PH.[66] In the human condition, 2ME2 treatment can attenuate proliferation in both control hPASMCs and lung fibroblasts[59] and in PAH hPASMCs, where it may induce proapoptotic effects.[65] Further work is required to elucidate the 2ME2-associated protective mechanisms in the pulmonary vasculature, and potential clinical benefits.

SEROTONIN AND SEX IN PULMONARY HYPERTENSION

The serotonin pathway first was implicated in the development of PAH after appetite suppressants, aminorex, fenfluramine, and chlorphentermine, which are indirect serotonergic agonists,[67] were shown to cause the disease. This led to the serotonin hypothesis of PAH. Pulmonary tissue normally is exposed to low levels of serotonin as most serotonin is stored in platelets. Platelet pool storage disease, however, can elevate levels of free serotonin and this can be associated with PAH.[68] In the pulmonary circulation, serotonin promotes pulmonary arterial smooth muscle cell (PASMC) proliferation, vasoconstriction, and thrombosis, processes involved in the development of PAH.[69]

Serotonin synthesis has been associated with the development of PH in the Sugen/hypoxia,[70] and ablation or inhibition of tryptophan hydroxylase 1, the rate-limiting enzyme in the synthesis of serotonin in the periphery, can protect against or reverse experimental PH.[71–73]

The SERT[+], S100A4/Mts1 (Mts1[+])[31,32] and dexfenfluramine mice[33,34] all demonstrate a PH phenotype only in female mice and exhibit increases in serotonin signaling pathways. In the SERT[+] female mice, the PH phenotype is prevented by ovariectomy and recovered by chronic administration of estrogen, indicating an essential function of this hormone in the development of the PH phenotype.[31] These findings suggest that serotonin facilitates and amplifies the effects of estrogen in the pulmonary circulation. Indeed, estrogen can increase expression of Tph1, SERT, and the 5HT$_{1B}$ (5-hydroxytryptamine receptor 1B) receptor in human PASMCs.[31]

Serotonin also can influence other pathways associated with PH potentially acting as a second hit. For example, exogenously administered serotonin uncovers a PH phenotype in BMPR2[+/−] mice.[74] Furthermore, female BMPR2 (R899X[+/−]) mice spontaneously develop PAH via 5-HT$_{1B}$–mediated effects thought to be regulated by inhibition of miRNA-96, mediated by estrogen.[75] Serotonin also may regulate estrogen metabolism as SERT overexpression and dexfenfluramine can increase CYP1B1 expression, which contributes to the pathogenesis of PAH.[50,76]

INFLUENCE OF SEX HORMONES ON RIGHT VENTRICULAR FUNCTION IN THE CLINIC

One of the key hypotheses for the sex paradox of PAH, in which women are more likely affected but men have poorer outcomes, is that there are inherent sex differences in RV compensation. Therefore, although PAH is observed more often in women, the female RV appears more capable of compensating during progression of the disease and this improves survival long term.[77]

In healthy study populations, women were found to have better RV function, in particular, higher RVEF than men.[78,79] Additionally, age-related decreases in RV mass are worse in men.[79] Exogenous E2 was found to be associated with this increased RVEF in postmenopausal women taking hormone replacement therapy, while increased testosterone was associated with larger RV mass in men.[78]

Even in the face of increased circulating estrogen,[43] male patients with PAH have been found to exhibit lower RVEF at baseline than female patients,[80] and this appears to decline faster in men over time[77] which may contribute to poor survival. In healthy men, higher DHEA-Sulfate levels were associated with higher RV stroke volume[78] whereas lower DHEA-S levels are associated with PAH in men.[43]

CLINICAL ASSAYS FOR QUANTIFICATION OF ENDOGENOUS ESTROGEN

The need to detect and quantify estrogens and estrogen metabolites in PAH patients is clear. Previous methods have been limited by the challenging chemistry of steroid hormones. Recent advances, however, allow more reliable measurement of estrogens, particularly at endogenous levels, in samples from human PAH patients. This will become invaluable in defining the role of estrogen metabolites in the disease.

Endogenous unbound estrogens in patient biofluids, most commonly E2, conventionally have been measured by enzyme-linked immunosorbent assay. In recent years, however, these increasingly are criticized due to cross-reactivity issues, particularly at low-level concentrations in male and postmenopausal study cohorts, resulting in overestimation of E2 concentrations.[81,82] Moreover, isomeric metabolite structures confound immunoassay measurements and drug treatments, such as fulvestrant. have structural similarities to E2, so interfere with immunoassay measurements.[83]

Hyphenated analytical approaches, which directly couple mass spectrometry with other analytical techniques, such as chromatography, now are coming to the fore owing to technological advances in the past 10 years to 15 years. Liquid chromatography–tandem mass spectrometry (LC-MS/MS) leads the way in terms of selectivity and low-level detection capabilities. Recent advances have described more accurate endogenous concentrations of estrogen and estrogen metabolites in PAH patients, confirming that previous studies have over-estimated endogenous levels of estrogens.[52,53,56]

Application of LC-MS/MS has shown that, in female iPAH patients, serum E1 concentrations decrease whereas 16OHE2 levels increase, potentially indicating increased conversion via CYP signaling.[52] Contrary to previous studies applying immunoassay, lower serum levels of E2 were detected in male iPAH patients. This may have been a cohort-dependent effect or a result of immunoassay over-estimating E2 concentrations, strengthening the requirement for continued development of LC-MS/MS methodologies in the clinical settings.[81,84–86]

Proof-of-concept clinical trials in PAH patients also have proved the suitability of both ERα and aromatase inhibitors as therapeutic targets in PAH. A randomized, double-blind, placebo-controlled study of anastrozole shows inhibition of aromatase displayed effective reduction of immunoassay measured E2 levels, which improved 6-minute walk distance in PAH patients.[35] A small open-label proof-of-concept study enrolling postmenopausal PAH patients treated with ERα antagonist fulvestrant since has analyzed plasma estrogen metabolites by LC-MS/MS. Fulvestrant treatment caused a trend toward reduction of 16OHE2 associated with a decrease in hematopoietic progenitor cells.[56] This study used the validated LC-MS/MS approach, discussed previously,[53] and represents the first to relate a decrease in estrogen metabolism to therapeutic response using LC-MS/MS. For future studies, LC-MS/MS approaches should be developed further to allow robust, high-throughput, and streamlined analyses. The development of automated sample preparation, better nonderivatized analyses and advances in mass spectrometry equipment will improve profiling of all estrogenic molecules. Analytical methods for androgens also should be explored to widen interpretation of metabolism in PAH. For estrogen analysis, development of capabilities to analyze the 2-hydroxylation and 4-hydroxylation pathways[87] and to distinguish between isomers in the 16-hydroxylation pathway[51,52,54] also is necessary.

To shed further light on sexual dimorphism in PAH, efforts should be concentrated on clinical studies to measure blood and site-specific levels of estrogen and estrogen metabolites using LC-MS/MS. Stratified analysis of the estrogen metabolism pathway in men and women would answer key questions surrounding the association of

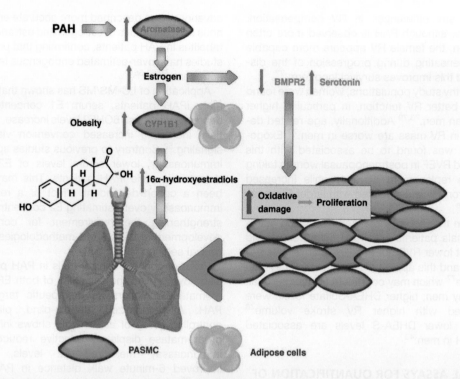

Fig. 3. Estrogen synthesis and metabolism in PAH. Aromatase expression is increased in the pulmonary arteries of patients with PAH leading to increased estrogen synthesis. Estrogen can decrease BMPR2 signaling and increase serotonin signaling leading to oxidative stress and increased proliferation of PASMCs. CYP1B1 expression also is increased in the pulmonary arteries of patients with PAH, leading to increased metabolism of estrogen. There is an accumulation of circulating 16-hydroxyestradiols, such as 16α-hydroxyestrone (structure shown) and 16α-hydroxyestradiol. These can act in a paracrine fashion to induce oxidative stress and increased proliferation of PASMCs. In obese patients, there may be increased estrogen synthesis and metabolism in adipose tissue, leading to further accumulation of 16α-hydroxyestrone, which contributes to PASMC proliferation.

estrogens with age, body mass index, contraceptive medicines, menstrual cycle, pregnancy, and disease severity in PAH.

SUMMARY

Clinically, female sex is a risk factor for PAH due to interactions between estrogens and *BMPR2* and increased penetrance in BMPR2 mutation carriers. Estrogen is pathogenic in the pulmonary circulation and PAH is associated with dysfunctional estrogen metabolism resulting in increased levels of 16OHEs, which exert pathogenic effects. Adipose tissue-derived 16OHE1 may and contribute to PAH in obese patients. Estrogen also can upregulate serotonin signaling, which also may contribute to the pathogenesis of PAH. These conclusions are summarized in **Fig. 3**. More clinical investigation is required to fully elucidate the effects of estrogens on the RV to determine if these influence sex differences in RV compensation. The role of other sex hormones in PAH deserves further investigation. Refined LC-MS/MS
techniques for the measurement of sex hormones in clinical and preclinical research undoubtedly will improve knowledge in this field.

DISCLOSURE

None.

REFERENCES

1. Kovacs G, Dumitrescu D, Barner A, et al. Definition, clinical classification and initial diagnosis of pulmonary hypertension: Updated recommendations from the Cologne Consensus Conference 2018. Int J Cardiol 2018;272s:11–9.
2. Humbert M, Morrell NW, Archer SL, et al. Cellular and molecular pathobiology of pulmonary arterial hypertension. J Am Coll Cardiol 2004;43(12):13S–24S.
3. Dresdale DT, Schultz M, Michtom RJ. Primary pulmonary hypertension. I. Clinical and hemodynamic study. Am J Med 1951;11(6):686–705.

4. McGoon MD, Miller DP. REVEAL: a contemporary US pulmonary arterial hypertension registry. Eur Respir Rev 2012;21(123):8–18.

5. Escribano-Subias P, Blanco I, Lopez-Meseguer M, et al. Survival in pulmonary hypertension in Spain: insights from the Spanish registry. Eur Respir J 2012;40(3):596–603.

6. Hoeper MM, Huscher D, Ghofrani HA, et al. Elderly patients diagnosed with idiopathic pulmonary arterial hypertension: results from the COMPERA registry. Int J Cardiol 2013;168(2):871–80.

7. Skride A, Sablinskis K, Lejnieks A, et al. Characteristics and survival data from Latvian pulmonary hypertension registry: comparison of prospective pulmonary hypertension registries in Europe. Pulm Circ 2018;8(3). 2045894018780521.

8. Shapiro S, Traiger GL, Turner M, et al. Sex differences in the diagnosis, treatment, and outcome of patients with pulmonary arterial hypertension enrolled in the registry to evaluate early and long-term pulmonary arterial hypertension disease management. Chest 2012;141(2):363–73.

9. Kjellstrom B, Nisell M, Kylhammar D, et al. Sex-specific differences and survival in patients with idiopathic pulmonary arterial hypertension 2008-2016. ERJ Open Res 2019;5(3). 00075-2019.

10. Ventetuolo CE, Praestgaard A, Palevsky HI, et al. Sex and hemodynamics in pulmonary arterial hypertension. Eur Respir J 2014;43(2):523–30.

11. Auchus RJ. Steroid 17-hydroxylase and 17,20-lyase deficiencies, genetic and pharmacologic. J Steroid Biochem Mol Biol 2017;165:71–8.

12. Kisselev P, Schunck W-H, Roots I, et al. Association of CYP1A1 polymorphisms with differential metabolic activation of 17β-estradiol and estrone. Cancer Res 2005;65(7):2972–8.

13. Simpson ER, Clyne C, Rubin G, et al. Aromatase–a brief overview. Annu Rev Physiol 2002;64:93–127.

14. Austin ED, Cogan JD, West JD, et al. Alterations in estrogen metabolism: implications for higher penetrance of FPAH in females. Eur Respir J 2009;34(5):1093–9.

15. Mair KM, Yang XD, Long L, et al. Sex affects bone morphogenetic protein type ii receptor signaling in pulmonary artery smooth muscle cells. Am J Respir Crit Care Med 2015;191(6):693–703.

16. Mair KM, Wright AF, Duggan N, et al. Sex-dependent influence of endogenous estrogen in pulmonary hypertension. Am J Respir Crit Care Med 2014;190(4):456–67.

17. Austin E, Hamid R, Hemnes A, et al. BMPR2 expression is suppressed by signaling through the estrogen receptor. Biol Sex Differ 2012;3(1):6.

18. van der Bruggen CE, Happé CM, Dorfmüller P, et al. Bone morphogenetic protein receptor type 2 mutation in pulmonary arterial hypertension: a view on the right ventricle. Circulation 2016;133(18):1747–60.

19. Yan L, Cogan JD, Hedges LK, et al. The Y Chromosome Regulates BMPR2 Expression via SRY: a possible reason "why" fewer males develop pulmonary arterial hypertension. Am J Respir Crit Care Med 2018;198(12):1581–3.

20. Ge X, Zhu T, Zhang X, et al. Gender differences in pulmonary arterial hypertension patients with BMPR2 mutation: a meta-analysis. Respir Res 2020;21(1):44.

21. Rabinovitch M, Gamble WJ, Miettinen OS, et al. Age and sex influence on pulmonary hypertension of chronic hypoxia and on recovery. Am J Physiol 1981;240(1):H62–72.

22. Xu D, Niu W, Luo Y, et al. Endogenous estrogen attenuates hypoxia-induced pulmonary hypertension by inhibiting pulmonary arterial vasoconstriction and pulmonary arterial smooth muscle cells proliferation. Int J Med Sci 2013;10(6):771–81.

23. Taraseviciene-Stewart L, Kasahara Y, Alger L, et al. Inhibition of the VEGF receptor 2 combined with chronic hypoxia causes cell death-dependent pulmonary endothelial cell proliferation and severe pulmonary hypertension. Faseb J 2001;15(2):427–38.

24. Tofovic SP. Estrogens and development of pulmonary hypertension: interaction of estradiol metabolism and pulmonary vascular disease. J Cardiovasc Pharmacol 2010;56(6):696–708.

25. White K, Johansen AK, Nilsen M, et al. Activity of the estrogen-metabolizing enzyme cytochrome P450 1B1 influences the development of pulmonary arterial hypertension/clinical Perspective. Circulation 2012;126(9):1087–98.

26. Dean A, Gregorc T, Docherty CK, et al. Role of the Aryl hydrocarbon receptor in sugen 5416-induced experimental pulmonary hypertension. Am J Respir Cell Mol Biol 2018;58(3):320–30.

27. Chen X, Austin ED, Talati M, et al. Oestrogen inhibition reverses pulmonary arterial hypertension and associated metabolic defects. Eur Respir J 2017;50(2):1602337.

28. Chen X, Talati M, Fessel JP, et al. The estrogen metabolite 16alphaOHE exacerbates BMPR2-associated PAH through miR-29-mediated Modulation of Cellular metabolism. Circulation 2016;133(1):82–97.

29. Morrell NW, Yang XD, Upton PD, et al. Altered growth responses of muscle cells from patients pulmonary artery smooth with primary pulmonary hypertension to transforming growth factor-beta(1) and bone morphogenetic proteins. Circulation 2001;104(7):790–5.

30. Machado RD, Pauciulo MW, Thomson JR, et al. BMPR2 haploinsufficiency as the inherited molecular mechanism for primary pulmonary hypertension. Am J Hum Genet 2001;68(1):92–102.

31. White K, Dempsie Y, Nilsen M, et al. The serotonin transporter, gender, and 17 beta oestradiol in the development of pulmonary arterial hypertension. Cardiovasc Res 2011;90(2):373–82.

32. MacLean MR, Deuchar GA, Hicks MN, et al. Overexpression of the 5-hydroxytryptamine transporter gene - effect on pulmonary hemodynamics and hypoxia-induced pulmonary hypertension. Circulation 2004;109(17):2150–5.

33. Dempsie Y, Nilsen M, White K, et al. Development of pulmonary arterial hypertension in mice over-expressing S100A4/Mts1 is specific to females. Respir Res 2011;12:159.

34. Dempsie Y, MacRitchie NA, White K, et al. Dexfenfluramine and the oestrogen-metabolizing enzyme CYP1B1 in the development of pulmonary arterial hypertension. Cardiovasc Res 2013;99(1):24–34.

35. Roberts KE, Fallon MB, Krowka MJ, et al. Genetic risk factors for portopulmonary hypertension in patients with advanced liver disease. Am J Respir Crit Care Med 2009;179(9):835–42.

36. Dean A, Nilsen M, Loughlin L, et al. Metformin reverses development of pulmonary hypertension via aromatase inhibition. Hypertension 2016;68(2):446–54.

37. Kawut SM, Archer-Chicko CL, DeMichele A, et al. Anastrozole in pulmonary arterial hypertension. a randomized, double-blind, placebo-controlled trial. Am J Respir Crit Care Med 2017;195(3):360–8.

38. Teichmann J, Schmidt A, Lange U, et al. Longitudinal evaluation of serum estradiol and estrone in male patients infected with the human immunodeficiency virus. Eur J Med Res 2003;8(2):77–80.

39. Muxfeldt ES, Margallo VS, Guimarães GM, et al. Prevalence and associated factors of obstructive sleep apnea in patients with resistant hypertension. Am J Hypertens 2014;27(8):1069–78.

40. Schneider G, Kirschner MA, Berkowitz R, et al. Increased estrogen production in obese men. J Clin Endocrinol Metab 1979;48(4):633–8.

41. Mair KM, Harvey KY, Henry AD, et al. Obesity alters oestrogen metabolism and contributes to pulmonary arterial hypertension. Eur Respir J 2019;53(6):1801524.

42. Baird GL, Archer-Chicko C, Barr RG, et al. Lower DHEA-S levels predict disease and worse outcomes in post-menopausal women with idiopathic, connective tissue disease- and congenital heart disease-associated pulmonary arterial hypertension. Eur Respir J 2018;51(6):1800467.

43. Ventetuolo CE, Baird GL, Barr RG, et al. Higher estradiol and lower dehydroepiandrosterone-sulfate levels are associated with pulmonary arterial hypertension in men. Am J Respir Crit Care Med 2016;193(10):1168–75.

44. Lahm T, Albrecht M, Fisher AJ, et al. 17 beta-estradiol attenuates hypoxic pulmonary hypertension via estrogen receptor-mediated effects. Am J Respir Crit Care Med 2012;185(9):965–80.

45. Lahm T, Frump AL, Albrecht ME, et al. 17beta-Estradiol mediates superior adaptation of right ventricular function to acute strenuous exercise in female rats with severe pulmonary hypertension. Am J Physiol Lung Cell Mol Physiol 2016;311(2):L375–88.

46. West J, Cogan J, Geraci M, et al. Gene expression in BMPR2 mutation carriers with and without evidence of Pulmonary Arterial Hypertension suggests pathways relevant to disease penetrance. BMC Med Genomics 2008;1(1):45.

47. Cohen-Solal JF, Jeganathan V, Grimaldi CM, et al. Sex hormones and SLE: influencing the fate of autoreactive B cells. Curr Top Microbiol Immunol 2006;305:67–88.

48. Nicolls MR, Voelkel NF. The roles of immunity in the prevention and evolution of pulmonary arterial hypertension. Am J Respir Crit Care Med 2017;195(10):1292–9.

49. Ventetuolo CE, Mitra N, Wan F, et al. Oestradiol metabolism and androgen receptor genotypes are associated with right ventricular function. Eur Respir J 2016;47(2):553–63.

50. Johansen AK, Dean A, Morecroft I, et al. The serotonin transporter promotes a pathological estrogen metabolic pathway in pulmonary hypertension via cytochrome P450 1B1. Pulm Circ 2016;6(1):82–92.

51. Hood KY, Montezano AC, Harvey AP, et al. Nicotinamide adenine dinucleotide phosphate oxidase-mediated redox signaling and vascular remodeling by 16alpha-hydroxyestrone in human pulmonary artery cells: implications in pulmonary arterial hypertension. Hypertension 2016;68(3):796–808.

52. Denver N, Homer NZM, Andrew R, et al. Estrogen metabolites in a small cohort of patients with idiopathic pulmonary arterial hypertension. Pulm Circ 2020;10(1). 2045894020908783.

53. Denver N, Khan S, Stasinopoulos I, et al. Derivatization enhances analysis of estrogens and their bioactive metabolites in human plasma by liquid chromatography tandem mass spectrometry. Anal Chim Acta 2019;1054:84–94.

54. Chen X, Talati M, Fessel JP, et al. Estrogen metabolite 16alpha-hydroxyestrone exacerbates bone morphogenetic protein receptor type ii-associated pulmonary arterial hypertension through MicroRNA-29-Mediated Modulation of Cellular Metabolism. Circulation 2016;133(1):82–97.

55. Fessel JP, Chen X, Frump A, et al. Interaction between bone morphogenetic protein receptor type 2 and estrogenic compounds in pulmonary arterial hypertension. Pulm Circ 2013;3(3):564–77.

56. Kawut SM, Pinder D, Al-Naamani N, et al. Fulvestrant for the treatment of pulmonary arterial hypertension. Ann Am Thorac Soc 2019;16(11):1456–9.

57. Dubey R, Tofovic S, Jackson E. Cardiovascular pharmacology of estradiol metabolites. J Pharmacol Exp Ther 2004;308(2):403–9.

58. Tofovic S, Salah E, Mady H, et al. Estradiol metabolites attenuate monocrotaline-induced pulmonary hypertension in rats. J Cardiovasc Pharmacol 2005;46(4):430–7.

59. Tofovic S, Zhang X, Jackson E, et al. 2-methoxyestradiol attenuates bleomycin-induced pulmonary hypertension and fibrosis in estrogen-deficient rats. Vascul Pharmacol 2009;51(2–3):190–7.

60. Tofovic SP, Hu J, Jackson EK, et al. 2-Hydroxyestradiol Attenuates Metabolic Syndrome-Induced Pulmonary Hypertension | C28. SEX, DRUGS, AND PULMONARY HYPERTENSION. Paper presented at: American Thoracic Society 2015 International Conference2015; Denver, Colorado.19th May, 2015.

61. Boudíková B, Szumlanski C, Maidak B, et al. Human liver catechol-O-methyltransferase pharmacogenetics. Clin Pharmacol Ther 1990;48(4):381–9.

62. Schendzielorz N, Rysa A, Reenila I, et al. Complex estrogenic regulation of catechol-O-methyltransferase (COMT) in rats. J Physiol Pharmacol 2011;62(4):483–90.

63. Xie T, Ho S, Ramsden D. Characterization and implications of estrogenic down-regulation of human catechol-O-methyltransferase gene transcription. Mol Pharmacol 1999;56(1):31–8.

64. Wang L, Zheng Q, Yuan Y, et al. Effects of 17β-estradiol and 2-methoxyestradiol on the oxidative stress-hypoxia inducible factor-1 pathway in hypoxic pulmonary hypertensive rats. Exp Ther Med 2017;13(5):2537–43.

65. Docherty CK, Nilsen M, MacLean MR. Influence of 2-methoxyestradiol and sex on hypoxia-induced pulmonary hypertension and hypoxia-inducible factor-1-alpha. J Am Heart Assoc 2019;8(5):e011628.

66. Tofovic S, Zhang X, Zhu H, et al. 2-Ethoxyestradiol is antimitogenic and attenuates monocrotaline-induced pulmonary hypertension and vascular remodeling. Vascul Pharmacol 2008;48(4–6):174–83.

67. Rothman RB, Ayestas MA, Dersch CM, et al. Aminorex, fenfluramine, and chlorphentermine are serotonin transporter substrates - implications for primary pulmonary hypertension. Circulation 1999;100(8):869–75.

68. Herve P, Drouet L, Dosquet C, et al. Primary pulmonary hypertension in a patient with a familial platelet storage pool disease: role of serotonin. The Am J Med 1990;89(1):117–20.

69. MacLean MMR. The serotonin hypothesis in pulmonary hypertension revisited: targets for novel therapies (2017 Grover Conference Series). Pulm Circ 2018;8(2). 2045894018759125.

70. Ciuclan L, Hussey MJ, Burton V, et al. Imatinib attenuates hypoxia-induced PAH pathology via reduction in 5-HT through inhibition of TPH1 expression. Am J Respir Crit Care Med 2013;187(1):78–89.

71. Morecroft I, Dempsie Y, Bader M, et al. Effect of tryptophan hydroxylase 1 deficiency on the development of hypoxia-induced pulmonary hypertension. Hypertension 2007;49(1):232–6.

72. Morecroft I, White K, Caruso P, et al. Gene therapy by targeted adenovirus-mediated knockdown of pulmonary endothelial Tph1 attenuates hypoxia-induced pulmonary hypertension. Mol Ther 2012;20(8):1516–28.

73. Aiello RJ, Bourassa PA, Zhang Q, et al. Tryptophan hydroxylase 1 inhibition impacts pulmonary vascular remodeling in two rat models of pulmonary hypertension. J Pharmacol Exp Ther 2017;360(2):267–79.

74. Long L, MacLean MR, Jeffery TK, et al. Serotonin increases susceptibility to pulmonary hypertension in BMPR2-deficient mice. Circ Res 2006;98(6):818–27.

75. Wallace E, Morrell NW, Yang XD, et al. A sex-specific MicroRNA-96/5-hydroxytryptamine 1B Axis influences development of pulmonary hypertension. Am J Respir Crit Care Med 2015;191(12):1432–42.

76. Dempsie Y, Morecroft I, Welsh DJ, et al. Converging evidence in support of the serotonin hypothesis of dexfenfluramine-induced pulmonary hypertension with novel transgenic mice. Circulation 2008;117(22):2928–37.

77. Jacobs W, van de Veerdonk MC, Trip P, et al. The right ventricle explains sex differences in survival in idiopathic pulmonary arterial hypertension. Chest 2014;145(6):1230–6.

78. Ventetuolo CE, Ouyang P, Bluemke DA, et al. Sex hormones are associated with right ventricular structure and function: the MESA-right ventricle study. Am J Respir Crit Care Med 2011;183(5):659–67.

79. Kawut SM, Lima JA, Barr RG, et al. Sex and race differences in right ventricular structure and function: the multi-ethnic study of atherosclerosis-right ventricle study. Circulation 2011;123(22):2542–51.

80. Kawut SM, Al-Naamani N, Agerstrand C, et al. Determinants of right ventricular ejection fraction in pulmonary arterial hypertension*. Chest 2009;135(3):752–9.

81. Stanczyk FZ, Jurow J, Hsing AW. Limitations of direct immunoassays for measuring circulating estradiol levels in postmenopausal women and men in epidemiologic studies. Cancer Epidemiol Biomarkers Prev 2010;19(4):903–6.

82. Stanczyk FZ, Xu X, Sluss PM, et al. Do metabolites account for higher serum steroid hormone levels measured by RIA compared to mass spectrometry? Clini Chim Acta 2018;484:223–5.

83. Owen LJ, Monaghan PJ, Armstrong A, et al. Oestradiol measurement during fulvestrant treatment for breast cancer. Br J Cancer 2019;120:404–6.

84. Cross TG, Hornshaw MP. Can LC and LC-MS ever replace immunoassays? J Appl Bioanalysis 2016;2(4):108–16.

85. Faupel-Badger JM, Fuhrman BJ, Xu X, et al. Comparison of liquid chromatography-tandem mass spectrometry, RIA, and ELISA methods for measurement of urinary estrogens. Cancer Epidemiol Biomarkers Prev 2010;19(1):292–300.

86. Handelsman DJ, Newman JD, Jimenez M, et al. Performance of direct estradiol immunoassays with human male serum samples. Clin Chem 2014; 60(3):510–7.

87. Denver N, Khan S, Stasinopoulos I, et al. Data for analysis of catechol estrogen metabolites in human plasma by liquid chromatography tandem mass spectrometry. Data in Brief 2019;23: 103740.

Moving?

Make sure your subscription moves with you!

To notify us of your new address, find your **Clinics Account Number** (located on your mailing label above your name), and contact customer service at:

Email: **journalscustomerservice-usa@elsevier.com**

800-654-2452 (subscribers in the U.S. & Canada)
314-447-8871 (subscribers outside of the U.S. & Canada)

Fax number: **314-447-8029**

Elsevier Health Sciences Division
Subscription Customer Service
3251 Riverport Lane
Maryland Heights, MO 63043

*To ensure uninterrupted delivery of your subscription, please notify us at least 4 weeks in advance of move.